THE TEENAGE BODY BOOK

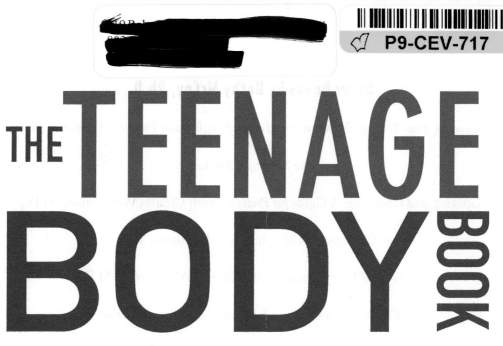

Kathy McCoy, Ph.D., & Charles Wibbelsman, M.D.

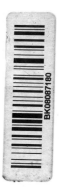

Other Books by Kathy McCoy, Ph.D.

Understanding Your Teenager's Depression: Issues, Insights and Practical Guidance for Parents

The Secrets of My Life

Growing and Changing: A Guide for Preteens (with Charles Wibbelsman, M.D.)

Life Happens (with Charles Wibbelsman, M.D.)

Crisis-Proof Your Teenager (with Charles Wibbelsman, M.D.)

Changes and Choices: A Junior High Survival Guide

Solo Parenting: Your Essential Guide

Coping with Teenage Depression

The Teenage Survival Guide

The Teenage Body Book Guide to Sexuality

The Teenage Body Book Guide to Dating

Purr Therapy: What Timmy and Marina Taught Me About Love, Life and Loss

Aging and Other Surprises

Making Peace With Your Adult Children

For more information, go to www.drkathymccoy.com

THE TEENAGE BODY BOOK

Kathy McCoy, Ph.D., & Charles Wibbelsman, M.D.

Illustrations by Bob Stover and Kelly Grady Callarman

Hatherleigh Press is committed to preserving and protecting the
natural resources of the Earth. Environmentally responsible and sustainable
practices are embraced within the company's mission statement.

Visit us at www.hatherleighpress.com and register online for free offers,
discounts, special events, and more.

Library of Congress Cataloging-in-Publication Data
available upon request

ISBN 978-1-57826-643-2

The Teenage Body Book is available for bulk purchase, special promotions, and premiums.
For information on reselling and special purchase opportunities, call 1-800-528-2550
and ask for the Special Sales Manager.

Interior design by Pauline Neuwirth, Neuwirth & Associates, Inc.
Cover design by Carolyn Kasper

10 9 8 7 6 5 4 3

Printed in the United States

DEDICATION

To Bob Stover, who has given so much to *The Teenage Body Book* over the years, and to Tim Schellhardt, whose help this time around was invaluable, we dedicate this new edition, with much gratitude and love.

Acknowledgments

Our special thanks to . . .

- Tim Schellhardt, a dear friend and an award-winning journalist. For this edition, Tim graciously stepped in to lend his research skills and resources to our efforts. He also offered warm encouragement and advice—as a father of four and grandfather of three—for this and earlier editions.
- Bob Stover, the artist for the original edition of this book in 1979 and for all subsequent editions. His creative talents, hard work and generosity in volunteering to double as a proofreader as well as artist have been much appreciated and have contributed significantly to the book's success.
- Kelly Grady Callarman, for her wonderful additional artwork, and Jennifer Rourke for her illustration on page 166.
- Our now retired agent, Susan Ann Protter, for believing in us and this book from the beginning and through the years.
- Our editor Anna Krusinski for her inspiration and support in the process of creating this new edition.
- Elizabeth Canfield, an extraordinary health educator and human being, who thought we might work well together and introduced us many years ago. Loving thanks, Liz!
- The 'TEEN Magazine "alum" group who have supported us warmly over the years: Mary Connolly Breiner, Betty Price, Roxanne Camron, Carole Ann Lyons, Andrea Cleghorn, Rita Warren, Daina Hulet, Jane Fort, Laurel Finnerty, Marilyn Frandsen, Jay Cole, Maureen Donaldson, Pamela Van Daalen, Leora Glass, and Marina Muhfriedel. We also want to express love and gratitude to Louise MacLeod, the widow of 'TEEN's long-time publisher and wonderful career launcher Robert MacLeod, who has continued to cheer us on to the present day.
- Special friends and family who have helped in so many ways as we dealt with deadline pressure: Mary and John Breiner, Mike McCoy, M.D., Jinjuta McCoy, Maggie

McCoy, Henry McCoy, Tai McCoy, Nick McCoy, Ryan Grady, David Hyman, Richard C. Holihan, M.D., Pat Hill, Sr. Rita McCormack, Sr. Ramona Bascom, Caron and Raymond Roudebush, Marsha Morello, Pat and Joe Cosentino, Kim Tuomi, Nora Valdiviezo, Vivian Wung, Jeanie Croope, Dee Ready, Mary Kate Schellhardt and Matt Palko, and Eliza and Chris Yarbrough and their daughters Lucy and Leah (who keep us smiling!)

Contents

Introduction

A NEW EDITION—JUST FOR YOU!

You're part of a very special generation of teens: you and your friends are the first teens to be born in the 21st century (or just at the turn of the century)!

As young people in a new century, your lives are unique.

While it's true that some aspects of teen life and health are timeless, your lifestyle—your choices and your challenges—are quite unlike those of previous generations. And so, we're changing to meet your needs and answer your questions about coming of age in these changing times.

■ *You're the most connected generation in history.* According to the latest studies from the Pew Research Center, 95% of teens ages 12–17 are online. 78% of you have cell phones, many of these smartphones. Some 24% of you report being online via your smartphone or computer every waking hour! You connect with each other (most often by texting). And, when looking for the latest information about health, you're looking for it online. According to a 2015 Northwestern University study of teens, health and technology, some 84% of you have sought health information online.

■ *You're very careful about the reliability of your health information.* Your generation doesn't accept information from just any site. According to the Northwestern study, teens are careful to seek out government, university or medical center sites most often when looking for health information online. You're unlikely to ask a question or seek answers on a social networking site. But, despite all this new technology, you rely mostly on information from your parents and from school health classes. You are less likely than previous generations to look for information in a book (though *The Teenage Body Book has* changed to be more relevant to this new generation). This will be the first edition to come out as an e-book as well as in print. And, as always, we are committed to giving you up-to-date information that you can discuss with your parents or in a school health class. Our Appendix has also changed to give you online sources of help.

- *You're part of the most diverse, multicultural teen population ever.* As such, this new edition will reflect more of the realities, needs and challenges of your life today.
- *New discoveries can change your life.* Medical advances are being made all the time — and you can benefit! In this book, we'll give you up to date medical information as well as reliable sources for continuing life and health-enhancing breakthroughs.
- *You have the power to change the direction of your generation.* There are so many good and positive things about teens today. But you're facing at least one serious challenge: your generation could well have shorter, less healthy lives than those of your parents! Because so many teens today are overweight or obese and inactive, you are at a higher risk of major health problems. You can start turning that around by taking good care of your body and your health. We're here to help with lots of information about healthy eating, exercise and self-care.

All that said, some aspects of being a teen *have* stayed the same since the first edition of this book was published nearly 40 years ago: the timing and facts of physical development, the pain of feeling different or losing a love, the risks of substance abuse, the challenge of living with a chronic medical condition, the responsibility of making decisions about sex that are right for *you.*

But, in so many other ways, your life is totally different.

So this is not *The Teenage Body Book* your parents might have read when they were young.

This one is for *you,* as you shape your unique, connected, diverse life. We're here to help in all ways possible as you face the exciting new possibilities of being a young adult in this new century.

We know it isn't always easy to be a teen. These years can be painful, exciting, boring, fun and challenging. They probably will not be the best years of your life (no matter what anyone says) but they can be very important to your whole life.

Now is the time when....

- You get to make a choice — either actively or passively — about how much education you will get and which general career direction your life will take. Choices you make now can affect your life for years to come — positively or negatively.
- You set a health pattern for your life. Your eating and exercise habits are often set during these years. Similarly, those who will be habitual smokers or problem drinkers in adulthood often start these behaviors in the teen years, establishing patterns that are harder to break than behaviors started in adulthood. Those who are active and maintain a normal weight in adolescence are less likely to get certain cancers and to experience obesity in later life. Young women who exercise regularly in their teens and young adult years build strong bones that can be a real benefit in older age. So what you do now is important — not only for today, but also for years to come.

- You become your own person—or not. Developing a strong sense of the unique person you are and what you want can be a vital step towards both greater independence and the capacity to have truly intimate relationships (because you have a strong sense of self and don't have to worry about losing yourself in a relationship).

We're excited to be here, and ready to help with your health and fitness concerns, your feelings, your relationship issues, your questions about sexuality, your plans and dreams for the future.

We're here for you in all the changes and challenges you're facing—today, and in the years to come!

CHAPTER ONE

Am I Normal?

What's normal? Good question. In fact, that's the one question teens have asked us over and over, in many different ways, over the years. This may be *your* most pressing question as you:

- Find yourself making quiet comparisons between you and your friends, calculating how you compare in your growth and development, and wondering who's normal and who's not.
- Feel uncomfortable about the way you look.
- Wonder if your feelings—such as loving and hating your parents at the same time, or feeling up and feeling down more than you used to— are normal or a sign that something is secretly (or, worse yet, very obviously) wrong with you.

If you've ever wondered "Am I normal?" you have a lot of company.

Most teens ask "Am I normal?" in the following ways:

IS MY GROWTH NORMAL?

You may wonder this for a lot of reasons. Boys may watch girls tower above them in junior high and wonder if things will always be this way. Girls may notice that one classmate begins to look like a teenager in third or fourth grade while another may still look like a kid when starting high school—with everyone else somewhere in between. And, strange as it may seem, everyone is normal!

The fact is, normal rates of development vary widely and are based, in part, on your genetic heritage. Ask your parents about their adolescent changes and you may discover some important similarities. For example, it's quite normal for many African Americans to start showing very normal signs of puberty at age 8 or 9. And, as a teen of the 21st century, your normal rate of development is quite different from that of teens a century ago. Then, it was normal for young people to start puberty in the mid-to-late teens! Now, due to better general health and nutrition, both boys and girls are larger and become physically mature at earlier ages.

IS MY BODY NORMAL?

Besides the changes of adolescence, young people worry a lot about how they look: whether they're too fat, too thin, too tall, or too short and whether they're attractive. Teasing by classmates or looking in the mirror and knowing, without a doubt, that you'll never look like the media ideal of beauty or hunkiness can cause a lot of pain. If you worry about your body, you're far from alone. Very few people look like models or movie stars. There are a number of different and quite normal body types. You can be healthy and attractive whatever body type you have.

ARE MY FEELINGS NORMAL?

Feelings are a big concern with teens wondering whether or not they're normal and fit in.

New feelings come as your body and your social world change. You may have very different feelings about the opposite sex these days, with boys (or girls) looking a lot more interesting to you than they used to. And you find yourself having mixed, often confusing feelings about the parents you once admired without question. Maybe they've turned totally embarrassing at times, wise and comforting at other times. You admire them one minute and can't stand them the next. What's going on?

It's all part of the normal passage of adolescence. Due to hormonal changes, you may have fairly dramatic mood swings— feeling on top of the world one minute and completely upset and depressed the next. And, in your changing world, relationships aren't as simple as they used to be. You both love and hate, have a desire for independence from and a longing to stay attached to your parents. Your friends are more important than ever—but friendships, too, can have their definite ups and downs. And because you're beginning to *look* like an adult, people expect more of you. You're growing up faster and facing more challenges at an earlier age than your teen counterparts of a century ago.

There are times when you feel quite different from your friends and family; times when you feel very much alone, wondering if anyone else feels the way you do and, painfully, whether you would be accepted or rejected if you were to tell your friends or family about these feelings. So you keep some of your thoughts and feelings secret because you want so much to fit in, to have friends and just be normal like everyone else.

But feeling different doesn't mean that you're not normal. What's normal for you may be different from what's normal for your best friend. "Normal" is a very individual matter. And you may find when you're all a little older and feeling more secure, that your feelings were (and are) shared by some of your friends—all of you feeling different and a little bit lonely during the years of so much change and so much wondering.

IT'S NORMAL TO BE CHANGING IN ALL WAYS!

Change is the natural order of things in adolescence and young adulthood. In fact, the Latin root of the word *adolescence* is *esco*, which means "becoming." This period of becoming is a long transition time between childhood and adulthood. This is a time of life when there can be dramatic differences between you and your friends. It's a huge temptation to look at someone who is your age and say to yourself: "That person seems to be normal. But I'm different. So I'm not normal."

The fact is, you can be both different and normal. Normal covers an incredibly wide range. The physical changes of adolescence are quire distinct and universal, but the *timing* of these changes is entirely your own. And how other changes happen is unique to you, too. For example, some people mature socially and emotionally before they have any signs of physical maturity—and you see a young adult in a child's body. The opposite is true, too: Some people grow physically into young adults before their social and emotional development has had a chance to catch up—and so you see an adult-sized child. And there are a lot of people somewhere in between as you enter junior high and high school.

At this time of life, feelings of confusion and self-consciousness and fears about being normal or not normal are common. It can help a lot to share these fears.

What are some low-risk ways to do that?

- Ask your parents about their own growing up experiences—and let yourself be reassured that, even though they came of age in a whole different era, some feelings and fears are timeless. And if your parents remember feeling self-conscious because their physical development seemed to be a lot earlier or later than that of their friends, that could be a clue for you about your own physical development timetable. The timing of adolescent development can have a genetic component.

- If you wonder whether your body is normal, find a doctor or school nurse to ask. If you're not comfortable with any medical professionals you know, look to see if there are any special teen clinics in your area where staff are particularly sensitive to teen concerns.

- Talk with your friends!! Sometimes it can be a real relief to know that other people worry about the same things you do—and what seemed abnormal is starting to look more normal all the time.

If talking with others seems too risky right now, try this: sit back in the privacy of your room or wherever you are and read this book. You'll discover what other teens are thinking and asking. You'll read letters from hundreds of teens we've met in schools, clinics and interviews, or who have read previous editions of this book and sent us additional questions.

As you read their letters and comments, you'll realize that you're both normal *and* unique. Once you see that you're as normal as the next person, then you can begin to appreciate ways that you are truly special. You may begin to give yourself permission *not* to be perfect. You may begin to appreciate who you are and who you may grow to become.

Most important, you will realize that you're not alone!

AM I NORMAL?

✔ Teens worry about whether their physical changes, body size and shape and feelings are normal. There is a very wide range of normal—especially in adolescence.

✔ The timing of your physical changes is linked to genetics: You may mature at the same rate your mom or dad did. Ethnicity can be a part of that. For example, if you're African American, you may quite normally begin puberty before your white classmates. Health and nutrition can play a part, too: a century ago, young people looked like kids until they were in their mid-to-late teens. Today's adolescents generally show signs of young adulthood much sooner.

✔ Ups and downs in relationships are a normal part of adolescence—and of life. You may have conflicting feelings of love and hate with your parents as you struggle for independence, with friends who can help you soar or take you down quick with a look or a word, and with a special person with whom feelings of love and anger can co-exist. Ambivalent feelings are a normal part of everyday life, no matter what your age!

✔ Talking with others can help to reassure you that you're normal. If you can't deal with talking with an adult—a parent, your doctor, a counselor, a favorite aunt or uncle or an older cousin—seek help and reassurance from trusted friends. If talking with anyone at all seems too daunting right now, just read on and see what other teens are asking us. You'll see as you read through this book that you're both normal and unique!

CHAPTER TWO
From Girl to Woman

FROM GIRL TO WOMAN

I used to feel good about being me, but now I'm not so sure. My body has changed a lot in the last year (I'm almost 13) and I got my period two months ago. I feel so different and embarrassed about how I look and having my period isn't as cool as I thought it would be. How can I start feeling better about myself?

Ashley

Even if you've looked forward to it, change can be unsettling. If you have mixed feelings about your changing body, you're far from alone!

You might feel proud of looking more adult, but self-conscious when people notice and comment on your physical changes, especially if they make embarrassing comments. You may know that puberty reshapes your body contours, but may feel fat with all those new curves.

With all these changes going on, your body may have become something of a mystery.

This chapter will help to clear up this mystery and help you to understand more about your body and the way it works. Knowing and understanding your anatomy, the process of physical change, and the common problems and concerns that young women have may help you to feel more comfortable and normal.

FEMALE ANATOMY

Maybe these illustrations and the terms for parts of the female anatomy are totally familiar

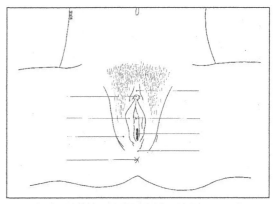

External Female Genitalia

to you. Or maybe not. If not, you might want to read this section especially carefully (and maybe even examine yourself with a mirror in the process).

The external female genital area, called the *vulva*, includes the *labia majora*, which are covered with hair if you have reached a certain stage of development, and which protect the genital area within. Inside are the *labia minora*. Sometimes these lips protrude from the outer lips and may be wrinkled or smooth. They may vary in color from pink to brown. The *clitoris* is located at the juncture where the labia minora connect. The clitoris is tiny but very sensitive and plays a vital role in a woman's sexual arousal and pleasure.

Below the clitoris is the *urethra* or urinary opening. Beneath that is the *vaginal opening*. This may be ringed or partially covered by the *hymen*. The hymen may be very evident or hardly visible. It may have one opening or several.

The presence or absence of a hymen is not indicative of whether you are—or aren't—a

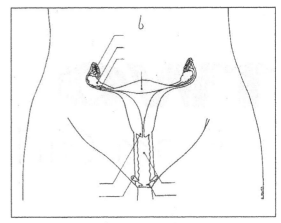

Side View of Female Reproductive System

virgin. Some women who are virgins are born without a noticeable hymen or may have stretched the hymen during vigorous sports activities or masturbation. Other women who are having sexual intercourse may have intact, though stretched, hymens. Only in very rare instances is there no opening in the hymen. This condition, called *imperforate hymen*, is very rare, is most often discovered early in life and requires surgery to create an opening.

The vaginal opening is the point connecting the external and internal genitals. What is beyond this opening? First, of course, is the *vagina*, a canal that stretches from the vaginal opening to the *cervix* or neck of the uterus. In the center of the cervix is the *os*, or opening, which feels like a small dimple. This tiny opening can open (or dilate) large enough to allow a baby to pass through, but, under ordinary circumstances, it is so small that it makes the upper end of the vagina seem closed. This fact may give some comfort to those who fear that tampons or other objects can get lost inside them. They can't. They have nowhere to go unless you remove them or expel them from your vaginal opening.

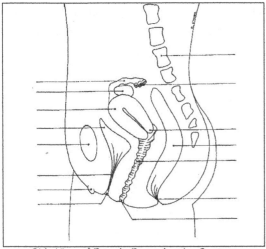

Side View of Female Reproductive System

The *uterus* is small, muscular, and pear-shaped. It's amazingly elastic—with the cavity in the non-pregnant state slimmer than the width of your little finger. After expanding to many times its original size during pregnancy, the uterus becomes quite small again after the baby is born.

At the upper portion of the uterus are the *Fallopian tubes*, passageways from the uterus to the *ovaries*, which hold the egg cells. Each month, an egg cell is released from one of the two ovaries in a process called *ovulation* and it then begins its journey to the uterus. If the egg is met by a male's sperm and fertilized (a process called *conception*) this is the beginning of a baby. This tiny collection of cells will travel on through the tubes to the uterus where it will attach itself to the rich *endometrial walls* (lining of the uterus) to grow and develop.

The unfertilized egg, on the other hand, disintegrates, as does the endometrial tissue that has been building up in anticipation of receiving a fertilized egg to nourish. This material makes up the menstrual flow.

We've been describing the anatomy and monthly cycle of the mature female. As an adolescent female, you're in the process of maturing and this process can cause a lot of concern for many teens.

PHYSICAL DEVELOPMENT

What is the normal age for body changes like getting breasts and your period? I have two friends who got their periods and were wearing bras in fifth grade, others who began to look like teenagers last year in seventh grade, and then there's me—almost 13 and nothing. Well, actually I do have very small breasts and I've grown a lot in the past year, but I don't have my period yet! My friend Madison, who is 13 and doesn't have her period either, and I are worried. Among the friends I've told you about, who's normal?

Kelsey J.

All of the people Kelsey describes fall within the range of normal. Everyone has his or her own special biological timeclock that dictates when the various stages of puberty will occur. There is a very wide range of normal. One person might begin puberty as young as 8 and another might be in junior high or even high school before she notices any physical changes. In both cases, the timing of these changes is entirely normal.

Why do normal people vary so in the timing of their physical changes?

Sometimes this variation is due to ethnic differences. For example, studies show that nearly *half* of African American girls begin the changes of puberty at the age of 8 (compared with 15 percent of white girls). At age 8, 48.3 percent of African American girls and 14.7 percent of white girls had begun developing breasts, pubic hair or both. We don't know why such differences occur. There are some theories that exposure to chemicals that mimic the female hormone estrogen or actual estrogens (which are used in some hair products made primarily for African Americans) may play a role. Other studies, notably those by Anne Petersen at the University of Minnesota, show that high stress can bring on puberty early. (And an argument can be made for the fact that being African American in a still-racist society is inherently stressful.)

STAGES OF PUBERTY IN GIRLS

Stages	Ages	Internal	Breasts	Growth	Pubic Hair	Menstruation
One	8–11	Ovaries are enlarging and making the hormone estrogen	None	Nothing Unusual	None	None
Two	8–14	Estrogen is quite evident in bloodstream	Breast buds: nipples elevated and tender	Rapid growth; hips broaden; fat deposits give softer, rounder shape	First signs: fine, straight and sparse	None
Three	9–15	Vagina is enlarging; chemistry of vaginal secretions is changing	Breasts continue to grow; areola (around nipple) enlarges.	Height and weight increase	Hair becomes darker and coarser but is still sparse	First menstrual period may occur at the end of this stage
Four	10–16	Ovaries enlarge; ovulation may begin	Nipple and areola form separate mound	Still growing	Pubic hair looks like an adult's, but covers smaller area; underarm hair appears	First menstrual period now if not at end of Stage Three; most periods at this stage don't involve ovulation
Five	12–19	Fully mature ovaries; regular ovulation	Full breast development	Full (or near) adult height	Full adult pattern	Regular menstruation with ovulation

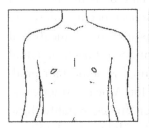

1. Breast buds begin.

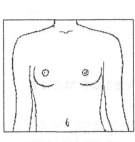

2. Breast areola grow.

3. Nipple and areola form separate mound, protruding from breast.

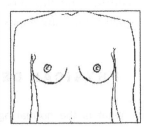

4. Areola rejoins breast contour and development is complete

AGE RANGE OF CHANGES OF PUBERTY IN GIRLS

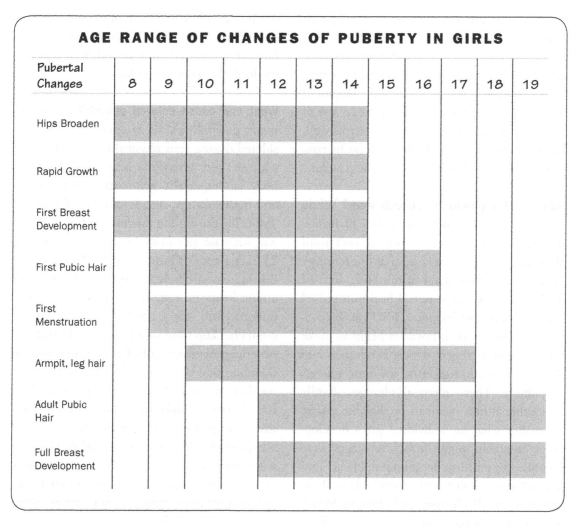

Pubertal Changes	8	9	10	11	12	13	14	15	16	17	18	19
Hips Broaden	▓	▓	▓	▓	▓	▓	▓					
Rapid Growth	▓	▓	▓	▓	▓	▓	▓					
First Breast Development	▓	▓	▓	▓	▓	▓	▓					
First Pubic Hair		▓	▓	▓	▓	▓	▓	▓				
First Menstruation		▓	▓	▓	▓	▓	▓	▓				
Armpit, leg hair			▓	▓	▓	▓	▓	▓	▓	▓		
Adult Pubic Hair					▓	▓	▓	▓	▓	▓	▓	▓
Full Breast Development					▓	▓	▓	▓	▓	▓	▓	▓

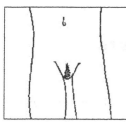

1. Initial pubic hair is straight and fine.

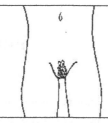

2. Pubic hair coarsens, darkens and spreads

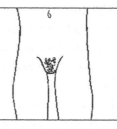

3. Hair looks like adults' but limited in area

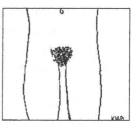

4. Inverted triangular pattern is established

Girls who are significantly overweight or obese may begin puberty earlier than their peers. Some studies, too, have found that those with diets high in protein or low in fiber may begin showing signs of physical development at an earlier age. Some wonder if heavy use of soy products can trigger early puberty as well, but more research needs to be done to confirm—or deny—that soy may also be a factor.

How does the process of puberty work? While a baby girl is born with thousands of immature eggs (ova) in her ovaries, it isn't until about age 8 (on the average) that the *pituitary gland*—the master gland of the body, located in the brain—sends a special hormone called *follicle-stimulating hormone* (FSH) to the ovaries. The long-dormant ovaries begin to make the hormone estrogen, which is released into the blood stream, triggering the long process of puberty. These physical changes, hardly noticeable at first, occur in predictable stages, no matter what an individual girl's development timetable might be. These stages were identified by a British doctor named J. M. Tanner, who noted that within each stage there are many small changes and steps in breast, genital, and pubic hair growth as well as changes in height and weight. By recognizing the changes characteristic for each of the five stages of puberty, you and your doctor can tell where you are physically in your adolescence and what is likely to happen next

The following charts will give you a map to the different stages of puberty (Chart 1) and the normal age range for each stage (Chart 2).

When should you worry about lack of development? Most physicians feel that if you're 15 or older and have no signs of puberty, such as pubic hair and breast development or if you haven't yet started your period by this age, a medical checkup is in order.

What can cause delayed puberty? There are many possibilities, all of which will be considered during your physical exam. Some girls who are very physically active and have low body fat, especially gymnasts, ballet dancers and figure skaters, may have delayed puberty. Typically, during the process of puberty, a girl will increase her body fat from 8 percent to 21-22 percent. Those who don't experience this increase in body fat due to restricted diets and/or heavy exercise may experience delayed puberty. Still, it's a good idea to get a thorough checkup from your physician. In fact, the American Academy of Pediatrics is now recommending that young people age 11 and older see their physician for an annual physical. This is a chance to make sure that all is well and, just as important, an opportunity for you to ask questions. Also having a complete checkup with your doctor will give you the opportunity to receive the three new vaccines for pre-teens: vaccines for protection against Pertussis, Meningitis, and the HPV virus.

BREASTS

What is normal breast size? I'm skinny and my breasts are small and everyone teases me. What can I do? Do those bust developers that are advertised in magazines really work? Help!

Embarrassed

Again, there is a very wide range of normal when we talk about normal breast size.

Heredity plays a major role in determining what *your* normal size will be. Time can also be a factor. The average white American teen doesn't reach the final stage of breast growth until age 17 or older, while African American and Asian American teens typically reach this stage a year or so earlier. Also, weight can be a factor in the size of your breasts—and gaining weight at any time in your life can increase breast size. But it is heredity more than weight that is the major actor in determining breast size. Heredity and skin tone can also affect the color of the *areola*, the area around the nipple. Teens with light skin tend to have very light pink areolas, while those with darker skin have brown-toned areolas. Those of any ethnicity who have been pregnant may notice a darkening of the skin of the areola. This is a normal change of pregnancy and is often permanent.

The breast is made up of fat and milk glands/ducts as well as nerves, arteries, veins and lymph channels. Connective fibers help to give the breast its rounded shape, a shape it may not assume until late adolescence. There are no muscles in the breast itself, but there are pectoral muscles just beneath the breast on the chest wall. Any exercise you do—with or without "bust development" devices—will not increase actual breast size. The most exercise can do is to develop the pectoral muscles underneath the breast.

Some women notice a slight breast swelling while taking birth control pills, but this increase is typically very small and doesn't happen to everyone. In most cases, small breasts are the result of heredity, not hormone deficiency, so hormone therapy has little to offer.

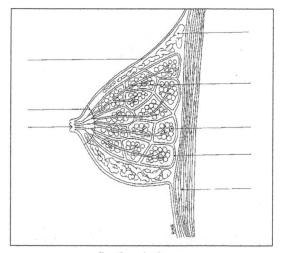

The Female Breast

Padded and uplift bras can make breasts look larger, but the best way to long-term comfort with your breasts is to accept and learn to love the uniqueness of your own breasts, whether you're small, large or somewhere in between.

My breasts are a different size. My left breast is quite a bit smaller than my right one. I feel lopsided and really embarrassed. Will they ever be the same size?

Lopsided

It's quite common, while breasts are growing and developing, to have one breast develop at a faster rate than the other. Generally, the slower breast will catch up. But breasts are rarely a perfect match, however. In most women, one breast may always be slightly larger than the other.

In rare instances, due to a congenital condition, one breast will remain undeveloped. In these cases, after the girl has reached full maturity, she may choose to have cosmetic surgery to increase the size of the undeveloped breast. However, such surgery should not be done during adolescence while one or both breasts are still developing.

I have gross nipples. They're hardly nipples at all because they're inverted and look like little slits. Why does this happen and what can I do about it?

Dana Y.

Inverted nipples—nipples that turn inward instead of outward—are not uncommon and can appear in male or female breasts. This condition is usually caused by a foreshortening of the milk ducts, with fibrous tissue strands binding the nipple down.

This condition is usually present at birth, but becomes most noticeable later in life.

Sometimes the enlargement of breast tissue during puberty will cause one or both of the nipples to turn out after having been inverted since birth. This can also happen during pregnancy. Even if it doesn't and a woman with inverted nipples wants to breast feed her baby, there are special shields that can be used on the breast to make it possible to breast-feed.

Can inverted nipples ever be a problem? Hygiene may be a special challenge, since secretions may dry and cake in the nipple crevices, and infections are also common. Some physicians recommend massage to help correct inverted nipples, but this usually isn't effective nor is surgery always successful. In surgery, the nipple is put in its normal position, but in the process, vital nerve fibers may have to be severed, causing the loss of some physical sensations in the breast.

If your nipples have always been turned out and then suddenly become inverted, this can be a sign of an underlying tumor and it's important to seek medical help immediately.

I have some dark hairs around my nipple. My mom said that pulling them out would cause cancer. How can I get rid of this hair?

Sue

Hair around the nipples is quite common and may be influenced both by ethnic origin and hormonal balance. It isn't necessarily the sign of underlying problems. The only cause for some concern would be if the hair appeared suddenly along with a number of masculine traits. Otherwise, if you have some hairs around your nipple that you find annoying or embarrassing, it's perfectly fine to remove them. There is no danger of cancer!

What happens if you get hit in the breasts by a soccer ball? I got hit last week and have a really bad bruise.

Leslie

Generally, breasts are pretty resilient, whether they are bruised by sports activities, accidents, or squeezing during sexual activity. However, a more severe injury—caused by very hard squeezing or pinching—can cause some hemorrhage into the tissues. If such injuries happen over and over this could result in chronic irritation of the breast tissue. Protecting your breasts—by speaking up for more gentle treatment if a lover is rough with them—or wearing a sports bra or protective padding if you're active in sports—can help keep such chronic irritation from happening.

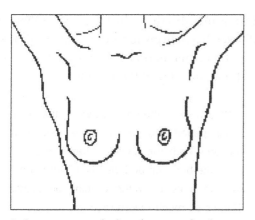

1. Raise your arms, look in the mirror for changes in contour, skin texture, or color.

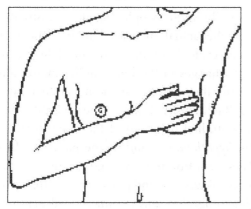

2. Examine your breasts, using a circular, clockwise motion to check for lumps.

Breast Self-Examination

Am I supposed to be doing breast self-examination? I saw a flyer my mom brought home from the doctor's office showing how to do it. How old do you have to be to do that exam? And how old do you have to be to get breast cancer?

Ashleigh K., 16

Many women, including teens, worry about breast cancer.

Medical guidelines currently don't recommend breast self-examination for teens because breast cancer is extremely uncommon in adolescents and constant examination of still-developing breasts may cause needless worry. However, if breast and ovarian cancer tend to run in your family, your doctor may want you to do breast self-examination beginning when you are 18–21 years old. Without a family history, making breast self-exams part of your self-care routine by your mid-twenties (primarily just to get into the habit) makes sense

Even though breast cancer is not especially common in teenagers, it's a good idea to check with your doctor if you notice a lump in your breast tissue or you have a discharge from your nipple. While it's quite likely that the lump is non-cancerous and the discharge may be a sign, not of cancer, but of an underlying infection, it's wise to get this checked out.

One very common breast condition during puberty is an *adolescent nodule*. This is an enlargement and swelling, usually under the nipple, making the nipple very tender. It can happen in both males and females. No one knows for sure what causes it, but it may be due to an increased production of hormones. It will usually disappear in a short time. It should never be surgically removed. To do so could interfere with future breast development in a young girl.

Another breast condition that many women experience is called *fibrocystic disease*. It isn't really a disease, but a combination of breast changes, influenced by hormones, that results in fluid-filled cysts that enlarge, sometimes painfully, around the time of your menstrual period. Some women, after consulting with their doctors, find some relief in diet management. Abstaining from caffeine (found in colas, coffee, tea and all forms of chocolate) as well as stopping smoking, can help. Your physician may also prescribe drug or vitamin therapies.

Moles can also occur on the breasts. These should be watched. If they begin to change color, increase in size, or bleed, they should be surgically removed.

Other breast changes you would need to let your doctor know about:

- A dimple or pucker in the breast
- A previously normal nipple that has become inverted
- A change in skin texture and color
- Scaly skin around the nipple
- A change in breast shape
- A noticeable discharge from the nipple
- Swelling or redness in the breast
- A feeling of heat in the breast

MENSTRUATION

Menstruation isn't a curse or an illness. It's a positive sign of health, one of the best barometers you have to show that your body is healthy and functioning normally.

For centuries, there have been superstitions and myth about menstruation: that it's dirty, that one shouldn't bathe or swim during menstruation, that exercise is not advisable during the menstrual period. None of this is true. It's important to keep your routines as normal as possible during your period whether this means bathing regularly, pursuing your usual exercise regimen, or doing any other things you enjoy. You don't have to put life on hold

during menstruation. In fact, some Olympic athletes have given top performances during their menstrual periods. So you can be at your best, too, *any* day of the month!

"What's the difference between the menstrual period and the menstrual cycle? Or are they both the same? What is the normal time between periods? Is it ever normal to skip a period without being pregnant? There's so much I need to know!"

Sheri A.

While most people equate menstruation with the actual menstrual period, the menstrual cycle is continuous—involving ovulation, changes in the lining of the uterus, and, finally, the monthly shedding of that lining via the menstrual flow. The monthly cycle is controlled by a part of the brain known as the *hypothalamus* and by the *pituitary gland*. These control the rise and decline of hormones—*estrogen* and *progesterone*—that cause girls to develop during puberty and that regulate the menstrual cycle. A regular cycle varies from one person to the next. While a 28-day cycle might be considered *average*, a 21-30 day or even 60-day cycle may be normal for you. You can figure out your cycle length by counting the first day of your period as Day 1. The average period lasts three to seven days. At this time, your estrogen level is low and some women feel a little less energetic than usual.

After the menstrual period ends, your estrogen level starts rising again, preparing the lining of your uterus to receive and nourish a fertilized egg. With this surge in your hormonal level, you may feel renewed energy and sense of well-being.

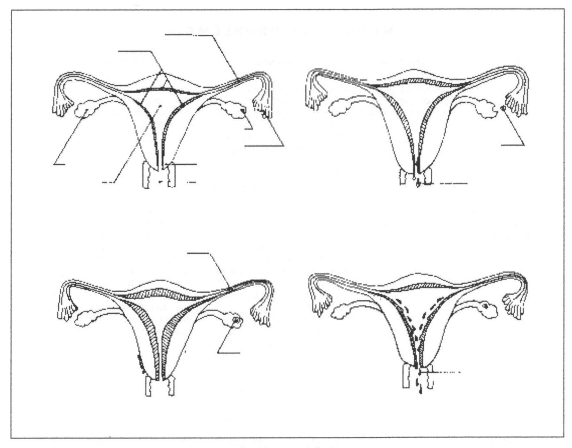

The Menstrual Cycle

Around mid-cycle—typically day 14 or 15—a second hormone, progesterone, joins estrogen in preparing the uterine lining for a fertilized egg. The egg itself has ripened and now receives the hormonal signal to leave the ovaries and begin its journey through the Fallopian tubes to the uterus. It's during this four to six day journey to the uterus that the egg is most likely to be fertilized. If you have sex during this time, you're much more likely to get pregnant than at other times. (Though relying on a calculation of more or less fertile times, especially in the teen years when your cycle may be quite variable, is a very risky form of birth control!) It's always wiser to assume that if you're having sex, even occasionally, and don't use a reliable form of birth control, you could get pregnant anytime of the month. (See Chapter 13 for information about birth control.)

At mid-cycle, as your hormonal levels peak, you may feel unusually good. After about day 20, these levels begin to drop if your egg has not been fertilized. The egg will begin to disintegrate and the lining of the uterus will start to break down. About day 28, this will begin to pass from your uterus, through your cervix, and out through your vagina. This is the menstrual flow.

MENSTRUAL PROBLEMS

Problem	Symptoms	Causes	What To Do
Irregular Periods	Skipping periods or spotting between periods	Most common cause is puberty itself: it can take several years for a regular cycle to get established. Other causes: stress, jet lag, or an underlying physical problem. Spotting is also a common side effect of birth control pills. It can also be a symptom of an ovarian cyst.	Keep track of your periods and any other symptoms you might have and discuss all this with your doctor.
Suddenly having no periods (Secondary Amenorrhea)	After having had menstrual periods, you suddenly stop	1. Pregnancy 2. Severe Stress 3. Heavy exercise (like elite training in gymnastics, ballet or long-distance running.) 4. A major weight change, up or down, a weight change of 10–15% of total body weight can affect cycle 5. Eating Disorder such as anorexia due to malnutrition and iron deficiency 6. Use of drugs—abuse of tranquilizers can affect cycle. Also, birth control pills can causer lighter periods or an occasional skipped period.	See your doctor. If your doctor finds that your condition is not due to prescription drugs, pregnancy or a physical problem like an ovarian cyst he or she may give you a medication to bring on your period or prescribe birth control pills to regulate your cycle for perhaps three months until the cycle is established again.
Endometriosis	Pelvic pain, prolonged periods	Overgrowth of uterine lining outside uterus—may be due to irregular ovarian function, or, perhaps, heredity	See your doctor. Endometriosis can be treated with painkillers, hormone therapy, birth control pills or, in severe cases, with laser surgery that does not harm the uterus or ovaries.

Problem	Symptoms	Causes	What To Do
PMS	Headaches, fatigue, increased appetite, mood changes with increased irritability. In severe cases, Premenstrual Disorder symptoms impair your ability to function at school or at work.	Experts are still unsure. There may be multiple causes.	1. Keep track of symptoms and periods to discover patterns. 2. Eliminate foods and drinks that may make PMS worse—like coffee, tea, chocolate and colas. These increase your prostagladin activity and that can trigger cramps, breast tenderness and nausea. Avoid salty or high sodium foods as well to help prevent pre-menstrual bloating. 3. Manage stress. Keep calm with music, meditation or other things you enjoy 4. Exercise regularly. This helps to manage mood swings involving anxiety and depression 5. See your doctor if symptoms persist.
Menstrual Cramps (Dysmenorrhea)	Pain in abdomen, legs and back.	Primary dysmenorrhea, the most common, is often caused by an over-production of prostagladins, hormone-like substances found throughout the body, including the lining of the uterus. These substances cause the uterus to contract, sometimes painfully. In the bloodstream, prostaglandins can cause muscles in the stomach and intestines to speed up contractions, causing nausea and diarrhea. Secondary dysmenorrhea, much less common, is caused by an anatomical disorder, infection, ovarian tumor or endometriosis.	1. Try over-the-counter remedies like Motrin, Advil, Nuprin, Naprosyn or Ponstel. Some feel Ponstel is most effective as it inhibits prostaglandin production. 2. If these don't help, see your doctor for prescription strength medication or for birth control pills that can decrease or eliminate periods. Your doctor will also determine whether you may have an underlying condition, like endometriosis that needs treatment. 3. Exercise. Walking, cycling or swimming all release substances called endorphins, which tend to diminish pain.

BUT DO I EVEN HAVE TO HAVE A PERIOD?

Please tell me what to do. Some of my friends take pills so that they have only few periods a year instead of one every month. And one girl I know takes a pill so she never gets a period! Is that safe? Can it make you not able to have children? I'm scared about taking pills and my mom says it's healthy to have regular periods and it's a way to tell that my body is working the way it should. I don't have cramps or anything terrible that happens with my period. I'm 15 and have had my period for almost three years, if that makes any difference. What should I do?

Brit B., 15

Today's teens are the first generation to be faced with menstruation as a choice, not as a monthly inevitability. However, having a monthly period is entirely healthy and normal. Especially if you don't have severe cramps or heavy bleeding that leads to anemia, it may not make sense to tamper with your cycle.

The pills that Brit mentions in her letter are synthetic hormones that are the same as or very similar to birth control pills. In fact, some birth control pills like Loestrin 24 Fe enable users to have light monthly periods of about three or four days.

A pill called Seasonale is taken for 91 days (instead of the 28 day cycle of many birth control pills) and eventually results in a woman having about four periods a year. However, there is a time of adjustment after a woman begins to take Seasonale where breakthrough bleeding—unexpected menstrual bleeding—may occur.

Since Seasonale is expensive, you might choose to take a low-dose estrogen/progesterone birth control pill like Sprintec-28 or Levora-28 for three months at a time, skipping the placebo pills in the last row of each packet and going on directly to the next packet. Again, you would take a pill every day for three months, and then have one of four periods a year before taking another three-month cycle of pills. The newest oral contraceptive that also regulates periods is called Lybrel and eliminates menstrual periods entirely for up to one year.

These pills are as safe as birth control pills and can be a real help to women who suffer severely from menstrual cramps or heavy periods. While they function as birth control pills and may be even more effective in preventing pregnancy when taken continuously over a year (because taking that daily pill may be easier to remember), they do not appear to impair long-term fertility. Advocates for these pills point out that today's women have many more periods than their ancestors, who spent most of their younger adult years either pregnant or nursing and thus not having periods—and so having uninterrupted menstrual periods over a number of years isn't necessarily natural to the species.

As with any medication, however, these pills are not risk-free. If you smoke, if you have a history (or family history) of blood clots, if you have high blood pressure or migraines with a pre-headache aura, it would be best to avoid any of these synthetic hormones.

You might think twice, too, if, like Brit, you don't have any particular problem with your periods and aren't in need of a birth control pill at this time. Menstruation isn't a disease to be cured or a problem to be fixed. You might choose to leave your periods alone for that monthly reassurance that all is well.

SANITARY PRODUCTS

I recently started my period and want to use tampons but my mom won't let me because she says tampons give you a fatal disease and make you not a virgin anymore. Is any of this true or just crazy mom talk?

Jana K.

Teens today have much better choices in sanitary products than their moms had—and sometimes that's what causes the disconnect when moms try to advise their daughters.

Pads today are much thinner, more absorbent and convenient than they were in your mom's youth. Tampons, too, come in a greater variety of sizes, including extra slim and can be comfortable for young girls just beginning to menstruate.

What about some of Jana's mother's concerns? They reflect common myths or misunderstandings about tampons.

You can, in fact, be a virgin and still wear tampons. You cease to be a virgin when you have sexual intercourse. The hymen is elastic and stretches easily, in most cases, to allow the use of a tampon.

Some fear that a tampon can "get lost" inside the vagina, but that can't happen. The cervical os, at the far end of the vagina, is much too tiny to permit the passage of the tampon into the uterus.

Many new users of tampons find that those with applicators are easier to use, at least initially, than the ones inserted with a finger.

The menstrual cup—called Instead—is a soft, flexible cup that is inserted into the vagina to fit over the cervix. At first, its insertion may be a little more difficult than that of a tampon. The advantage of the cup is that it gives you more protection time. For example, if you have to change a tampon every two hours, you can go about four hours without a change with Instead.

However, it's important to change whatever form of sanitary protection you use before the maximum time. This is especially true of sanitary protection that you wear internally—like tampons and, possibly, Instead. Which brings us to Jana's mom's other point of concern: a condition called *toxic shock syndrome*. This is a very rare, but sometimes fatal disease caused by a bacterium that is most often found in surgical wounds, cuts, skin abscesses or highly absorbent tampons left in the vagina for a long stretch of time. TSS was a greater danger in the Eighties, when your mom might have been a teen, than it is now that tampons have been redesigned in response to the threat, using somewhat less absorbent materials.

You *can* use tampons safely, but need to keep the following safety tips in mind:

- Change tampons frequently—at least every three to four hours, even when the menstrual flow is light.
- Use tampons with the lowest possible absorbency. Even on heavy flow days, you might consider using a regular tampon with a mini-pad.

- Consider using tampons during the day and pads while you sleep.
- Avoid using tampons with petal-shaped plastic ends. Some of those have sharp edges that could scratch your vagina.
- Always wash your hands before inserting a tampon to make sure that you don't introduce bacteria into your vagina.
- Don't use tampons to absorb non-menstrual vaginal secretions.
- If you're having your period and notice flu-like symptoms (a sudden fever of 102 F or higher, vomiting and diarrhea, headache, dizziness, sore throat, muscle aches, and a sunburn-like rash, most commonly seen on the hands and feet), remove your tampon and seek medical help immediately.

VAGINAL HEALTH

What should I be doing as far as feminine hygiene goes? I'm not even sure what it means. But I heard my mother and her friend talking about douching and I don't know what that is and if I should be doing it, too. How can I prevent odors? I haven't noticed any myself, but I keep hearing about the in commercials. Help!

Andrea Y.

A daily bath or shower that includes washing your genital area with soap and water is the best possible safeguard against unpleasant odors. Body odors are most often caused by bacteria acting on perspiration and other normal secretions. Avoid clothes that increase perspiration such as nylon underwear or pantyhose—unless they have cotton or ventilated crotches. Keeping clean and wearing clean, well-ventilated underwear is really all you need to do.

Forget those "feminine sprays"—they can irritate the delicate tissues of the vulva and vagina and are no substitute for personal cleanliness.

Forget douching, too. Douching is a bad habit from the old days and involves cleansing the vagina with a solution of water and vinegar or a commercial douche preparation, using a douche bag or special squeeze bottle. This is useless and can even be harmful. First, the healthy vagina is self-cleansing, making douching unnecessary. Second, studies have found that excessive douching may actually make a woman more likely to get a vaginal infection by altering the normal acidic balance of the vagina. For example, researchers at the Mount Sinai School of Medicine in New York looked at 30 years of published research on the topic and found that women who douched had a 73 percent greater risk of pelvic inflammatory disease than women who did not. The only time a douche may be indicated is if it is a medicinal one prescribed by a doctor for some varieties of vaginal infections.

Vaginal Infections

Help! I think I have an infection because I have this discharge. How do I know whether I have an infection or not without going to the doctor?

Cammie K.

It's normal to have a clear, whitish, non-irritating vaginal discharge. This mixture of mucus, bacteria, and discarded vaginal cells may turn from clear or white to pale yellow as it is exposed to the air. This discharge can become more noticeable under certain circumstances—like during sexual excitement or during ovulation or in women who are taking birth control pills.

How do you know whether you might have an infection? A vaginal discharge is *not* normal if it is irritating, causes itching, is mixed with non-menstrual blood, has a foul odor, or is a different color from your normal discharge. These are usually symptoms of a vaginal infection and a sign that it's time to see your doctor. Don't try to self-treat a vaginal infection. Seek advice from your physician first.

The following chart will show you the most common types of vaginal infections, their symptoms and treatment.

MOST COMMON VAGINAL INFECTIONS

Infection	Cause	Symptoms	Treatment
Bacterial vaginosis	Vulnerable during times of stress or while taking antibiotics. May also be sexually transmitted.	Heavy, creamy, gray-white discharge that has a foul, fishy odor	See a physician. Treatment is usually prescription drug Flagyl (metronidazole) in pill form.
Candidiasis (yeast infection)	Imbalance of natural vaginal bacteria due to diabetes, tight clothing, prolonged use of antibiotics such as tetracycline, or birth control pills. Rarely sexually transmitted	Thick, odorless, white discharge with the consistency of cottage cheese. Itching of the vulva and vagina and white patches of fungus over reddish, raw areas. Painful urination.	See a physician for correct diagnosis rather than trying to self-diagnose. Treatment of choice is either Monistat or Lotrimin in cream or suppository form. These are now available over the counter, but a correct diagnosis from your physician is crucial.
Trichomoniasis	Caused by a protozoan organism spread via shared washcloths, towels, wet bathing suits, toilet seats. Often sexually transmitted.	A frothy greenish-yellow, foul-smelling discharge, vaginal itching, inflammation of the vulva. There may also be frequent, painful urination and, in some cases, severe lower abdominal pain.	See a physician. The treatment is usually Flagyl in pill form. There are also Flagyl suppositories. Both forms are available only by prescription. If you're sexually active, your partner also needs to be treated.

If you have persistent vaginal discharge that has not been diagnosed as an infection, you may just have a more copious than usual vaginal discharge. What can help? Try alternating baths with showers, wearing cotton underwear, and avoiding very tight jeans Also, don't sleep in confining clothes such as sweatpants or underpants.

If you have urgent, painful urination, this could be a symptom of a bladder or urinary track infection. Consult your physician.

If you have pain when you urinate, but don't

feel the urgency that characterizes urinary bladder infections, you may have a small cut on your labia or vaginal entrance that burns when the acidic urine touches it. If you have a small cut, dab some petroleum jelly on it to protect it and thus promote healing

Although various types of vaginal infections may be identified by a specific discharge, your doctor may need to do further tests to make absolutely sure you have that specific infection since treatments vary from one infection to another.

Also, if you're having sex, even only occasionally, you are at risk for sexually transmitted diseases and must see your doctor to rule out that possibility—or to get appropriate treatment. Some common sexually transmitted diseases such as chlamydia and gonorrhea must be promptly and correctly treated in order to preserve health and fertility. So if you have an unusual discharge or other troublesome symptoms, don't try to diagnose and treat yourself!

But What About the HPV Vaccine?

Hi! I'm 13 and have a question: what do you think about the new vaccine that girls as young as 9 are supposed to get to keep from getting cancer? Is this just a rumor or bogus or what? My mom says I don't need to get it because I'm not having sex yet (Huh? Does sex give you cancer???) I'm confused and I hate shots! But I also don't want to get cancer. What should I do?
—Madison A., 13

The vaccine that Madison is asking about is called Gardasil and it protects girls from four of the most common strains of the human papillomavirus (HPV) that cause cervical cancer and genital warts. These four strains include two types that cause an estimated 70% of cervical cancer cases and two other types that cause about 90% of genital warts.

This vaccine is safe (though if you have severe allergies, you may want to discuss with your doctor whether or not to get the vaccine series). Both the Centers for Disease Control and the American Academy of Pediatrics are recommending this vaccine for young women ages 9 through 26 years old. The most recommended age range for the injection series is between the ages of 11-13 before a girl becomes sexually active. Because HPV is a sexually transmitted disease, there is some controversy over making these vaccinations routine or even mandatory for girls entering middle school.

However, even if you're not sexually active or even planning to be anytime soon, routine protection against HPV makes sense. In fact, it makes the most sense to have it well before you ever become sexually active. HPV, which infects over 6 million people in the U.S every year, is the most common sexually transmitted disease in the nation and, yes, it can lead to cancer if one is infected with a cancer-causing strain. And think about it: it might be much less embarrassing to get vaccinated as part of your pre-middle school physical instead of waiting until sex looks like a real possibility and then trying to get in and see a doctor for the shot series. Besides, sometimes you don't have a lot of lead-time once you are close to being sexually active—and, to be fully protected, you need to have three doses of the vaccine over a six-month period.

We know that three injections over a six-month period is not exactly good news for people like Brit who hate shots, but this treatment works and is totally worth the effort—sooner rather than later!

GROWING FROM GIRL TO WOMAN

I feel ugly, not cute like my friends. They have boyfriends and I don't even though I like this special boy a lot. He doesn't notice me at all. I feel like a total loser and like there's something the matter with my body.

—Hannah N.

Cultural expectations can hit hard, especially in the early teens, when there's so much pressure to be pretty, thin, and popular that it's easy to lose one's sense of self.

Women of all ages have insecurities about their bodies and a lot of this is based on our society's unrealistic standards of beauty for women. Think about it: does a guy have to look perfect to be considered a hunk? But women are often held to near impossible standards. Who, in everyday life, looks like a supermodel? Not even the supermodels—minus makeup, lighting and photo touchups!

Your beauty as a woman and your value as a person are expressed in many ways—more through who you are than how you look according to society's standards. Girls can get distracted from this fact by comments and teasing from classmates or family about their changing bodies or by comparing themselves unfavorably with actresses and supermodels—and develop poor body image.

Having a negative body image can affect your life in many ways. Your confidence and self-esteem may suffer. You may feel insecure around guys –and not pretty unless some guy says you are. Your self-consciousness may keep you from doing things you enjoy. You may even begin to believe that you're less deserving of love and happiness than other people are.

If any of this sounds painfully familiar, what can you do?

- *Change your mind about your body before you try to change your looks.* You are loveable and valuable just as you are right now. Repeat this to yourself and believe it. Otherwise, no amount of cosmetic changes will make any real difference in how you feel about yourself. There are countless overweight people who lose lots of weight—but still feel fat. There are others who never get over feeling like awkward kids with crooked teeth, acne and thick glasses—even after braces have straightened the teeth, the acne has abated and the glasses have given way to contacts. If you can feel accepting and positive about yourself right now, you'll be able to take change in stride. See exercising and eating healthy foods as a reward you deserve not as a punishment because you're fat.

- *Realize that people who tease have their own insecurities.* Their comments have more to do with themselves than with you. Concentrate on what's right about you and your impressive array of good qualities. If you're stalled here, ask for help from your parents or a trusted friend.

- *Realize that in the real world, attractive people come in all shapes and sizes.* And what makes them attractive goes far beyond the shape of their nose or body or the color of their hair. Being active, friendly, kind, having a sense of humor, moving with confidence and grace, feeling at ease with yourself as you are—all of this can go a long way toward developing a positive body image and being an overall attractive person. Feeling good about yourself can do more for your appearance than all the cosmetic treatments put together!

Part of your growth as a woman is to find inner peace and self-acceptance of who you are physically and emotionally. In the chapters to come, we'll be sharing some useful ides to maximize your body's health, fitness and vitality. But it's up to you to discover your own unique beauty. That has nothing to do with being a certain weight or bra size and everything to do with good health, loving self-care of your body and emotional needs and your growth as a loving person. When you're able to love, accept and appreciate yourself, others will, too!

QUICK SCAN ✓

A WOMAN'S BODY

✔ *There are many variations of normal when it comes to development.* Your own timetable is based on your genetic and ethnic heritage. For example, if you're African-American, it is normal to develop somewhat earlier than friends of other ethnicities.

✔ *If you're very physically active with low body fat, your development may be slowed despite your genetic heritage.* This is particularly true for those heavily training in ballet, gymnastics or figure skating where body fat tends to be very low. But if you haven't started menstruating by age 16 or so, it's essential to see your physician to make sure all is well.

✔ *Learning how to manage stress can help to ease PMS and menstrual cramps.* Other aspects of a healthy lifestyle—like eating lots of fruits and vegetables and getting regular exercise—can help a lot, too.

✔ *Don't self-diagnose vaginal infections.* Always see a doctor for correct diagnosis.

There are steps you can take to decrease your chances of getting a vaginal infection: Don't wear tight clothing or nylon underwear. Don't share towels or damp bathing suits. And make personal hygiene (regular baths or showers) a priority.

CHAPTER THREE
From Boy to Man

My school sex ed class is, in a word, lame. My parents are too embarrassed to talk to me about anything personal and there are some things I'm too embarrassed to ask. But I have lots of questions. Like is it normal to have a hard-on a lot of times, off and on, throughout the day? What about the fact that I'm 14 and look pretty much like a man while my friend Eric, who is my age exactly, still looks like a little kid? Is there something wrong with him? I wonder about all the stuff what's going on with my body. Can you help me figure this all out?

Michael S.

Michael has lots of company. The changes of adolescence are dramatic and not always easy to understand. There is a much greater variation in male physical development from start to finish. One 14-year-old by may be, indeed, still be a boy, while his taller, more physically mature classmate may look very much like a man. Becoming a man is a complicated process. The better you understand the changes that your body is experiencing and what is normal, the more readily and completely you will begin to understand and accept yourself.

MALE ANATOMY

There are three parts to the male reproductive system. First, there are the organs of production—the *testicles*. At the beginning of puberty, on a chain-reaction signal from the *hypothalamus*, *pituitary* and *pineal* glands, the

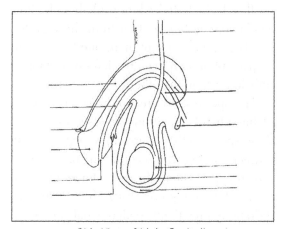

Side View of Male Genitalia

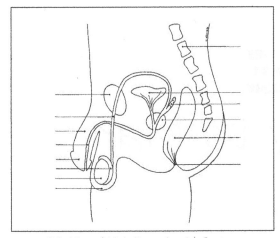

Side View of Male Reproductive System

testicles begin to produce the male hormone *testosterone*. This hormone triggers the common changes of adolescence such as enlargement of genital organs, growth of pubic hair, and deepening of the voice. As puberty progresses, the testicles also begin to mature and to produce sperm cells that, if united with a female's ovum, or egg, will produce a baby.

The two testicles are encased in the *scrotum*, which hangs under the penis. It is quite common for one testicle to hang somewhat lower than the others. (There is a biological reason for this: If the testicles hung side-by-side, they would get constant friction from the legs. So, in a large percentage of men, one testicle—in 70 percent of such men, the left one—hangs a little lower than the other.)

The sperm cells are produced in a series of tiny chambers within the testicles, and as these sperm cells mature, they begin a long journey through the second part of the male reproductive system: the ducts for storage and transportation of sperm. First, there is the *epididymis*, a long, tightly coiled canal (uncoiled, it would stretch about 20 feet!) that lies over each testicle. Next, the sperm travel to the *vas deferens*, a shorter continuation of the epididymis. This brings the sperm from the scrotum to the abdominal cavity, passing to the back of the bladder and joining the seminal vesicles, forming the ejaculatory duct where sperm is stored.

The *prostate gland*, which lies against the bottom of the bladder, secretes much of the *seminal fluid*, which, combined with fluids from the seminal vesicles, carries the sperm from the body. The prostate gland enlarges dramatically during the changes of puberty. Other secretions come from the *bulbourethral glands*, two tiny structures on either side of the *urethra*, the passageway through which both urine and seminal fluid pass out of the penis. During sexual excitement, the bulbourethral glands produce a clear, sticky fluid that is thought to coat the urethra for the safe passage of the sperm. This is not seminal fluid, but it may contain a few stray sperm.

The third part of the male reproductive system is the *penis*.

When a mature or maturing man is sexually excited, he may ejaculate his seminal fluid out of the penis in a series of throbbing spurts. The total volume of this thick white *ejaculate* is, on the average, about one teaspoon and is made up mostly of secretions from the prostate gland and the seminal vesicles. Although sperm make up only a small part of the total ejaculate, they are impressive in number. There may be about *400 million* sperm in one ejaculation! Obviously, the sperm cells are tiny. They are so small, in fact, that 400 million of them could fit on the head of a pin!

Another bit of sperm trivia: Your testicles may produce 200 million or more sperm cells in a day! Obviously, only a few sperm cells, in any average lifetime, end up fertilizing an egg and producing a baby.

A lot of people think that the penis is a skin-

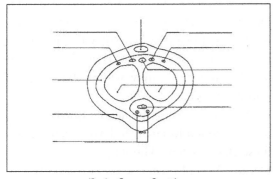

Penis Cross Section

covered cylinder. That isn't so. The penis is made up of spongy tissues interlaced with large blood vessels (see cross-sectional illustration). There is a constant flow of blood in and out of the penis, which, despite a wide normal deviation in size among men, *averages* three to four inches long and one and one-quarter inches in diameter—in the *flaccid*, or soft, state—in the mature male.

When a man becomes sexually excited, however, this even blood flow stops. The blood vessels expand, bringing more blood into the penis. Valves in the veins retain this blood under pressure, causing the spongy walls of the penis to expand and become hard. This is called an erection or hard-on.

The skin of the penis is loose to allow for expansion during erection. In some males, there is the *prepuce* or *foreskin*, which covers the head, or *glans*, of the penis. Although all males are born with this foreskin, many have it

surgically removed, usually soon after birth, in a procedure called *circumcision*.

All Jewish boys are circumcised for religious reasons, but it has been common practice in this country until quite recently for the majority of hospital-born male infants to be circumcised. The practice today is becoming somewhat controversial, with some doctors questioning the automatic nature of this procedure and calling circumcision an option rather than a necessity. (In response to this changing feeling about circumcision, some insurance companies no longer cover the costs for this procedure, and the percentage of circumcised boys in this country is dropping.)

The circumcised and uncircumcised penis may look a bit different from each other in the flaccid state. Otherwise, each functions normally and there is no concrete evidence that circumcision—or lack of it—sharpens sexual response. The uncircumcised male, however, must take special care to keep his penis clean, since a foul smelling substance called *smegma* may collect under the foreskin if the penis is not washed daily. Circumcised males don't

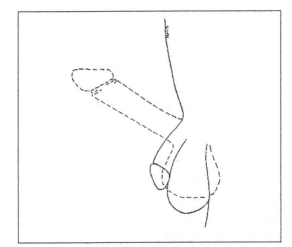

Penis During Erection

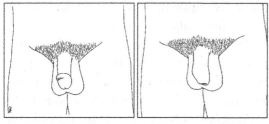

Circumcised Penis   Uncircumcised Penis

experience this accumulation of smegma, and, according to some medical studies, may have a lower incidence of urinary tract infections.

As we mentioned earlier, circumcision is usually performed in the first few days of life. However, some teen boys and adult men elect to have this done, often due to a particularly tight foreskin—a problem we'll be discussing later on in this chapter.

We have just been describing the reproductive system of the mature male. It is important to know how your body is working—or will work. For some, it is the process of growing to manhood that is of most concern.

PHYSICAL DEVELOPMENT

When is the normal time to start maturing? I'm almost 14 and I still look like a kid and get teased a lot. Should I see a doctor? Is something wrong with me?

Kevin T.

Males, as well as females, have their own highly individual biological time clocks. The changes of puberty in the male may begin as early as age 8 or as late as age 15. Puberty may finish between ages 14 and 18. Therefore, some very normal 13- or 14-year olds appear to be grown

men, while some of their equally normal classmates still look like boys.

Slow development—often an inherited genetic characteristic—may be even more worrisome for a boy than for a girl. Girls tend to start puberty about a year or two earlier, on the average, than their male classmates. So the late-blooming male may feel really left behind. In most cases, however, the so-called late bloomer is entirely within the range of normal.

What are some of the age ranges for a boy's development into a man and what sequence do these changes flow? The stages of puberty were identified by a British doctor names J. M. Tanner, who noted that within each stage there are many small changes and steps in growth, genital development, and pubic hair development. There are many variations, of course, but the major changes follow a basic pattern shown in the following charts.

SPECIAL PROBLEMS

Short Stature

Please help me. I'm short and I get teased all the time. Is there anything I can do, like a treatment, that can make me taller?

Sean A.

There is a wide range of height among teen boys, but those on the lower end of the range may wonder whether they will always be shorter than average.

Heredity is a factor. If you're well along in your development and have shorter-than-average parents, you're likely to be relatively short,

STAGES OF PUBERTY IN BOYS

Stage	Ages	Internal	Genitals	Growth	Hair	Other
One	9–12	Male hormones are becoming active	No obvious change; testicles are maturing	Some start rapid growth late in this stage	No pubic or other body hair	None
Two	9–15	Hormonal changes cause new muscle tissue and fat to be added to body, changing the shape of the body	Testicles and scrotum are enlarging, but penis is not increasing much in size at this stage	Rapid growth, in height and in changing physique	Pubic hair appears at the base of the penis; will be straight and fine	The areola, the circle of darker skin around each nipple on the chest increases in size and darkens a little.
Three	11–16		Penis grows mostly in length; testicles and scrotum still growing	Adding more muscle tissue; still growing; shoulders broaden	Pubic hair is getting darker and coarse, spreading along the base of the penis; first traces of hair on upper lip	Voice starts deepening due to growth of larynx
Four	11–17	Sperm production begins; first ejaculation	Penis grows in width; testicles still growing		Underarm and facial hair increases; pubic hair looks more adult	Voice gets deeper and skin becomes more oily
Five	14–18	Full development	Adult in appearance	Near full adult height	Adult pubic hair; full beard	May get chest, body hair later

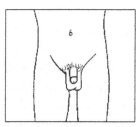 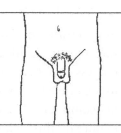 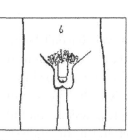 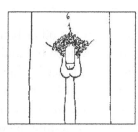

1. Straight hair appears at penis base. Testes increase in size and skin of scrotum reddens.

2. Pubic hair becomes curly and coarse. Penis grows in length.

3. Pubic hair is full, but limited in area. Penis grows in width.

4. Development of pubic hair and genitals is complete.

AGE RANGE OF CHANGES OF PUBERTY IN BOYS

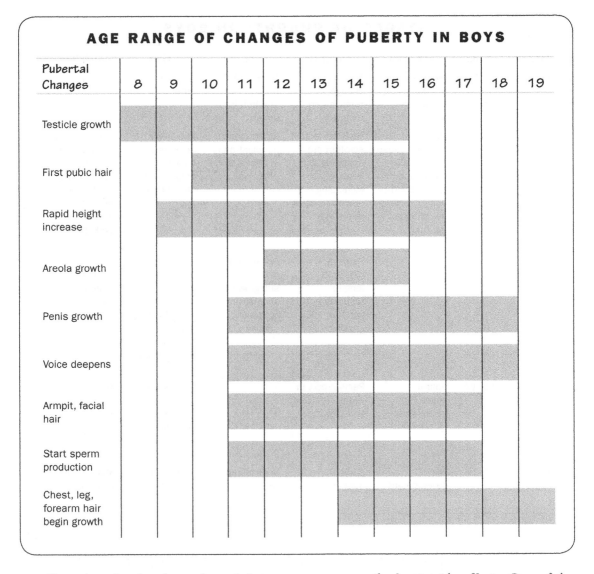

Pubertal Changes	8	9	10	11	12	13	14	15	16	17	18	19
Testicle growth	▓	▓	▓	▓	▓	▓	▓	▓				
First pubic hair			▓	▓	▓	▓	▓	▓				
Rapid height increase		▓	▓	▓	▓	▓	▓	▓	▓			
Areola growth					▓	▓	▓	▓	▓			
Penis growth				▓	▓	▓	▓	▓	▓	▓	▓	
Voice deepens				▓	▓	▓	▓	▓	▓	▓	▓	
Armpit, facial hair				▓	▓	▓	▓	▓	▓	▓		
Start sperm production				▓	▓	▓	▓	▓				
Chest, leg, forearm hair begin growth							▓	▓	▓	▓	▓	▓

too. If on the other hand, you haven't begun much development and have a tall parent or parents you may be due for a lot of growing.

Just to make sure all is well, check with your doctor for a complete physical, including thyroid testing, blood and urine analysis, and X-rays to determine bone age. While hormone therapy can speed up a delayed puberty, physicians are reluctant to use this unnecessarily due to side effects. One of the side effects, ironically, in speeding up the process of puberty is that accelerating growth may cause a boy to be shorter as an adult than he would have been had he been allowed to mature on this own timetable. For this reason and others, many physicians prefer to let natural development take place in its own time whenever possible.

Society tends to value tall men. However, like a number of other societal expectations, this "tall, dark and handsome" measure of desirable manhood is a myth. There are many very loving—and loved—men who are none of the above. Real men come in all sizes and physical types. You can be attractive even if you're far from tall or handsome. A lot has to do with how you develop your personality, your social skills, and your own good feeling about yourself.

Adolescent Nodule/Adolescent Gynecomastia

What does it mean when you have swelling on your chest under the nipple area? It almost looks like I'm getting breasts. I'm too embarrassed to tell my parents or my doctor. Is something wrong with me?

Travis T.

Several conditions can cause breasts swelling in the adolescent male. First, there is the *adolescent nodule*. This small but firm swelling under the nipple may occur in one or both breasts. It has been linked to increased secretion of the male sex hormone just before puberty begins. Although this nodule may be tender and cause some concern, it doesn't require treatment. Most of these nodules go away within a year.

Second, and perhaps most common is a condition called *adolescent gynecomastia*. This breast enlargement, which looks much like female breast development, seems to be caused by an increase and, perhaps, a slight imbalance in the amount of hormones during early puberty. Less common types of

this condition are found in boys with undescended testicles (who have, as a result, too few hormones in the bloodstream), and in boys with certain birth defects. It has also been linked with prolonged and heavy use of amphetamines (uppers) and even heavy use of marijuana. In its most common form, gynecomastia tends to subside as the teen boy progresses in his physical development, usually running its course within sixteen months. Several studies have found that several drugs—including Danazol—can be somewhat effective in reducing the size of a boy's breasts when symptoms of gynecomastia persist beyond sixteen months. However, more research needs to be done about the effectiveness and possible side effects of such drug therapy.

Prostatitis

I've been having a problem with pain when I piss. And I seem to be going to the bathroom a lot more than usual. I know it isn't any sexual disease because I'm not having sex. I'm more into weight lifting and sports in general. What should I do?

Brad C.

Brad's complaint sounds very much like prostatitis, and the cause may be his weight lifting. The symptoms? Frequent urination, often with pain. Since several sexually transmitted diseases have similar symptoms, it's always a good idea to see a physician for a correct diagnosis. Besides, prostatitis doesn't just go away. It requires treatment with antibiotics for several weeks—and swearing off weight lifting during the period of recovery.

Pink Pearly Papules

Can you have a disease without having sex? I'm 16 and haven't ever had sex but I just noticed these bumps in a circle around the head of my dick and I'm nervous that something serious may be wrong. This isn't something I can ask my mom about. What's going on?

Jared P.

What Jared is describing is called *pink pearly papules*. These benign lesions of the penile *corona* (the raised area of skin that separates the tip of the penis from the shaft of the penis) are not at all related to sexual activity and are not a disease of any kind. They usually grow in one to five rows along the corona of the penis and are pearly white in color. Uncircumcised males are somewhat more likely to have pearly papules. These are most likely to occur in the midst of the major changes of puberty. About 15 percent of all adolescent males have these papules. They're completely harmless and no treatment is indicated.

However, especially if you are sexually active, it's important to see a doctor to confirm the fact that these are, indeed, pearly papules, since some sexually transmitted diseases show up as growths or lesions on the penis. Although all of these look quite different from the harmless papules, it may take a physician's practiced eye to tell the difference.

Undescended Testicle(s)

Is it true if you have an undescended testicle, you can get cancer? That's all I want to know: is it true?

Brandon H.

It's true that an undescended testicle is 10 to 40 percent more likely to become cancerous than a properly placed one. And testicular cancer does happen in young men.

What is an undescended testicle and how do you know if you have one? When a baby boy is developing in the womb, both of his testicles are in the abdomen. These usually descend into the scrotum before birth. However, in some cases, a boy may be born with one or both testicles undescended.

In many cases, this condition is detected right away and, if the testicle doesn't descend on its own between birth and puberty, medical intervention will be used to make sure it does get into the scrotum where it belongs. Only 1 boy in 500 will have a testicle still undescended by the time he starts puberty.

You can't always tell, simply by looking, whether your testicle is undescended. Some boys have testicles that move up into the groin area and then back to the scrotum from time to time. This is called *a floating testicle*. If you have this condition—or if you think or know that you have an undescended testicle—please see your doctor.

Some require plastic surgery to correct this condition. Even if surgery means removing one testicle, that isn't going to interfere with your normal functioning as a male. You'll still be able to have sex and have children as easily as anyone else. You can manage just fine with one testicle. You don't even have to look different. Your doctor can put something called a *sialastic implant*, a special material made the size of a testicle, into your scrotum to make it look as if you have two testicles.

Testicular Cancer

I heard from a friend recently that people my age (16) can get testicular cancer, and that scared me. Is that true? How can I keep from getting it?

Scared in Spokane

According to the American Cancer Society, testicular cancer is one of the most common cancers in men between ages 15 and 35. It occurs in about 6,300 men each year, with 350 deaths. With early detection, however, the survival rate for the most common forms of the disease is almost 100 percent; for all types of testicular cancer, there is a 78 to 85 percent five-year survival rate. Those with the best chance of survival are those whose cancer is discovered very early.

It's important, once you're well into puberty—generally between ages 13 and 15—to make a habit of examining your testicles about once a month. This is an important safeguard for your health and will take only about three minutes once you get used to doing it. It's best to do this self-exam after a warm bath or shower, when the scrotum is relaxed.

How do you do the testicular exam? First, hold your scrotum in the palm of your hand, feeling one testicle at a time. Gently roll the testicle between the thumbs and fingers of both hands for several minutes. Then check the epididymis. This cord is behind your testicles. It will be a bit tender to the touch. That's normal. Next, check the vas deferens, which is above the epididymis and feels like a smooth, firm tube. Examine these cords on both sides.

It's important to get to know the feel and shape of your testicles. If you notice any nodules,

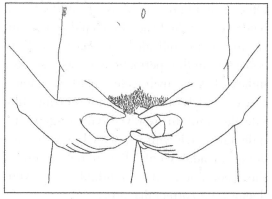

Testicular Self-Examination

lumps, swelling, or a severe, knifelike pain in the groin or testicles, see your doctor immediately! And, when you have regular physical exams, ask your doctor to examine your testicles as well. (This may be embarrassing the first time, but it's an important part of your exam, so be sure to speak up if your doctor doesn't include it in the exam process).

Benign Scrotal Masses

I felt my balls when I was showering last night and felt something different like a bag of worms or something on the left side. Does this mean I have cancer or something horrible? Please answer me fast

Todd L.

There are several benign conditions that can feel scary when you first notice them. One is a *varicocele*, which is what Todd is describing. It is due to the dilation of the veins in the scrotum and usually occurs on the left side. Surgery is done only in extreme cases where there is a major enlargement of the scrotum accompanied by pain. About 10 to 15 percent of adolescents experience this condition.

Other conditions such as *spermatocele* (a benign cyst at the head of the epididymis with no treatment indicated), *hydrocele* (a fluid collection in the spermatic cord, with surgery indicated if the hydrocele persists in adolescence), and *hernia* (a protrusion of intestine into the scrotum, resolved with surgery) are quite rare, each with less than 1 percent incidence in adolescents. If you notice any of these conditions, it's important to see your doctor for a correct diagnosis.

Foreskin Problems

I'm not circumcised and that's never been a problem for me until recently, when it has become harder to pull my foreskin back all the way when I wash. What can I do?

Clive K.

Clive—and anyone else who is suddenly having trouble pulling his foreskin back—should check with his doctor. It's possible that a physician could correct this by loosening the foreskin. This condition often develops because of poor hygiene. The foreskin needs to be pulled back daily to wash the head of the penis. This is an important preventive measure.

If you find that your penis is swollen and painful *and* you're unable to pull back your foreskin, seek medical help immediately. This condition, known as *paraphimosis*, and another condition called *phimosis*, where the foreskin adheres to the head of the penis and can't be pulled back at all, are best corrected by circumcision. Although circumcision in the adolescent or adult male may be more involved than it is for an infant, it is still a safe and minor surgical procedure.

Pain in the Groin

What does it mean when you have pain in your groin? I guess what I mean is, how serious is it?

Cameron J.

If you have pain in your groin, see your doctor immediately. The problem could be minor—or it could be major—and only your doctor can tell for sure. The reason we suggest *immediate* action is that severe, knife-like pain in the groin can be a symptom of *testicular torsion*. If this condition is not diagnosed and treated within a few hours of the onset of symptoms, the affected testicle will die, eventually shriveling to the size of a marble and becoming useless. In rare, but tragic cases, this has happened to some boys and men, at different times, in both testicles and was not treated in time for either testicle to be saved.

How does testicular torsion happen? The testicles, by necessity, are quite mobile, moving closer to or away from the body in response to heat or cold in order to maintain a constant temperature for the developing sperm. In some instances, however, a testicle may twist around its blood supply cord, trapping blood in the testicle and causing it to swell suddenly and massively as well as causing pain in the groin. A boy or a man may also experience nausea and vomiting.

The twisting may take place during strenuous activity or even during sleep. If this happens, don't just turn over and try to get back to sleep while waiting for the pain to pass. (The pain may pass, but only as the testicle dies—

which can happen very quickly, within four to eight hours.)

Surgery for testicular torsion is quite simple. The testicle is untwisted and then fixed into place with a few stitches so that it will no longer be susceptible to torsion. If this surgery has been prompt enough to avoid any tissue damage to the testicle, fertility is generally not diminished. If the testicle has died, the surgeon may remove it and, at the same time, surgically anchor the surviving testicle so it will not be vulnerable to the same twisting.

Pain in the groin doesn't always signal testicular torsion. There are other common causes as well. One of these is hernia, which occurs when abdominal contents bulge through a spot in the abdominal wall. This can signal that the blood supply to that area has been reduced, which could be serious. Seek medical help immediately. Surgery is the usual method of treatment.

Swollen glands could be another cause of groin pain. Lymph glands in the groin region may become infected and swell painfully. Treatment with antibiotics will usually alleviate this problem.

Another cause for pain in the groin, which does *not* require medical attention, will happen when you have experienced sexual arousal and a prolonged erection without the release of semen — a condition commonly called "blue balls". This is caused by prolonged engorgement of blood in the penis and pubic area. It will go away without intervention — medical, your partner's, or your own — and with no harm done.

Ejaculation Problems

What if you get sexually excited, get an erection and everything, but then can't come? This has happened to me several times—once when I was masturbating and once when was messing around with my girlfriend. Is this a sign that something serious is wrong with me?

Ryan K.

Inability to ejaculate during shared sex or masturbation is not unusual. It happens for a variety of reasons. Perhaps you were just not turned on enough to ejaculate. Maybe the setting or the other person wasn't right. Maybe you were feeling too self-conscious or guilty or pressured to perform. Inability to ejaculate can also be caused by the use of some commonly abused drugs (see Chapter 8).

Whatever the causes in your particular case, you may be reassured after discussing the matter with your physician. Chances are, especially if this happens only occasionally, you simply need to pay attention to what feels right for you and what doesn't in terms of partners, activities, location, and timing.

In the last two days, I've had pain in my penis and something that looks like milk comes out. I'm scared. I know it can't be anything sexually related because I haven't had sex, but what can it be?

Marty S.

Marty's problem is seen frequently in adolescent males. His penis pain and milky discharge is probably cause by *retrograde ejaculation*, which occurs when an ejaculation (release of semen) is incomplete or prevented from happening. This may happen when a guy is masturbating, but reluctant, for any number of reasons, to ejaculate. So, as he feels ejaculation about to occur, he places a thumb over the head of his penis to prevent the ejaculate from escaping. Or he may be ready to ejaculate while kissing or petting with a partner, but the semen is held back by tight pants or, again, by a thumb over the opening of the penis.

In any case, the ejaculate may be backward into the prostrate gland, causing engorgement and, at times, *prostatitis*, or infection of the prostate. In this condition, the symptoms may include pain felt at the base of the penis or in the testicles and a small amount of clear or milky discharge from the penis. (However, prostatitis is not invariably linked to retrograde ejaculation or the sex practices just described.)

What can you do about retrograde ejaculation?
Consult your physician. It may feel embarrassing, but doctors see this a lot and are likely to be very understanding and able to treat the condition. The best way to keep this problem from happening is to stop the practice of inhibiting ejaculation. However, if, unlike Marty, you are sexually active, a discharge from your penis may be a sign of a sexually transmitted disease: you need to be tested for that possibility as well.

This is embarrassing, but I'm worried enough to tell you about it. See, last week I noticed blood in my come. (I noticed it while jerking off. I don't have real sex yet.) For the next two nights, blood was still in my semen. Now it has stopped, but I'm still worried. What's wrong with me?

Dale C.

The condition that Dale describes, called *hematospermia*, is not uncommon in teenage boys. A very small blood vessel ruptures along the route which the semen travels—usually in the prostate gland or in the seminal vesicles. A tiny amount of blood is then mixed with the semen and may be evident for one or several ejaculation, which is why Dale noticed this for three nights and not again. The tiny break heals itself. This is quite common and not a sign of a serious problem.

What causes "wet dreams"? I've had a few and it's fairly embarrassing.

J.P.

"Wet dreams" (also called *nocturnal emissions*) are normal and involuntary (that is, you have no conscious control over them). These wet dreams are the release of semen during sleep and are most likely to happen in guys who don't masturbate much or have sex. These are not a sign that anything is wrong. It's just nature's way of releasing stored semen, which a man produces constantly.

GROWING FROM BOY TO MAN

While much has been said and written lately about the difficulty of growing up female, growing up male isn't exactly easy either. There are inevitable pressures from parents, peers, and society to look, act, or be a certain way. There can be a lot of self-inflicted pressure, too. Many guys have unusually high expectations of themselves and suffer when they fall short in some area of another. We'll be addressing self-esteem and other emotional issues in the next chapter, but just want to emphasize here that becoming a man is a journey unique, in many ways, to each individual.

Many men are take-charge, aggressive, strong, and tough: many equally masculine men are more low-key, gentle, and content to follow. Ideally, a man will have access to his full range of skills and feelings: expressing quiet, tender feelings as well as being decisive and assertive when necessary.

It's important to know, too, that healthy, masculine bodies come in all shapes and sizes. Taking care of yourself—getting enough rest, good nutrition, and sufficient exercise; avoiding harmful habits such as smoking and drug use; doing monthly testicular self-exams; and seeing your physician for yearly check-ups—starting at age 12—can help you get and stay in top form physically. Some new vaccinations are recommended for preteens. These include: the Whooping Cough (Pertussis) booster, the meningitis immunization, a second Varicella (Chicken Pox) vaccine (if you have only had one as an infant). An HPV vaccine for men is now available and is an important addition to your vaccine lineup as you begin adolescence.

You don't have to be a jock to be a real man. You don't have to be a leader or a sexual superman or dress or talk a certain way to be a real man. You are a real man just as you are: confident sometimes, scared sometimes; as likely to be shy and gentle as tough and assertive; straight or gay, athletic or not, tall or short. Being a real man comes down to just being you.

QUICK SCAN

A MAN'S BODY

✔ *Normal changes of puberty are highly variable.* These may begin as early as age 8 or as late as age 15 and finish between the ages of 14 and 18. Some very normal 13 and 14 year old guys look like adult men, while their equally normal classmates still look like boys. The timing of puberty is unique and may be determined genetically.

✔ *Monthly testicular self- exams are an important safeguard for your health.* Testicular cancer is one of the most common cancers in young men between the ages of 15-35. When should you start these exams? When you're well into puberty—usually between age ages of 13 and 15.

✔ *If you experience pain in your groin, see your doctor immediately!* It could be something relatively minor (such as a sports injury) or it could be major (such as testicular torsion) where timely treatment is essential. Only your doctor can tell for sure whether your problem is major or minor. Don't take a chance on guessing wrong: call your physician!

✔ *Masculine bodies come in all shapes and sizes.* Keep in top form by developing healthy habits— getting plenty of rest, eating good food, getting exercise, avoiding harmful habits, and getting regular medical checkups.

CHAPTER FOUR

Feelings

I think something is the matter with me. I cry at the least little thing and feel down a lot, but I also enjoy lots of stuff, too, especially with my friends. Sometimes I hate my parents and think how I can't wait to be 18 and go away to college or get a place of my own and sometimes I love them so much I cry at the thought of ever leaving them. Do people go through this at my age (14) or is something wrong with me?

Taylor B.

Does Taylor's experience sound just a little familiar? One thing's for sure: adolescence is a time of feeling strongly and deeply! You may feel alternately bored and excited, depressed and elated, yearning for independence while loving and needing your parents.

Some of your emotional ups and downs might be linked to all the changes you're experiencing, not just physically, but also at school (like adjusting to junior high or high school or getting ready for college), changes in your family as you become more independent and changes in your social life.

Some mood swings, too, can have physical causes. Some studies have found that certain teen behaviors can be linked to fluctuating hormone levels. We can't prove that hormones actually cause moodiness, but they can play a role in up-and-down feelings, especially in the early teen years when you're going through such dramatic physical changes.

Other strong feelings can come up as the result of important changes and milestones in your life. We're not talking just about things like graduation or important birthdays. We're talking about things like your changing relationship with your parents, the increased importance of friends in your life and those first, intense experiences with falling in love.

With all that's going on, you may find yourself loving and hating with almost equal passion, crying more than you used to, and feeling new hopes and new fears about all kinds of things. It's not at all unusual, while you celebrate your growing young adult competence and independence, to grieve a little for the past when life seemed so much simpler and people didn't expect so much of you.

As you grow through life, you encounter losses in the most unexpected situations: feeling a loss of childhood security even as you look ahead eagerly to going away to college; achieving a dream and, suddenly in the midst of your joy, feeling the loss of your dream, having achieved it. Of course, we're always in the process of finding new dreams to replace ones achieved or ones we've decided to let go. And there is joy in building new, often closer relationships with our parents as we grow up, or finding that we can handle our new independence just fine.

Losing the child part of yourself can be part of your mixed feelings at this age: you can't stand the idea of an adult or peer thinking you're a child in any way and, at the same time, it feels sad to think of leaving the child in you behind entirely. But not to worry: each of us, no matter how old we are, keeps a part of the child we once were inside. The child part of you can bring an openness, warmth and special joy as you grow into a practical, responsible, mature adult. And loving your parents and family as immensely as you did as a child—but with greater insights into who these important people really are—can enrich your relationships throughout your life.

FEELINGS ABOUT YOURSELF

I want to be the best I can be, but I'm not sure exactly who I am and I hate certain things about myself like my fat thighs and my bad temper. How can I be my best when I don't always like myself?

Hannah P.

As you grow and change, it's important to know both what you like and value about yourself— and what you'd like to change.

You're a special and complex person. Even if you're an identical twin, there will be some personality and life experience differences between you and your twin. How you make use of your special talents, what values you take from your family and friends and which ones you reject or embrace from outside people and experiences, the people you choose to love, the lifestyle choices you make that have a positive or negative impact on your health, the ways you spend your time—all of this adds up to the unique person you're growing to be. It's all, largely, your choice.

So how do you begin to develop a sense of who you are?

- *Act instead of just reacting.* Rebellion and making choices based on what is most likely to shock or disgust your parents or other adults are reacting. Make active choices about your life based on your own point of view. When you're very much your own person, with a strong sense of self, you can even agree with your parents in many areas without feeling that your independence is in jeopardy.

- *Make observations about yourself.* What kinds of observations? Maybe things like:

  ✔ What would I like to see happen in my life (and what can I do to make this happen?)
  ✔ When was the last time I really felt excited about something? What excites me or might excite me about my life?
  ✔ When I'm free to choose, how do I

spend my time? (If you spend most of your time in passive pursuits like watching television, you may not be too thrilled with life as it is right now. But you can change all that!)

- *Take inventory of your strengths and limitations, but don't get stuck in the latter.* It's true as you get older, you're more aware of yourself—what you do well and what is a challenge for you. Becoming aware of your limitations can be a real shock and you may have a tendency to criticize yourself harshly. But think about it. You're probably pretty tolerant of limitations you see in your friends. Practice being a friend to yourself and silence that harsh inner critic. Awareness is one thing, but beating yourself up for not being perfect—or having a particular talent—is quite another! You have a lot of strengths and talents you may not have discovered yet, possibly because you've been mired in a self-hate trap.

Seven Common Self-Hate Traps
(Take this test to see if you've fallen into at least one of them!)

1. *Beating yourself up emotionally for making mistakes.* Under most circumstances, a mistake is a learning experience. It doesn't doom you to total failure. In the middle of your embarrassment and chagrin, ask yourself what you can learn from this experience.

2. *Feeling like a loser—and rejecting others before they can reject you.* If you shy away from others because you fear they'll reject you immediately or when they find out that you have some flaws, life could be pretty lonely. The imperfect part of you is what some others may find most likeable. Think about it. We often love our friends for their very human qualities, yet berate ourselves for being just as human. It isn't fair! Give yourself a break. And don't deprive others of knowing you as you really are.

3. *Assuming that others are as aware of and as critical of your flaws as you are.* First, most people are so focused on their own concerns that they're not going to spend a lot of time thinking about what's right or wrong with you. Most people do tend to be fairly indifferent to each other until they get to know one another. If you feel that others dislike or ignore you, you may be acting in a way that increases your invisibility—and you can change this starting today. Make eye contact with others. Greet people warmly. Show an interest in what they're doing or saying. You may find other people's reactions to you change a lot as a result. If you're self-conscious about a physical characteristic and are sure that others hate you because you're overweight or have acne or one bad hair day after another, keep in mind that in the real world, people love other people for a wide variety of qualities. Being active, friendly, and kind; having a sense of humor; moving with confidence and grace (whatever your size) and feeling at ease with yourself as you are can go a long way toward developing a positive self-image. Your self-acceptance can make you very attractive to others.

4. *Telling yourself that if you're not the best, you're nothing.* This mindset often stems

from the "Winning is everything!" philosophy so prevalent in our culture. But it's wrong. You don't have to be Number One at everyone (or anything) to be a worthwhile and joyous human being. You can enjoy activities, hobbies or professional pursuits without having to be the best at what you do. You don't have to be a great writer to keep a comforting and insightful journal. You don't have to be a great musician to love and enjoy music. You don't have to make the swim team at school to enjoy swimming. Focus on what brings you joy—and do it, whether you're good at it or not!

5. *Being prejudiced.* Studies have shown that people who tend to be prejudiced against certain racial or ethnic groups or certain religious or socioeconomic groups are likely to have low self-esteem and attempt to put others down to build themselves up. It can't be done. You can't build self-esteem on the basis of hate, intolerance and scorn. This ugliness within will always prevent you from feeling good about yourself. Positive self-image grows from compassion, tolerance, and love; from being open and emotionally embracing; and from learning from and appreciating others who are quite different from you in many ways.

6. *Calling yourself hurtful names.* Do you call yourself "dumb" or "stupid" or "nerd" or "fat and ugly" or even worse? Stop tormenting yourself when you make a mistake or discover a limitation. Stopping those hurtful labels can help to stop the painful feelings that go along with them. Treat yourself as gently as you would a good friend in the same situation.

7. *Being a perfectionist.* If you constantly expect perfection, you're in for a rough time. It's great to have goals and dreams, but also important to realize that you're a valuable person who isn't perfect. We all make mistakes. We all say things we regret later. We all have embarrassing moments. Being imperfect is a normal part of life. You don't need perfection, prizes or great achievements to justify your existence. Start today to embrace, not only your wisdom and talents, but also the less perfect parts of yourself. All combine to make you the unique person you are. That doesn't mean that you can't change some behaviors or hone some talents. We're growing all our lives. But the most important part of that growth is self-love and self-acceptance right here and now.

FEELINGS ABOUT YOUR PARENTS

I have a 15-year-old son and during an argument the other day, he said, "I hate you, Mom!" Five minutes later, he came back with tears in his eyes and said he didn't mean it. I tried to tell him that it's O.K. to feel hate at times for people you love. I'm not sure he really believed me. I do know that I have suffered greatly because no one ever told me when I was young that I could dislike or even hate my mother at times and so these furies were buried, only to engulf me in later life. I think this whole love-hate thing is important for kids to know about and to feel O.K. about.

A Loving Mom

While polls show that today's teens love and respect their parents more openly than other recent generations, there still may be times when you have mixed feelings about your parents. You may love *and* hate them; yearn for independence yet still need your parents very much. You may be struggling to find your own values while feeling shaped and influenced by theirs. You may come to the conclusion that growing up means rejecting the values of your parents as a way of declaring your independence and separateness.

Rebellion isn't inevitable, though conflict is likely at times as you and your parents adjust to your growing up. Realizing that mixed feelings are normal can help. Respecting each other—even when your opinions and viewpoints differ—can help. To be truly independent is to accept and recognize that each person is different—and valuable. When you feel comfortable having your own point of view and respecting theirs as well, you may even feel free to agree with your parents without fearing a regression to childhood.

When you feel free to choose your own values, you will be free to express more positive feelings around your family, when you agree and when you disagree. You can have very different viewpoints and live very different lives—and still love each other very much.

FEELINGS ABOUT YOUR CHANGING FAMILY

Why do parents think teenagers don't care about them divorcing? I'm hurting a lot about my parents' recent divorce even though I'm 14 and have friends and all. Something that makes it hard is that Dad has a girlfriend he expects me to like and accept—like instantly. Mom just started dating a guy who has a six-year-old son who is a brat and who came along with us to Six Flags last weekend and spoiled everything! How can I convince my parents to get back together again? Things weren't nearly as bad before (even though they did fight pretty much) as they are now.

Briana C.

When parents are divorcing, it's very common to wish you could turn back time and live life as it used to be because life with divorced parents and the new people they bring into your life can be so complicated. But relationships, like time, can't be turned back to replicate the past. (Even when divorced partners reunite, the relationship invariably changes in some ways.) For most families, this means adjusting to a lot of changes: being single-parent-headed families or blended families with a sometimes awkward combination of stepparents, stepsiblings, and half-siblings.

You may find yourself torn between two warring parents you love very much—at a time when you need their united support as well as the security to begin to move toward independence in your own way and your own time. Suddenly, perhaps, you have too much responsibility thrust upon you as parents or stepparents assume that you can handle more responsibility for caring for yourself or your siblings or stepsiblings than you feel you can manage.

Maybe you're feeling incredible grief about the breakup of your everyday family and upset that your parents don't seem to be as upset about it as you do. It's important to know that many, though certainly not all, divorcing couples go through a lot of the grief process while making the decision to break up. For some, too, the final decision is a relief and a new beginning. For you, however, it can be a shock. You may be doing *your* grieving mostly after the fact. Grieving is an important part of healing and going on with your life. People do this in a number of ways, some more obviously than others.

Keep in mind that loving, though hurting, families can grow from all kinds of situations. It takes time and effort on everyone's part. It can help to talk with your parents about your feelings and what is comfortable for you and what isn't.

If, for example, a noncustodial parent expects you to spend every weekend with him or her and feels rejected if you don't, explain that you need time to spend with your friends and to have a social life, too, that this doesn't mean you don't want to be with him or her. Discuss possible compromises. Maybe your friends can join you and your parent for some activities. Maybe you can spend part of the weekend or every other weekend with your parent and then get together on a weeknight for dinner or special activity you both enjoy.

If a parent never spends any time alone with you (minus a girlfriend or boyfriend), let him or her know that you would treasure some time for just the two of you. (Keep it positive instead of sulking and complaining, "Why does *she*

always have to come along?") Some parents assume that you're at an age when time alone to talk doesn't matter as much to you—when, in fact, it can matter more. Some parents, too, get so caught up in a new relationship, eager to have you know and accept the new person, that they lose sight of the fact that you still need them to yourself sometimes. In these cases, it's up to you to tell them how you're feeling.

Accepting a new person in your parent's or parents' life can be a complicated process: you may feel grief for your parents' lost relationship, guilt over liking this new person (even a little), jealousy over the place this person may have in your parent's life and anger over issues that may exist between this new person and you –like the new stepfather who moves right in and starts giving commands, or a stepmother who feels hurt if you don't call her "Mom." Talk with your parent or parents about the fact that you're trying to keep an open mind and open heart, but need time to adjust to all the changes.

It can take some time, when you're part of blended families, to begin to feel like a united family. And, in the meantime, you may feel overwhelmed with all kinds of new expectations and responsibilities.

Maybe you're feeling upset because your parent seems to favor your new stepsiblings while expecting more of you. Or maybe you're expected to care for younger siblings or stepsiblings so much that you feel you have no free time. Let your parent know how you feel without making angry accusations and see if you can work toward a compromise.

If your parents have joint custody and you're beginning to feel like you're living out of a suitcase, think what kind of arrangement might work better for you and talk it over with both parents. You might decide spending longer stretches of time at each parent's home would work better for you than splitting each week between homes.

Compromise and good communication can help you to deal with a changing family. It's true that some families are closer than others, but you can build shared respect, cooperation, peace and some happy memories by keeping an open mind and heart.

LOVE

It really upsets me when my parents act like I don't know what I'm talking about when I say I love my boyfriend. They say I'm too immature to know what love is. I don't think that's fair. I'm almost 16 and am mature in a lot of ways. I think real love can happen at all ages. Am I right?

Lindsay B.

It's impossible to set an age limit on a person's ability to love. We love in different ways all of our lives. Love has no age limit. However, the character of love may change, depending not so much on your chronological age as on your emotional maturity and feelings about yourself.

Some older people, quite unfairly, label all young love as infatuation. Some emotionally mature young people are quite capable of mature love while some older people are chronically infatuated. What's the difference between love and infatuation and between mature and immature love?

Infatuation means being "in love with love," when being in love is more important than lov-

ing and giving to someone. This happens in people of all ages who are emotionally immature. If love takes over your live and makes you unable to function in other areas because you're constantly fantasizing about the other person, you may be infatuated. If you feel a need to cling, if you feel a lot of insecurity in the relationship, if you're more concerned with getting than giving, you're likely to be infatuated. Immature people of all ages fall in love with idealized images rather than real people—and when a real person doesn't live up to this vision, disillusionment sets in. You've seen it happen—or experienced it yourself: one day the person you feel you're in love with is the greatest, most awesome person in the world and the next day—when he or she shows signs of being hopelessly human—you're convinced your former love is a total jerk.

How is mature love different?

- *Mature love is accepting.* You are aware of each other as independent, real human beings. You allow each other the freedom to be yourselves without feeling the need to transform the other. You accept each other as you are and forgive what you are not, instead of constantly criticizing and blaming each other.
- *Mature love is energizing.* It means that you have more energy to give to all aspects of your life: your studies, your friendships, your family relationships, your special interests as well as your love relationship. All are enhanced by your good feelings, rather than ceasing to be important, overshadowed by your love.
- *Mature love can survive joy and pain.* You're strong enough and trust each other enough to be vulnerable, to cry as well as laugh together. You can be honest with each other and weather hard times, knowing that the

true test of love is not just how you're there for each other in the good times, but how you make it through sad, lonely or difficult times in your relationship. (And these times come to *all* relationships!)

- *Mature love means that there is more to your relationship than physical attraction.* You are, first and foremost, best friends. You treat each other as dear friends, not letting old expectations about what it means to be in love come between you.

- *Mature love is enhanced by time.* You know that, as you grow as individuals and as a couple, that your relationship will only get better, so who needs to rush anything? Real love takes time and growth. It's worth working and waiting for.

- *Mature love means neither instant fulfillment nor diminishment of who you are.* You have a solid sense of yourselves as distinct individuals. You feel that your partner is wonderful—but realize you're special, too! You have the security of knowing that if, for some reason, your love for each other would end, *you* could go on

The shock and sorrow of losing a love is familiar to all of us. What do you do when the worst happens?

For a time, let your pain and grief happen in non-destructive ways. Cry. Rage. Write in your journal. Talk with a caring friend or family member. Destructive methods of dealing with your pain—like trying to anesthetize your feelings with drugs, alcohol, frantic activities, an instant involvement with someone else, overeating (or not eating) or otherwise not taking care of yourself and your life—all leave you feeling even worse.

It's important to feel the pain in order to work past your grief and loss. Forgiveness, which will be possible in time, is also an important part of healing. Forgiving the person you lost frees you to love again.

The freedom that comes with forgiveness can let joy into your life again and allow you to appreciate what your previous relationship taught you about life and love. You may, at some point, quietly celebrate what was good in the relationship and then let go, little by little, of the pain you feel at losing it.

There may still be times of sadness—when you hear a song on the radio or come across it on your smart phone playlist—that used to mean a lot to the two of you or when pursuing an activity alone that you used to enjoy together. But, if you've grown with your grief, your sadness may be mixed with joy—joy not only because you lost this special love and yet survived, but also joy in the fact that you were able to love then and will, someday, find love again.

ANGER

I get really mad at some things people at school say or do and I've been in trouble for fighting. It's scary to fight at my school because, even though we're in a fairly nice area, there are gangs and you never know if someone has a knife or gun or if their friends will get you later on. What can I do when people are acting like shitheads so they'll leave me alone and not get myself in trouble?

Kyle H.

Of all the emotions, anger is the one most often denied, unexpressed or harmfully expressed. Unexpressed anger can seep out in strange ways. You may fly into a rage at someone over some minor annoyance or take your anger out on an innocent person. You might turn on yourself with destructive habits such as driving recklessly or eating or drinking too much. You may also get depressed—or turn on yourself in physical ways, with stomachaches or headaches.

Expressing anger can have its risks, too, in this age of increasing violence in the schools. Fights can escalate. Gangs are a presence nationwide. It isn't safe these days to tell someone off or get into a fight at school, no matter how intensely angry you are.

So how can you deal with anger in a way that doesn't make your situation worse?

- *Report how you feel rather than attacking the person who makes you angry.* This can defuse a variety of situations—from a peer who's ragging on you to a parent with an opinion that differs considerably from your own. It's better to say, "I'm upset about what you just said" instead of "You're a jerk!" or "You don't understand me at all."

- *When you can't express yourself directly, look for constructive ways to deal with the anger.* If, to protect yourself at school, you've needed to ignore taunts, or if a parent has said "I said 'No!' and I don't want to hear any more about it!," expressing your anger directly isn't possible. So what can you do with all that unexpressed anger? Why not:

- ✔ *Get physical!* Exercise can be a great anger release. Play tennis or any sport with hitting. Or run until you're exhausted.

- ✔ *Take a long walk.* This helps you blow off steam—and has the added advantage of lightening your mood as you notice beautiful or interesting things along the way.

- ✔ *Pound your bed pillows or scream into them.* This can help to discharge some of that angry energy.

- ✔ *Write a letter.* Express how you really feel in this letter. Then tear it up.

- ✔ *Try some hard physical work.* Scrub a bathroom or floor. Pull weeds in your family's garden. Mow the lawn. You'll get rid of angry tension—and accomplish something, too!

- ✔ *Cry.* This doesn't have to be a public display. Crying can be very therapeutic.

- ✔ *Talk to someone.* Talk about your feelings with someone who will listen, care and help you get some perspective—without telling the world.

These are just some suggestions. You may find your own best ways to deal with anger. Just remember: don't let it simmer. Unexpressed anger can cause depression and physical symptoms. It can also block out feelings of happiness. Dealing with your anger in ways that are best for you will help clear the air for joy.

SHYNESS

I miss out on a lot because I'm so shy. Howe can I be more normal when meeting people so I can have friends and fun like everyone else?

Scott J.

People describe themselves as shy for a variety of reasons. Some are socially isolated and have trouble talking with anyone they don't know well. Others are shy with the opposite sex only. Some are fine in social situations but get weak in the knees at the thought of speaking in public—and would rather pretend they don't know the answer to a teacher's question than to speak up in class.

Why are you shy? Some researchers are exploring the possibility that a tendency toward shyness can be inherited, just like blue eyes or red hair. Some experts feel that shyness can also have its roots in childhood experiences. Maybe your parents have always expected a lot of you. If you've been held to impossibly high standards by your parents, your extended family or even just yourself, you may find yourself afraid to try new things or to meet new people. You may feel that if you're not the best at something, you're a total failure . . . which isn't true at all!

How can you begin to conquer shyness?

- *See risk-taking in a different way.* Fear of making a mistake may be keeping you tongue-tied. But all of us make mistakes, say the wrong thing or face rejection at times. That's just part of life. Seeing all this not as a catastrophe but as a learning experience may ease some of your fears. And risk-taking doesn't have to be major. Start small by reaching out in ways that make you least uncomfortable and build up to the scarier challenges.
- *Take your conversational cues from listening to others.* You don't have to be a brilliant speaker or an incredible wit to have a good conversation with someone. Listen and ask questions. Laugh. Comment on what another has said. These are all ways to show signs of life in a conversation or in a relationship. If you can get away from your own fear for a time and get interested in what another has to say, you might just surprise yourself!
- *Set a goal and a deadline.* You might say hello to five people this week. Just "Hello." Start small. This will help you get in contact with others and build your confidence little by little.
- *Don't expect the world to change when you take the first step.* It takes time for others to get past indifference to the point of wanting to know you. It takes time for you to get to know and feel comfortable with others. Don't overburden yourself or others with high expectations. You can still be friendly no matter how others respond to you at first. And change will happen gradually. Be patient with yourself and with others and don't stop trying to reach out just because you don't see instant, dramatic results.
- *Accept yourself as a normal and unique person.* As such, you'll make mistakes at times. At worst, you'll make a mistake and learn from it. At best, you'll learn and feel the joy of connecting with others. So the risks you take here aren't really so great. Knowing this can give you a new sense of power and control in your own life.

BOREDOM

I live in this horrible small town where nothing ever happens and life gets really boring. What can I do to stop being so bored with life?

Rick G.

Boredom, which can be closely tied to

depression, can come from a variety of causes. Some of these causes are: non-participation in life due to lack of confidence or motivation; fear and a sense of hopelessness because goals and dreams seem so far away; the inability to make your own fun and joy in life when your general environment isn't especially stimulating.

What can you do if you're bored all the time?

- *Ask yourself WHY you're so bored.* How long has this been going on? When did it start? What feelings are you not expressing? Which goals and dreams seem impossibly far away? (Maybe if you're living too much in a fantasy future, the present time can't possibly measure up.)
- *Remember that if you're bored, you're boring!* This is a favorite saying of psychologist and author Dr. Sol Gordon—and it's so true! Dr. Gordon actually has a list of the five most boring things you can do (these do double-duty, adding to your own boredom and making you boring to others): running yourself down; telling your friends how terrible you are; telling people you're horny; bragging about things everyone knows you haven't really done; and watching TV for more than an hour and a half a day. Just avoiding boring behavior can take you an important step away from boredom!
- *While planning the future, don't forget to live fully in the present.* Long-term dreams and goals are great. So are intermediate and short-term versions. If long-into-the-future dreams are the only source of your pleasure and excitement today, no wonder you're bored! Focus on today. Think of the least boring thing you can do—and then do it! Volunteer

for a worthy cause. Spend time with someone who is lonely. Get a part-time job. Take a course just for fun at a local community college. Keep a list of things you can do right now that might be fun. Action of any kind can break that paralyzing cycle of boredom.

- *Be open to new experiences, and vow to learn one new thing everyday.* Learning something new every day—a word, a fact, a skill—can help you feel in touch with the world and to grow in exciting new ways. Be open to new people and experiences. Listen eagerly to opinions that differ from yours. Curiosity, joy and diversity can enrich your life immeasurably.
- *Make a list of things you love in life.* Just thinking of things to include can help lift you out of boredom and the blahs. If you can't think of anything right now, think of what you used to enjoy or could still enjoy if you'd let yourself. The more you think about what you love in life, the more you will rediscover the joy and excitement of simply being alive.

FEELINGS AND CYBERSPACE

My parents are bugging me because I spend so much time on the Internet, but they're too clueless about computers to understand how great it is. I especially enjoy chat groups. These have really helped me because I'm gay and just came out to my family but haven't told anyone at school, so chat groups are a safe way to talk about my feelings with guys who are older and more experienced and who can help me in a way my family can't. How can I make my family understand?

Jon P.

The Internet can be fascinating, rewarding and fun for people of all ages. As in all good things, however, moderation is in order. If you find that you're online so much that you're not seeing much of friends and family, or having time for homework, hobbies and healthy exercise, your life may be a bit out of balance.

It's important to know, too, that while chat groups can be interesting and helpful, you need to use caution. There are people who victimize the young and vulnerable or the gullible of all ages. Be very careful to protect your identity. Don't agree to meet an adult who befriends you in a chat room. The situation may be entirely harmless or potentially risky, and you may have no way of knowing which. In Jon's case, the chat groups may be useful to a point, but when he's ready to talk face-to-face about his coming out, it could be much more to his advantage to find and join a support group for gay teens or for him and his family to become involved in a group such as PFLAG (see Appendix) than for him to risk direct contact with any of his chat room buddies.

In summary, the same rules of common sense—moderation in all things and the importance of protecting oneself from con artists and predatory strangers—apply to new technology as much as traditional socializing.

I am so upset, I don't know what to do. These girls from school are spreading lies about me online and making fun of me and people I don't even know are reading their comments and adding to them! I don't want to go back to school and feel like killing myself if my parents make me because I'm scared everyone will believe what they're saying and hate me and make fun of me.

Alli J., 13

Cyber-bullying is a lot worse than traditional bullying: it can be read by millions and can take on a life of its own. It isn't a joke or a prank. It can be life-threatening. A number of young people have killed themselves after they have been humiliated, harassed or tormented via the Internet or text-messaging. In fact, smartphones and other mobile devices are prime territory these days for cyberbullying. This makes it extra hard to get away from since, if you're like most teens, your phone goes everywhere with you.

If you are bullied online by another teen or if you bully a peer using cyberspace, it is called "cyber bullying." If an adult bothers you online, it might be called harassment or stalking or, when the adult's intent is sexual, it would be called exploitation by a sexual predator.

If you are bullying or thinking of bullying someone online, think again.

- *If your online behavior is seen as a problem by the victim or the victim's parents, you could lose your ISP or IM accounts.* Most cyber bullying, from hurtful blogs, harassing emails, humiliating pictures or websites, stealing passwords and the like, violate the ISP's terms of service.
- *If you're mad at someone, don't use the Internet to strike back.* Instead, try some anger management—deep breathing, a brisk walk, screaming into a pillow, counting to ten once and maybe again. Talk to or yell at the person you're upset with. But don't take your grievances online.
- *Online pranks are far from funny.* Some of these might include: disguising your identity and sending fake email or flooding someone's inbox with spam, particularly porn spam; or sending text messages or emails that frighten

another. There are so many better ways to spend your time and your energy!

If you're the victim of a cyber-bully, take action to protect yourself. This can mean:

- *Ignoring the online comments.* Like playground bullies, cyber bullies are trying to get to you and provoke a strong reaction. If that doesn't happen, the thrill of bullying is largely gone.
- *Ask for help.* Many teens hesitate to tell their parents about cyberbullying, especially if it involves bullying via their phones, because they're afraid that their parents will opt for the instant solution of taking their phones away. But if you're being hurt relentlessly by such mobile bullying, it's important to let parents know. Your principal or school counselor or a trusted teacher can be a protective measure if some of your tormentors are other students and the harassment continues in person and on school property.
- *Warn and/or block the sender.* Clicking on a button on the IM to warn the sender can create a history that leads the ISP to warn the sender or close his or her account. Blocking a sender can also stop some cyber bullies.
- *Get extra help and guidance online.* WireSafety.org helps victims find their tormentors or stalkers and, in some instances, to prosecute them. Going to stopcyberbullying.org can give you invaluable information for handling cyber bullying whether you're a tween, a teen or a parent.
- *Get help to improve your cyber-judgment:* This could be as simple as a new software program, developed by a teen for teens.

It's called ReThink, and it came about in 2013 when then 13-year-old Trisha Prabhu read about an eleven year old Florida girl committing suicide because of relentless cyberbullying. Trish was shocked, saddened and outraged—and determined to do something to make sure that other teens wouldn't be bullied literally to death. So she developed ReThink, which gives young people a chance to pause and to reconsider a comment before posting. In an international study, this award-winning program was found to have prevented 93% of those using the program from sending bullying comments. The program can teach you to make better choices—both online and off!

SEXTING AND CYBERSPACE

Help! I don't know what to do and I'm too afraid and ashamed to tell anyone my problem, which is: my boyfriend threatened to break up with me if I didn't sext him and so I did and now he's saying he's going to break up with me and put my sexting picture online for everyone to see! What can I do???

Madison Y.

Many teens feel pressure from their boyfriends to sext. In fact, a recent Indiana University study revealed that one in five young adults who have sexted have done so because of pressure from a partner. While this is fairly common, that doesn't mean it is okay. Pressuring a person to sext is abusive, a new phenomenon called "digital sex abuse."

We have one word for you about sexting—and it's probably something you've already heard from parents and teachers—DON'T!

The minute you take an explicit picture of yourself and hit "Send" you lose all control of what will happen. What is likely to happen is that this will not be a private sharing between you and your boyfriend. Just assume that, no matter what he says, it will be shared—and the more it is shared, the more out of control the situation as it becomes shared over and over by recipients. It may exist in cyberspace forever. You may go viral in a way you never anticipated nor wanted.

No one has the right to insist that you put yourself at such risk. That is not a sign of love, but rather the mark of an abuser who sees no problem in pressuring you to do something that just doesn't feel right to you. You have a right to say "No" to putting yourself at risk for cyber humiliation.

If, like Madison, this warning comes too late and an ex-boyfriend is threatening you with "revenge porn", you can turn to a legal advocate who can work with you to come up with an action plan. Contact loveisrespect.org for more information, or go to http://www.endrevengeporn.org/revenge-porn-laws. You can also find help in getting revenge porn pictures taken down via undox.me (http://www.undox.me)

STRESS

I feel so stressed out. I dread getting up in the morning. It's like I'm on this treadmill of school, community service, work, homework and all the time feeling the pressure to make good grades so I can get into a top college and later get a good job. I don't have time just to be young and enjoy life. My friends feel the same way. What can we do? Doing less isn't really an option right now.

Elizabeth A.

The teen years are full of stresses. You may feel stress from your parents to measure up to their expectations of you. There also may be pressures from your teachers and from your peers.

The greatest pressures, however, tend to come from within as you grow, and sometimes struggle, to become your own person.

What can you do when stress is getting to you in a major way?

- *Be aware:* Keep a stress diary to determine what stresses you out and when. Be very specific about the sources of stress in your life. Which of these can be changed? Which can't? And what can you do right now to try to alleviate a little of the stress or change your attitude about a stressor in a way that will help you to feel calmer? Focusing on what you can change or can deal with right now can help cut down the feelings of being helpless or overwhelmed.
- *Set realistic goals.* When you're starting to stress out about something you want or feel pressured to do, ask yourself two questions: First, is this a possible, attainable goal for me? And, second, do I really want it? For example, if you hate science and your grades reflect your distaste, medical school probably isn't in your future, no matter how you or your parents may wish it. In another instance, if you want to be popular, a reality check is in order: you can't please everyone. Even if you could be liked by everyone, you

might find yourself having to give up important parts of yourself to fit in with other people's expectations—and that could cause you even more stress than not being quite so popular. Another part of setting realistic goals is starting small, one challenge at a time. If you try to take on too much all at once, you can get immobilized by anxiety and frustration. One challenge at a time is do-able.

- *Put your stresses in perspective.* Have you ever put stress on yourself by saying things like "If I don't pass this test, that's IT." The fact is, IT—your worst case scenario—may be uncomfortable, inconvenient, embarrassing or even devastating at the moment, but it isn't the end of the world or even life as you know it. The world is full of happy and successful people who didn't get into their first-choice colleges—and who subsequently had great experiences at their second or third or fourth choice schools. Faced with a stressful event, ask yourself how much this will matter in one year or ten years or 100 years. The pain or anxiety might be very much present right now, but knowing that this won't be forever or doom you to a life of unhappiness or failure may take some of the heat off. Whatever happens, you'll get through it and the stressful time will pass.

- *Realize that you and only you can change your life.* Only you can choose to be nervous or to alleviate some of your stress. Taking responsibility for your own nervousness makes it possible for you to do something about it. Think about the difference between saying "I get nervous when I'm around strangers" instead of "Strangers make me nervous." When you acknowledge that the feelings of discomfort are coming

from you, then you're in charge and you can change your reactions.

- *Be good to yourself.* Eat a healthy diet and cut down drastically on or even eliminate junk food and beverages that contain caffeine (such as coffee, tea or colas). Beverages with caffeine can make you even more jittery and irritable. Be sure you get enough sleep every night. Take a warm bath or shower just before going to bed and try to go to get to bed and get up at the same times every day whenever possible.

- *Make time for fun.* Enjoying hobbies, relaxing times, friends, meditation, a long walk or other exercise (exercise is a great stress reducer!) can help you manage stress and tension. Laugh heartily and often. Cultivate a sense of humor. It can help you put things in perspective and laughter has physical benefits as well. It's true! Blood flow to the brain increases when we laugh and we release hormones called endorphins that help us to feel better and reduce the levels of stress hormones in our blood.

- *Take action on your own behalf.* This may mean making a decision—even a small one—instead of staying mired in stressful indecisiveness. It may mean taking a stand and letting people know what you want and how you feel. Write about your feelings in your journal. Call a friend. Do whatever it takes to help yourself actively face down your stress.

- *Discover your stress-busting pleasures and DO them!* Do what relaxes you—and that doesn't cause stress down the road. Listen to or make music. Take a warm bath or shower or go swimming (water can be very relaxing). Take a walk and notice all the beauty around you. Close your eyes and travel back in time to a moment when you felt very relaxed. Breathe deeply and let that feeling of deep contentment and relaxation fill you completely right now.

- *Reach out to others.* It's a real temptation to isolate yourself when you're feeling stressed. Don't do it! Share your feelings with those you trust. This can help you to feel less alone and may also help you test reality. If conflict with another is causing you stress, talk to that other person or persons and work things out as much as you can so you don't have to worry about it anymore. If you're feeling stressed out about everything in your life, enlist the aid of a friend, parent, teacher, school counselor or professional psychotherapist in sorting out all your stresses and exploring your choices.

No matter how impossible or hopeless a situation seems to be, there is hope and there are choices. And no matter how alone you feel right now, there are people in your life who care and who want very much to help you—if you'll let them!

SELF-DEFEATING BEHAVIOR

I hate my life. My dad left my mom for another woman and my mom yells at ME all the time and I never see my dad anymore. I hate both of them and am getting back at them by skipping school and not doing homework. They always put pressure on me to make good grades so I could go to a top college and my grades have been very good, but now I'm getting C's and D's in most of my classes and may even get an F in algebra (I hate the teacher because he reminds me of my dad!). When my mom finds out about this, she will go ballistic, which would be worth it to me and maybe my dad won't even care...I still feel miserable. What can I do?

Steve T.

Defiant, self-defeating behavior usually comes from a lot of stress and anger in your life. You may feel backed into a corner by circumstances and feel like lashing out—even if it hurts you most of all. As Steve is discovering, you may be able to get to a parent or someone else who cares about you by doing things that are harmful mostly to yourself. The person may recognize this as a cry for help and positive attention—or he or she may not, acting in a punishing rather than nurturing way.

What can you do if you find yourself in this situation or one very similar?

- *Recognize that the person you're hurting most is yourself.* You may upset your parents by self-defeating behavior, but it hurts you—immediately or long-term—most of all. Your parents won't feel the consequences of your actions nearly as much as you will. So if you get back at education-conscious parents by messing up at school, you're the one who may have fewer options in the future. If you get back at weight-or-health-conscious parents by gaining weight, you're the one who will have to live with the social stigma (however unfair) and the health risks of being overweight or obese. If you lash back at puritanical parents with wild behavior that is shocking even to you (if you stop and really think about it), you're the one taking the potentially life-changing or even life-threatening risks. Instead, expressing your anger directly, in words, to a parent or parents can save you a lot of heartbreak.

- *There are better ways to let your parents know that you're angry or unhappy with them.* Talk to them. Write them a note or talk with a trusted adult relative, friend or teacher who can help you express what you're feeling to your parents.

- *Encourage your parents to seek family counseling where all of you can express what you're feeling in a safe environment with a professional who can help you resolve your situation.* Even though it can be very hard to seek professional help—both parents and teens may be embarrassed about talking with a stranger, worried about what family or friends might think—it can be well worth the effort. It isn't an admission that you're crazy or a horrible family or incompetent people. It can be a sign that you love each other and are committed, as a family, to making things work better for everyone. It's well worth a try.

FEELINGS ABOUT THE "ISMS"

I'm 16 and am an African American living in a mostly white suburb. I have friends at school but sometimes I feel lonely and angry because they can't understand how things are for me at times. My parents, who are well off because my dad is an attorney and my mom is a teacher, bought me a used BMW for my birthday and I couldn't tell you how many time the police follow me or stop me when I'm driving just because it's a nice car and I'm black and they think I stole it. And some of my friends' parents don't treat me like just a normal friend either. Either they ignore me or they're overly nice if you know what I mean. And lots of people at school, especially girls, if they didn't know me, would cross the street or not get into an elevator if they were to encounter me as a stranger, but no one wants to admit the little bit (or more) of racism they have inside. Everybody always says I should be grateful for the good life I have. I AM glad to be growing up in my family and having what I do, but there are times I wish I could just relax with people who really understand what it still means to be black in this country no matter who you are or how much money or other stuff you have.

Alex J.

People at school make fun of me because I'm fat and ugly. I weigh 200 pounds, wear glasses and have bad skin. People tease me all the time about how I look and I cry every day at school and then come home and eat. I hate getting up and going to school in the morning. My parents tell me not to pay any attention to the teasing, but that's impossible! What can I do to make them stop or to feel better?

Courtney B.

"Isms" such as racism, sexism, or "lookism" are hurtful not only to the people being singled out for discrimination or ridicule, but to us all. These ways of thinking and acting diminish and divide us. Often, those who are most prejudiced against others have very little going for them personally, low self-esteem or limited life experience outside their own ideologies. Of course, that in no way excuses any of their hurtful attitudes and behavior. Some people try to build themselves up by tearing others down instead of looking within to see how to improve their own lives and realizing how much we can all learn from each other.

What can you do if you're feeling besieged by an "ism"?

- *Look for ways to educate others.* Especially for someone who is a racial minority, this may seem a wearisome, never-ending task. But you don't have to be alone in your efforts. Enlist the aid of a teacher or an organization at your school. Perhaps the school could sponsor awareness days or intercultural workshops or other events that will raise people's levels of consciousness about others who are different in some way.

- *Let others know how you feel.* We aren't necessarily suggesting that Alex bare his soul to the police, but when you see signs of unfair assumptions, racism or sexism in people you know, let them know how this affects you. Many people don't realize how ingrained the "isms" are in our society and how we all have pieces of these buried within. If people can begin to hear how what they're saying or assuming is affecting you, they may be motivated to change their way of thinking. It's important for others to know that hurtful teasing, thoughtless comments or racist or sexist assumptions are not OK with you. Or, if you have simply misunderstood each other, this can be a chance to clear things up instead of living with hurt.

- *Find safe places of solace.* If you're being teased or excluded or discriminated against, you're likely to have feelings that you don't feel safe sharing with others you're not sure will understand. Think about people with whom you feel safe to be yourself: family, close friends, a special teacher, a counselor, a church group, or a special-interest group. It's important to be able to express your hurt and anger to someone or some group who can listen with understanding and who can offer emotional support.

- *Make a truce with your world—and with yourself.* The pain of being different in some way and being the target of an "ism" can make you bitter or it can make you stronger and wiser. Life isn't fair a lot of the time. Racism, sexism and "lookism" unfairly hurt and sometimes limit the potential of many good, talented and deserving people.

Accepting the fact that this unfairness exists does not means saying it's OK or accepting limits on yourself. It means that you decide to make a difference in your own life by not letting bitterness and frustration kill your spirit. You can use your pain and your anger in positive ways—to strengthen your resolve to have a happy, productive life and making an effort to do your part in trying to change old ways of thinking that perpetuate life-limiting "isms."

PHYSICAL, EMOTIONAL AND SEXUAL ABUSE

My parents are always hitting me and telling me they wished I was never born, mostly when they're drunk. Even when she's sober, my mom is always criticizing how I look (she thinks I'm ugly) and my dad yells at me for never doing anything like schoolwork or housework as good as he thinks I should. I hate my life. What can I do?

J.J.

Abuse at the hands of family members, especially parents, can be a devastating experience, and each type of abuse—physical, emotional, sexual—has its own kind of pain. You may fear for your safety and even your life. You may feel guilt, sometimes blaming yourself for your family's problems. You may feel confused about conflicting feelings of love and hate for the person who is abusing you. You may feel isolated and alone, feeling so different and so certain that no one else shares your situation. You may be terrified that friends and others at school will find out and, at the same time, you may long for help and support from others. You may be afraid to tell anyone for fear you will be blamed or not believed or that your family will be torn apart. You may feel angry, frightened, and used. You may feel shame, yet strong family loyalty.

My Dad has been forcing me to have sex with him several times a month since I was 10 (I'm now 13). I tried telling my mother hundreds of times, but she says she doesn't want to know what she calls my "dirty little lies." I feel like I'm walking around with compartments in my mind. At school, I'm friendly and outgoing. With my mom, I'm angry and upset. With my dad, I'm just numb. Does this mean I'm going crazy?

M.T.

How can you deal with these feelings and begin to heal?

- *Realize that you're not alone.* The pain of isolation can increase the pain of abuse. It's important to know that you're not alone. There are more people than you could ever imagine who have experienced some sort of abuse at home. It doesn't make you or your family uniquely horrible. It is a sign of significant family problems, but no matter how complicated and painful your situation is, it's not hopeless. Help is available.

- *Realize that you're not to blame.* Even if your behavior hasn't been beyond reproach and you've done things such as talking back to a parent or defying rules, this still doesn't justify a beating or consistent emotional abuse. Even if you've had sexual fantasies about a family member or even flirted a bit, this is not a reason or justification for incest. It's the adult's responsibility to use his or her power in a positive way—whether it's admonishing you or punishing you for inappropriate behavior or whether it's steering your relationship clear of overt sexual activities.

So abuse, whether physical, sexual or emotional, is a sign of a problem with the adult. A healthy parent will punish in ways that do not crush the spirit. He or she will encourage better judgment or behavior the next time. Abuse is attacking, not teaching. It harms the body and the soul. Deep down, you can feel and know the difference.

- *Get help for yourself and your family.* That's a tough but necessary step to take. Abuse represents family problems that are too seriously and complex to be handled or resolved within the family. Professional help is necessary.

Right now, you may feel that finding help is too scary and overwhelming or getting your family to agree to go for help an impossibility. Take a small step and ask your school counselor, a teacher or a hotline for help. It's important to know that some professionals, such as teachers and counselors, are bound by law to report abuse of minors. It's possible that social and legal agencies may intervene. But remember that the abuse isn't likely to stop until others step in to help. Your first priority must be to protect yourself and stop the abuse. That may mean living outside your family setting for a time—or it may not. It may certainly mean counseling for you and your parents and other involved family members. There are no quick or easy solutions, but there can be an end to your abuse and, eventually, to your pain.

- *Healing means making a choice to survive and to live for you—not for them.* While some people live lives scarred by pain and bitterness as a result of their early abuse, others survive horrible home situations to live happy, productive adult lives. You can, too. Your courage in facing your present crisis and in resolving your feelings with the help of therapy can have a very positive impact on your life in years to come.

The healing process can be long and painful. You may go through a period of grief for a childhood of pain and for a family so troubled. You may feel a combination of anger and great sadness. In order to be free, you need to resolve these feelings and then grow past this traumatic time. If possible, you might think about forgiving your parents sometime in the future. This doesn't mean saying what happened was right or OK. It's more for you than for them. Prolonged feelings of anger and revenge can keep you tied to the past. Forgiving your parents sets you free to value yourself and live for you—not them. In time, with forgiveness and supportive therapy, you will find new freedom to be yourself, to value your separateness and uniqueness, to reach out to others, to trust and to love.

DATE RAPE

As a 19-year-old college student, I am just now finding out there is one area of sex education that I wish my parents had been more explicit about: sexual assault. I believe that most people in my generation have the attitude that women and men can do exactly the same things in the world. In many cases, that is true, but women do need to be especially careful to prevent sexual assault. I received my education about this unexpectedly when my roommate was raped. I have since read many books on rape and learned that one in four women is raped at some point in her lifetime. This is not a topic to be taken lightly and more people need to be informed about it.

Laurie T.

Laurie is absolutely right. Unfortunately, one in ten teenagers experience physical violence, often date rape, in their dating relationships.

Date rape is about not respecting another person's right to say no and to control her own body. It is more about power than sex, and more about control than caring.

How can you avoid becoming yet another statistic?

- *Be selective in your dates.* That popular athlete or that incredibly cool fraternity guy can be big trouble. Recent studies show that young women most at risk for date rape are those who are in high school or who are college freshmen, who date athletes or men who belong to college fraternities, and/or who drink on dates. This doesn't mean that you should never go out with an athlete or frat man, but it does mean that you should be careful. Don't let yourself get into vulnerable situations when you're with them.

- *Don't mix alcohol and dating.* Abstaining from alcohol is a good idea no matter *who* your date happens to be. Alcohol can lower your inhibitions and decrease your ability to stand up for yourself or to see warning signs before the situation becomes a crisis. It's important to know that alcohol plays a major role in date rape.

- *Be aware of club drugs.* These drugs—such as CHB and Rohypnol—are sedatives that can lead to unconsciousness, immobility and, in the case of Rohypnol, amnesia so that you can't remember anything that you did or that was done to you while you were under the influence of the drug. But you're not into drugs, you say. You would *never* think of taking a drug like this. The truth is, many girls take these drugs without knowing what's happening. When you're in a club or even just at someone's house with a group of people or a guy you don't really know all that well, don't leave a drink unattended and be aware of the people around you. Some people who wouldn't dream of taking a drug voluntarily end up ingesting a club drug that is slipped into their drink.

- *Avoid troublesome situations.* You know what they are—being at a fraternity party where everyone is drinking, being alone with a guy in his dorm room or in his room at home when no one else is around. Don't set yourself up for trouble, especially with a guy you don't know well.

- *Let him know that no means no.* This means being very clear about what you will do and what you won't do, and that when you say no, you mean it. No one deserves to be raped. It isn't justifiable—ever! But you *can* put yourself in danger by wavering back and forth between "Yes" and "No," or teasing him sexually. He may not believe you really mean "No!" Don't put yourself in that position. Set your boundaries firmly and mean it!

What to Do If You Are Raped

Whatever the circumstances, rape is a crime and it's *not* your fault. Whether the rapist is a stranger or a guy you thought you knew and liked a lot, no one has the right to force you to have sex against your will. No one has the right to take advantage of your being under the influence of alcohol or drugs to have sex with you when you're in no condition to give your consent. (A note for boys: if you have sex with a girl who is too drunk or wasted to know what's going on, you could well be accused—and convicted—of rape. Not only is this a risk not worth taking, but it is also a crime and a terrible thing to do to another human being.)

No matter what mistakes you might have made—like making poor choices about being alone in a secluded spot with a guy or drinking too much—the rape still isn't your fault. Some girls and women who have been raped suffer even more or delay getting help because they feel what happened was their own fault, and they don't want further pain inflected on them by disapproving family, friends or officials.

So what can you do?

- *Find someone you feel safe with to help you decide what to do.* That person might be a parent or other family member or a friend. Or, if you don't feel safe with anyone you know, call the National Sexual Assault Hotline for help and advice (1-800-656-HOPE (4673)). When you call this number, you'll be routed to the nearest affiliate to you, based on the first six digits of your phone number. (If you're calling from a cell phone that has a different area code from where you are, you have the option to enter the zip code of your current location in order to more accurately locate the nearest sexual assault crisis help center.) Know that this service is safe and totally confidential. You can also find help online 24 hours a day via www.online.rainn.org.

- *If you want to report the rape to police or think you might want to in the future, go to a local hospital emergency room right away without changing your clothes, washing or taking a shower first.* Washing all the evidence away is a natural emotional reaction to a sexual assault, but this evidence is necessary to show that you have been raped and to identify the rapist conclusively via DNA evidence.

- *Even if you don't plan to report the rape, consider getting immediate medical help at a hospital emergency room, clinic or rape treatment center.* This can be especially important if you have been injured and/or in order to prevent an unwanted pregnancy. (You may elect to get a Plan B or "morning

after" oral contraceptive.) If you're certain that you don't want your parents to know about the rape, find out what the local policy is regarding parental notification. Many medical facilities give confidential rape treatment, but in some states and towns, parental notification is required. If that is important to you, find out what the policy is *before* you set foot in the medical facility. Ideally, if you're facing a crisis like a rape, you will have a loving, supportive parent by your side as you deal with the difficult aftermath. However, we realize that not everyone's life situation is ideal. Some facilities provide patient advocates to help you through the post-rape medical exam and talk about what your choices are if you don't have a family member or friend by your side.

- *Realize that rape can be a trauma that stays with you.* Your feelings about rape can be complicated, a mixture of guilt, betrayal, anger, sadness, numbness and grief. You may feel a sense of unreality, a disinterest in things you once cared about. You may find comfort in talking with people you love, or in talking privately with a counselor, or even participating in a group of women trying to heal from the trauma of rape. Group therapy, while it may seem scary and embarrassing, can actually help many people to heal. Think about it: these people will know more about what you have experienced and the complicated feelings that can happen after a rape than many of the people who are close to you, who haven't had such experiences. Every person heals in her own way. But keep your mind open to all the help that's out there.

When a Love Relationship Turns Abusive

I'm very confused and upset. My friends hate my boyfriend because they say he acts like a total tyrant, wanting to read every text I receive from friends on my phone, and doesn't like me to spend time just with my friends or my family. I haven't listened because I believed it when he said they were just jealous. But now I'm scared because he has started to pinch me really hard—and then say it was just a joke—and last night he got mad and slapped me and went on about how it was all my fault. I don't know what to do.

Emma C.

What Emma is describing is dating abuse, which can take several forms.

While it is estimated that about 1.5 million U.S. high school students of both sexes admit to being hit or otherwise physically assaulted in the last year by a dating partner, emotional and verbal abuse may be even more common and potentially harmful. This can begin as early as sixth or seventh grade and can end up with victims being more at risk for long-term problems like eating disorders, alcoholism, and suicidality.

Being abused can not only cause bruises and broken bones, but also can break a person's spirit.

Most people don't start off in a relationship abusing or being abused. A potentially abusive partner may, in fact, seem very in love and romantic, taking an interest in everything you do…even as they gradually start taking control of your life.

How do you know if you're in an abusive relationship if your date doesn't hit or physically threaten you?

Beware of someone who:

- Is extremely jealous and possessive, flying into rages or giving you an extended silent treatment if you even have a conversation with a friend of the opposite sex
- Takes all of your time and energy, isolating you from friends and family
- Has contempt for his or her parents, teachers and all authority figures
- Has no interest in school or career plans
- Is abusing drugs or alcohol
- Insists on listening in on phone calls or reading the texts your friends send you
- Is highly critical and always finding fault with you
- Minimizes your dreams, your talents and your achievements
- Humiliates you by putting you down in front of friends or family
- Ignores your opinions or preferences
- Is constantly checking up on you
- Has unpredictable moods—sometimes nice and then flying into a rage over something that seems pretty minor to you
- Blames you for his or her abusive behavior
- Says you can't do anything right and that you deserve to be abused (hit or yelled at or criticized)
- Seems to follow a cycle of abusive behavior, acting so nice and apologetic, doing and saying all the things you've hoped he would, and then getting tense, before becoming abusive again
- Makes you afraid much of the time, forcing

you to tip-toe around subjects that could set him or her off

If even a few of these symptoms sound familiar, it's time to take action to get out of the relationship, no matter how much you care about this person or how much he or she needs your love, because:

1. It's highly unlikely that he or she will change. Abusive behavior stems from deep-seated problems that you cannot solve, no matter how devoted you are to this person.
2. You do not deserve to be treated abusively—ever.
3. You have a long life ahead of you, with prospects for love that doesn't hurt, that encourages your emotional growth instead of stunting it. No matter how much you care, or how sorry you feel for this person, it's time to say "Goodbye."

Granted, that is sometimes easier said than done. You may be feeling so uncertain, with such a lack of confidence in your own judgment or so afraid of being physically harmed or harassed by this person, that breaking up seems impossible.

- Ask for help, even if you're embarrassed. Maybe your friends have been warning you about this person or making observations for months about the behaviors that are finally starting to upset you. Maybe your parents have voiced strong objections to this person and you've been determined to prove them wrong. But remember that these observations from friends and family come from a place of love and concern for you. It's especially important that your parents, a special teacher you can trust and/or your school counselor know what's going on so that they can help you and protect you through the process of breaking up with the abuser.
- Understand that tears and apologies, promises and protestations of love are all part of the abuser's arsenal to keep you attached, trapping you with him or her in the cycle of abuse.
- If you are feeling that you may be in danger, alert your parents and talk to local police about the situation and a possible restraining order. If the abuser is a classmate, school authorities should be aware of the threat or potential danger.
- You can feel sorry for the abuser's pain, but that pain has little if anything to do with you. You can feel bad for a person without taking on their problems and immersing yourself in them until his or her problems become yours.
- Don't let shame and embarrassment keep you silent. This is a particular danger for male victims of dating abuse and for gay, lesbian and transgender teens, especially those who are not out to their families or communities. If you're among these, you may fear not being taken seriously or worse. The fact is, emotional abuse of males by females can be as threatening to emotional well-being, even to one's life, as male-female abuse. A case in point: the girlfriend who urged her troubled boyfriend via texting to commit suicide. When he had second thoughts and got out of the truck he had rigged to kill himself via carbon monoxide poisoning, she sent him a series of texts making fun of his indecision and ordering

him sternly to get back into the truck and go through with it. He did and he died. Dating abuse doesn't get any worse than that.

- If you are gay or lesbian and need help in getting out of an abusive dating situation and feel you can't talk with your parents or teachers about this—at least not right away—there is help available. Check the Appendix for information about the GLBT National Help Center and The Trevor Project.

- Teens of all sexual orientations and gender identifications can find help from loveisrespect.org, which offers a 24-hour hotline as well as a texting helpline, and has partnered with Break the Cycle, a leading advocacy group for preventing dating abuse. (Contact information for these services is in the Appendix.)

- Give yourself time to heal. People who have been abused often have a variety of physical symptoms like headaches and stomachaches, anxiety, feelings of self-blame and worthlessness, and difficulty trusting others. If you find such symptoms persisting, seek help from your doctor or get a referral to a counselor. Asking for help doesn't mean you're crazy. It means that you're making a commitment to get better.

- Reconnect with friends and interests. After a relationship that took so much of your time and energy, there may be some friends who are gone forever, but many will come back to you. If you get out of the house and get active again in activities you love, you'll connect with some of these people and even make new friends. You may find yourself grieving the loss of "the dream of love" and connection at times, but remember that living your own life and reclaiming your dreams can feel wonderful.

- Know that love—real love—will come your way in time, especially if you have learned from your abuse experience to spot the warning signs and not get caught in the painful cycle again. You'll find that real love is trusting and respectful, a gentle pairing of true equals, with lots of space within the relationship for growth and friends and family.

DEPRESSION

I've been feeling really bad. At first, I thought it was depression over my parents' divorce, but things are better now and I still don't feel right. I have no energy. I get irritated with my mom AND with my friends for no good reason. My grades in school are falling because I just can't concentrate. What's wrong with me?

Caitlin O.

When people talk about depression, they can mean many different things. Crying and feeling down after the death of someone you love (whether a person or a pet) is grief. Feeling down after a romantic breakup or after not making a team could signal a depressed mood. A clinical depression is much more complex. Initially, it may spring from an identifiable event, but quite often it doesn't. For some, depression can be a lifelong illness that comes and goes in a recurring cycle.

Depression is, in short, often used as a catch-all phrase to describe a variety of symptoms. It is often the result of a complex mix of social, psychological and/or physical factors that can trigger sadness, hopelessness, feelings of inferiority, powerlessness, and helplessness.

Grief is a natural response to loss. A depressed mood is usually a relatively brief period (a few days or a few weeks) of feeling sad over a specific event. Clinical depression, on the other hand, is more persistent and severe.

There are several types of clinical depression as described the American Psychiatric Association. These include:

Major Depressive Disorder, Single Episode or Recurrent

To be diagnosed with major depressive disorder, you must have suffered from five or more of the following specific symptoms for more than two weeks in a way that interferes with your daily life. These symptoms include the following:

- Depressed or irritable mood most of the day, nearly every day
- Loss of interest or pleasure in activities you have previously enjoyed
- Significant weight loss (without dieting) or weight gain (a change of more than 5 percent of body weight in one month); diminished or increased appetite
- Insomnia (difficulty sleeping) or hypersomnia (sleeping too much) nearly every day.
- Feelings of restlessness or being slowed down
- Feelings of fatigue and loss of energy nearly every day
- Feelings of worthlessness or excessive or inappropriate guilt on a daily basis
- Diminished ability to think or concentrate or persistent indecisiveness nearly every day
- Recurrent thoughts of death (not just fear of

dying), thoughts of suicide with or without a specific plan and/or suicide attempts.

How long does a major depressive disorder last? Some people have one episode in a lifetime and never repeat this experience. Others have a number of depressive episodes (separated by at least two months in which the person does not have symptoms of a major depression).

Dysthymic Disorder

Teenagers with dysthymic disorder experience depressive symptoms that are long-lasting (for at least one year without having been symptom-free for longer than two months at a time), but this depression may not be quire as life-interrupting as major depressive disorder. Teens with dysthymic disorder may go through all the motions of everyday life and do all the things they are supposed to do, but without ever feeling free of depression for long. The symptoms, which must be present for most of the day, nearly every day, for a year or more, include the following:

- Poor appetite or overeating
- Sleep problems— sleeping too much or suffering from insomnia
- Low energy level and fatigue
- Low self-esteem
- Poor concentration or difficulty making decisions
- Feelings of hopelessness

If you have dysthymic disorder, you may be cranky and irritable most days as well as being depressed. You may have trouble making friends with peers or talking to adults. You also tend to be a pessimist about life in general.

Bipolar Disorder

Teens with bipolar disorder have mood swings that go quite beyond the usual changeable moods of adolescence. If you have bipolar disorder, you will have moods alternating between highly energetic (manic) during which time you sleep very little, talk a lot, have a surplus of energy and feeling wonderful about yourself—and the inertia of major depression.

A chronic form of bipolar disorder is called cyclothymia. Here the teen has bipolar episodes for at least a year without more than a two-month respite from symptoms (either manic or depressive).

Some teens with this disorder don't always have the classic manic-depressive symptoms that are so evident in older adolescents and adults, and the dramatically changing moods may be mistaken for the ups and downs of adolescence. But there is a difference. Many people do well in school, have friends and generally get along with parents and siblings despite the normal mood fluctuations of adolescence. Those with bi-polar disorder usually have noticeable problems in school, with peers and at home.

What can you do if you're feeling depressed? It depends on the kind of depression you have.

If You're Grieving a Loss

- *Let your feelings happen.* You may be experiencing a confusing combination of feelings. You may feel angry one minute and profoundly sad the next. You may cry or be unable to cry. There is no right way to grieve—only your way. It's important to know, too, that tears can mean courage, not weakness. It takes courage, after all, to fully face and experience your pain.

- *Share your feelings with others.* This might be family or friends or an understanding adult, such as a teacher or clergyperson. Or it could mean joining a support group for teens who have experienced loss. Having a chance to talk and be truly understood and hearing that others share many of your feelings can be a huge step toward healing.

- *Realize that the grief process can mean zig-zagging emotionally between pain and healing.* It takes time to get through the grief process. You may have periods of feeling OK and then find yourself overwhelmed by a wave of grief again. You're not going crazy. It's a normal part of the process. Just remember that the pain-free moments, the times of laughter and enjoyment of life between your waves of grief, will give you strength to work through your pain and get on with your life.

If You're In A Depressed Mood

- *Change the pace of your life.* Go for a walk. Listen to upbeat music. Act as if you weren't feeling depressed and do things you would do if not depressed. Your dark mood may lift dramatically!

- *Resist the drug or alcohol "cure".* Don't try to deaden your pain with alcohol or drugs. This just postpones and sometimes even prevents life-affirming solutions.

- *Get daily exercise.* Even if you have to force yourself, do some kind of exercise every day. Studies have found that regular exercise and general physical fitness can help combat depression and anxiety.

- *Release feelings in ways that feel safe.* Sometimes unexpressed anger is an important part of a depressed mood. Try releasing angry feelings by pounding pillows, crying, writing in a journal or talking with friends.

- *Keep a journal or diary.* Studies have found that keeping a journal can help to alleviate stress and depression by helping you to express in writing the feelings you have difficulty expressing any other way. You may also come to understanding these feelings—and yourself—better by keeping a journal.

- *Give yourself something to look forward to every day.* This doesn't have to be something major, just something pleasurable to you: time spent on an interest or hobby; taking time to notice beauty around you; meditation; listening to music you enjoy; reading for pleasure; talking with someone you like or love; or taking a soothing bath. The point of this whole exercise is to give you a reason to anticipate rather than dread each new day.

If Your Depressed Mood Persists

- *Talk with your parents about seeking professional help.* If you can't talk with your parents about this, talk with someone who can help you get through to them—a relative, a teacher or trusted adult friend. Getting help from a mental health professional—a psychiatrist (M.D.), a psychologist (Ph.D. or Psy.D.) or a psychotherapist (MFT or LCSW)—doesn't mean you're crazy. It can be an important step toward healing when there doesn't seem to be anything you, on your own, or those around you can do to make a positive difference.

- *Be open to help beyond talk therapy.* Much of the time, talking with a therapist (as well as family and friends) can help a lot in sorting out your feelings. But there are times when you need more help than that.

Some major depressive episodes may be severe enough to warrant the use of anti-depressant medication. If you have bi-polar disorder, medication can help to even out your mood swings. It isn't a matter of taking a pill so life will be perfect. But many health professionals now believe that some depression has chemical origins and that medication can restore your body's chemical balance, making you better able to cope with the ups and downs of life as well as making better use of therapy. Medications aren't appropriate for everyone who is depressed, but they can be real lifesavers for some.

It's important to be aware that there are so-called black box warnings on some anti-depressants like Prozac, Zoloft, Paxil, Celexa, Lexapro, Effexor, Remeron and Serzone. Parents and professionals alike need to be alert to signs of worsening depression or suicidal feelings or behaviors when a teen is taking these drugs. Among these, only Prozac, at this writing, has been approved for the treatment of depression in teens. Among teens with bi-polar disorder, medications that treat attention deficit disorder (ADHD) can make manic symptoms worse as can use of only an anti-depressant without a medication to stabilize the array of manic symptoms as well.

While no treatment is perfect, there is a treatment plan that can help you. With supportive therapy and, possibly, appropriate anti-depressant drugs prescribed by a psychiatrist, you can begin to leave the darkness and pain behind and rediscover hope.

SUICIDAL FEELINGS

I don't know why I'm writing this except to say maybe I'm looking for a reason not to kill myself. I think of dying every day because living is just too awful. I have parents who are fighting over their divorce, my best friend at school won't speak to me anymore, and now that I'm 14 and in high school, I'm nothing. I didn't make the soccer team and my grades aren't as good as they were. I mean, what's the point? I used to enjoy my life, but now I just want to die. Help!

Megan M.

Many teens feel as Megan does; depressed and despairing about life and looking for a way out of their pain. What many don't realize is they may not want to die as much as to live differently. But when you're feeling depressed and hopeless, it's hard to see how life might be different. Many teens like Megan cling to a tiny spark of hope and seek help. Tragically, many others do not.

Suicide is the third leading cause of death in adolescents. While boys are more likely to kill themselves, girls are more likely to attempt suicide.

However, according to a recent report from the Centers for Disease Control, there has been a sharp increase in the suicide rate of girls between the ages of 10-14. The rate of suicides in this age range increased 76% between 2003 and 2004. Suicide rates for girls 15-19 increased 32% during that same time period and the rates for teen boys increased 9% during that year. Some experts believe that this spike in suicides may have occurred as the result of doctors prescribing anti-depressant medica-

tions less frequently for children and teens in the wake of warnings that these drugs could increase suicidality, preventing some of these teens, who might have benefited from these drugs, from getting much-needed help.

Other experts point to the particular stresses of the middle school years, in particular, that can put some vulnerable teens into a severe depression. Some, too, have noted that suicide methods have changed for young girls—with hanging and suffocation being much more prevalent in recent years. These methods may be more accessible to young teens than a gun or pills.

Beyond statistics, however, every single loss of a young life to suicide is a tragedy. When a young person dies in this way, the people who knew him or her ask each other "Why?" Most often, there is no one answer to this. Some suicidal teens experience not one critical event, but a series of stressors in the areas of family, friends, school, and other important aspects of their lives. Mix a combination of stressors, depression, and perhaps some substance abuse (which can make depression worse) and you have a recipe for disaster. Suicide may begin to seem like the logical or the only solution.

If you have a friend or loved one in trouble, be alert for signs of suicidal feelings or behavior. Don't dismiss them as bids for attention or conditions that will pass. It may not be possible for a severely depressed teen to "just forget it". And if someone is seeking attention via suicidal threats or plans, this is a definite cry for help.

Some of the signs that your friend may be suicidal are:

- Severe depression that lasts months or years.
- Sudden elation or a burst of energy after a prolonged depression. (It's quite common for

a suicidal young person to find the energy to commit suicide after the most immobilizing part of the depression begins to lift.)

- Talking about dying or committing suicide. This is especially serious if he or she has a plan and a method in mind.
- Giving away possessions, especially prized ones.
- Sudden withdrawal from friends and family.

What can you do if someone you love is showing some or all of these signs?

- *Take all comments about death and suicide seriously.* Ask your friend directly whether he or she has thought of suicide and, if so, if he has a method in mind. The more thought and planning that has gone into this, the more immediate the crisis. Instead of dismissing such comments as attention-seeking tactics or a passing whim, urge your friend to get help—and offer to assist with this.
- *Show that you care.* Let your friend talk while you listen. Let your friend know that he or she is very important to you. Emphasize that, no matter how hopeless life seems right now, it can change. Even the worst pain and hurt imaginable diminishes with time—even though that might seem impossible right now.
- *If your friend won't seek help, get help for him or her.* Your friend may be furious, but there may be a life at stake here. Don't let yourself be part of a tragic conspiracy of silence. It's better to risk a friend's wrath than be mourning his or her death. This is a secret you must not keep! Tell one or both of your parents or your friend's parents. If that isn't possible, tell some other adult who

can help. It's worth risking a friendship to save a life!

If You Are Feeling Suicidal

- *Ask yourself whether you really want to die— or if you really want to live, but live differently.* Life can be different. It may sound like a cliché, but it's quite true: as long as there is life, there is hope. Some things that seem unchangeable now will change in time. Even serious depression doesn't last forever. No matter how appalling your life circumstances, help is available if you reach out to someone. While there are no easy or instant solutions to life's major problems, there are alternatives to the anguish you're feeling right now. You can—and you will—feel better.
- *Real life suicide is not tragically glamorous the way it may be depicted on television or in the movies.* There is no glamour or beauty in it at all. Many of your classmates, friends and acquaintances may feel sad for a while, but they'll go on with their lives, maybe even forgetting you in time. Those who truly love you will be devastated and their lives will never be the same. To society, you'll be just another statistic. And you will no longer be. That's the saddest, most tragic fact of all.
- *Remember that there are people who care, even if you're feeling very much alone right now:* Reach out for help. Let others know how you're feeling. If it doesn't seem possible to talk to people you know and love, call a special hotline (See Appendix)

There are people who are willing to listen and to help. You can change your life and your feelings. It may take time to turn things around. It may not be easy. But it's not hopeless.

FEELINGS AND YOUR HEALTH

Is it true that your feelings can make you sick? If you never feel anything, does that mean you'll live longer and be healthy? How can you go through your life and never feel anything? My dad never seems to feel anything and he has colds all the time.

Matthew Z.

Our health can be impacted both by feelings and by lifestyle choices. Some people, for example, smoke or drink or overeat when they're tense and stressed out. These feelings-related actions can and do contribute to health risks.

Of course, it's not possible to go through life without feeling. We suspect that Matthew's dad may feel a lot, but can't express these feelings. Keeping his feelings bottled up inside may indeed be making him more vulnerable to illness.

What have researchers found out about the role feelings play in health?

- Hostility can be a factor in heart disease. In fact, a Duke University study found that teens with hostile attitudes might develop high cholesterol levels while growing up, with high blood pressure and heart disease possibly shortening their lives.
- Sharing feelings with friends, family, or a diary can strengthen the immune system.
- Optimists have better physical health than pessimists, mostly because they handle stress better. This gives them a longer life expectancy and stronger immune systems.
- Depression can be a factor in disease. Various studies have shown that depression can

weaken immunity and, long-term, can make a person more likely to develop cancer.
- Loneliness can kill. Studies at the University of Michigan and Ohio State University found that loneliness impairs the immune system and that those with few friends have higher death rates.

So what can you do to deal with feelings and maximize your health?

- *Make and keep connections with others.* We all need love and trust in our lives. This love can come from a variety of people—from friends and family as well as from lovers. (Friends and family, in fact, may well be more reliable throughout your life than lovers!) You will also find that when you're kind and warm toward others, you'll feel better yourself. Be positive toward others. Most people are interesting if you give them a chance. Most want to be fair and kind—and they can teach you important lessons. You just need to be open to these lessons and to a variety of people.
- *Cultivate a sense of humor.* Humor puts life in perspective and takes the edge off your pain. It will also attract others to you and will make it easier to live with yourself. Laughter is a wonderful safeguard for both mental and physical health.
- *Accept the fact that you will have pain, disappointments, and setbacks.* These are all part of life. Let yourself experience and learn from the inevitable pain in your life instead of trying to avoid it at all costs.
- *Tell yourself (and really believe) that you're in charge of your own life.* You can make your own life, your own good luck, your own

choices, and your own love. Whatever your circumstances, you don't have to be a helpless victim. You can do more than you ever imagined. You can overcome terrible pain and loss if necessary. You can lose a special love and survive to love again. You can have a worthwhile, happy life without being a genius or a great beauty or super-talented or rich or famous. You just need to be the best you know how to be. You need to accept and learn to live with your feelings, your strengths and your limitations (without letting any of these overwhelm you). You can choose to be in charge of your life. And, if you choose, this life can be full and rewarding—with an abundance of love and growth and joy.

CHAPTER FIVE

Eating For Good Health

My health ed teacher at school said something about what you do as a teenager can make a difference in how healthy you are later in life. Are there some basic things I can do to stay healthy without spending a lot of time at it? The reason I'm asking is that I don't have a lot of free time between school and work and time with my friends. Some books and articles I've seen about healthy eating have all these complicated recipes that my mom doesn't want to make and I don't have time to make. What can you do if you want to be healthy but don't have lot of time?

Sarah H.

It's true that what you do now—how you eat, how you exercise (or not) can have a lifelong impact. A large part of this is developing healthy habits now that, if continued, can make a long, active healthy life possible.

There seems to be a correlation between health and happiness. It's hard to be happy if you're not feeling well. And, if you're feeling unhappy with yourself, you may tend to neglect your body and thus get caught up in a spiral of bad feelings, both mental and physical. If, on the other hand, you feel well physically, you're likely to do better in all aspects of your life. Your body *is* you and it's vital that you build a strong, healthy body to go along with your active, healthy mind.

Seven Steps to Lifelong Good Health

1. Eat a healthy balanced diet.
2. Get regular exercise.
3. Maintain a healthy weight for your height and build. If you're overweight, pay attention to what you eat (making health-minded choices), and get moving with a regular exercise program.
4. Don't smoke or take drugs.
5. Get regular medical checkups and inoculations as required, and visit your dentist at least once a year.
6. Get involved in work and/or a cause you believe in, or activities that help you feel good about yourself and of service to others.
7. Build strong friendships and love

relationships. Those who form warm, loving bonds with others tend to live longer, healthier, happier lives.

ARE YOU WHAT YOU EAT?

Yes! What you eat has a huge impact, not only on your physical health and appearance, but also on your emotions.

As you can see from the following Food Guide Pyramid illustration, a balanced diet requires a variety of food in four different categories. And as you will see from the charts after that, the vitamins and minerals required for optimal health also come from a variety of foods.

Three of the most common problem-eating patterns among teens are the following:

- Filling up with empty calories: sugary snacks, soft drinks, potato chips and crackers.
- Eating on the run with a high-fat fast-food diet. With a steady diet of fast food and/or high-calorie snacks, you can take in a lot of calories and gain weight and *still* be malnourished because you're not getting the nutrients you need.
- Dieting so stringently—often skipping meals or eating only a few varieties of food items—that important nutrients are missing from the daily food intake.

How do you build a balanced diet? Does it mean that you have to eat stuff you hate or never go to a fast-food place with your friends again? Balance doesn't mean deprivation or never having fast food or candy. It means paying attention to what you're eating and making

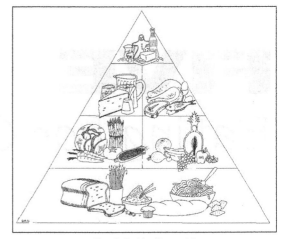

Food Guide Pyramid

sure that you're getting the vitamins and minerals you need.

The U.S. Department of Agriculture has issued nutritional guidelines over the years, mostly in the form of Food Pyramids (like the one pictured above). Their latest food guidelines, however, are in the form of a divided plate (which you can access via www. ChooseMy-Plate.gov). There are some reservations about the USDA Pyramids and Plates, which we'll discuss shortly, but they *are* useful for suggesting a balance of nutrients and helping to give you ideas about what your best food choices might be within the various food groups. For example:

- Milk products such as yogurt, low-fat cheese, or cottage cheese may be more to your taste than plain milk. Or you may choose to use milk in soups, casseroles, or puddings.
- You don't have to eat plain, recognizable eggs if you don't like them. Eggs can be ingredients in casseroles, soufflés, omelets, custards, and other dishes.
- If you hate vegetables, try new varieties or the same variety in different form. If, for exam-

VITAMINS YOU NEED FOR A HEALTHY BODY

Vitamin	How It Helps	Where to Get It
Vitamin A	Growth, healthy skin, teeth gums, eyes, digestive and urinary tract	Milk, butter, margarine, carrots, liver, eggs, fruit, dark green and yellow vegetables
Vitamin B-1 (thiamine)	Converts carbohydrates into energy. Promotes healthy eyes, skin, body tissues	Meat, fish, poultry, rice, whole-grain breads and cereals, fruits, vegetables
Vitamin B-2 (riboflavin)	Smooth skin, clear vision	Dairy products, enriched bread, cereal, eggs, poultry, fish, meat
Vitamin B-6 (pyridoxine)	Healthy skin, red blood cells, and nervous system	Vegetables, cereal, lean meat, milk
Vitamin B-12	Healthy nervous system; also safeguards against certain types of anemia	Eggs, liver, meat, milk
Vitamin C	Healthy teeth, gums, bones, and capillaries	Citrus fruits, cantaloupes, berries, tomatoes, green peppers, broccoli
Vitamin D	Helps body use calcium and phosphorus in building strong bones and teeth	Fortified milk, liver, eggs, and fish, especially salmon
Vitamin E	Theory is that this prevents abnormal breakdown of fat in body tissues and aids absorption of nutrients	Seeds, nuts, soybeans, wheat germ, leafy vegetables, whole-grain cereals
Niacin	Converts food to energy and aids production of certain hormones	Halibut, tuna, poultry, milk, eggs, whole grains, peanut butter, fruits and vegetables
Folic acid	Helps red blood cell formation and safeguards against anemia	Asparagus, broccoli, spinach, lima beans, liver
Pantothenic acid	Helps metabolize carbohydrates and fats	Broccoli, nuts, eggs

ple you find canned green beans totally disgusting, try steaming some fresh green beans with a touch of herbs. It's a whole different taste. Steaming fresh or frozen vegetables with subtle seasonings can make a big difference. A little cinnamon sprinkled on yellow squash can transform it into a delicious snack or side dish. A touch of lemon or apple cider vinegar can bring new zest to broccoli. If you still hate vegetables, try them in a stew or soup or stir-fried Chinese dish.

■ Cut down on red meat, substituting chicken, turkey, fish, seafood and tofu. There are many wonderful ways to prepare these—from salads to hot entrees.

If you're a vegetarian or thinking of becoming one, balance in your diet is vital, too. While vegetarians generally are less likely to suffer from heart disease or obesity (which are often linked with overconsumption of animal protein and fat), you still need to keep a balance of

MINERALS YOU NEED FOR A HEALTHY BODY

Mineral	How It Helps	Where to Get It
Calcium	Healthy teeth, bones, muscles; also helps blood clot normally.	Green leafy vegetables, shellfish, milk products such as yogurt and cheese.
Phosphorus	Helps get energy to body's cells	Meats, cheese, milk
Fluoride	Helps build and maintain strong, healthy teeth and bones	Lettuce, onions, soybeans, and specially treated water.
Potassium	Growth, a strong heart, and healthy nervous system; also helps regulate water balance in the body	Bananas, orange juice, leafy vegetables, dried fruits, lean meats
Iodine	Essential aid to the thyroid gland in regulating energy and metabolism	Seafood, iodized salt
Iron	Increases resistance to disease and prevents some forms of anemia	Dried fruits (especially raisins), whole-grain breads, cereals, liver, eggs, lean meat

fruits, vegetables, and proteins in your diet and not overdo it with sugars and starches.

Teens need to be particularly careful to get sufficient nutrients for their growing bodies. Protein-rich legumes (beans), milk, eggs, cheese, tofu, and perhaps fish and seafood can help a lot. In these growing years, you need protein and calcium, so nutrition experts tend to discourage teens from following a strict vegetarian diet.

Before beginning a new way of eating, make up a week-long menu and check it out with your physician, your school nurse, or a nutritionist to make sure that such a diet will be sufficiently balanced to meet your nutritional needs.

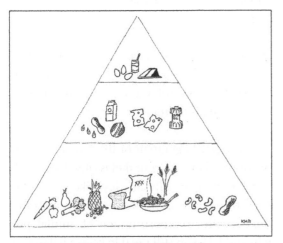

Vegetarian Food Pyramid

A WORD OF CAUTION ABOUT PYRAMIDS AND PLATES

While the USDA guidelines (presented through the Food Pyramids and MyPlates) *can* give you some idea of what it means to create a balanced eating plan for yourself, we have a few reservations about the nutritional guidelines themselves. First, it's important to know that these guidelines aren't entirely the product of good nutritional information, but are also—in part—the product of politics and lobbying by corporate agriculture. Thus, grains and dairy may get more attention than might be nutritionally optimal for you.

For example, the USDA guidelines for grains (suggested to be 30% of the daily diet in MyPlate) is too carbohydrate-heavy for teens struggling with obesity and/or diabetes. Similarly, the recommendation of daily consumption of dairy products may not make sense for many people of all ages who suffer from lactose intolerance.

It's useful to look at these as simply suggestions and then make a healthy food plan for yourself based on your needs and, to a certain extent, your preferences.

IMPROVING YOUR EATING HABITS (PAINLESSLY!)

Here are the best ways to start:

- Don't eat anything with high fructose corn syrup as an ingredient. Start reading labels and avoid products with this additive. This sweetening agent is added to many processed foods and is hazardous to your health and your waistline.
- Watch your sugar intake in general. It doesn't just mean making candy or cookies an occasional treat rather than a daily indulgence. It also means checking labels once again. For example, some packets of instant oatmeal are plain and have little or no sugar (and old fashioned oats in a canister or steel cut oatmeal is better still!) while some of the flavored instant oatmeal packets are loaded with added sugar. Cooking some plain oatmeal and adding berries or a banana to sweeten it makes more nutritional sense.

Also, be aware of how much sugar you're getting when you enjoy your favorite soft drink. Many teens get their biggest sugar blast from sodas. And diet sodas aren't the answer since artificial sweeteners are not healthy choices either. What to do? Try some club soda with a squeeze of fresh lemon or lime juice. Better still, try plain water with a lemon or lime slice. In time, you may find that you prefer it to the chemical taste of sodas.

- Start choosing real food over highly processed products: whole fruits instead of fruit juice, steamed vegetables instead of French fries, fish or chicken instead of deli meats and frozen dinners. A general guideline: if your great grandparents living 100 years ago would recognize something as edible, it's probably a reasonable food choice for you.
- Find ways to eat a healthy meal if you're out with your friends at a fast food place. Many of these places now offer salads, wraps and yogurt cups, and options for water or unsweetened tea instead of sodas. If you're embarrassed to order such things in front of your friends, think about it: you don't go to a fast food place for the great cuisine, but to be with and enjoy your friends. You can still do that and eat a healthy meal or snack, too.
- Eat at home with your family at least several times a week. Eating at home gives you more control over what is added to your food and also portion size. A recent study showed that teens who eat dinner with their families are better nourished and have healthier eating habits as young adults. If your parents are so busy working that they often come home with pizza, Chinese or fast food for dinner, offer to cook dinner for the family,

CUTTING DOWN ON DIET HEALTH HAZARDS

Food Hazards	How These Are Hazardous	Foods to Avoid or Cut Back	Good Food Substitutes
Soft Drinks/ Caffeine	Can add to stomach acidity Can add empty calories Caffeine can contribute to sleep disorders, heart rhythm disturbances	Sugary soft drinks Colas (no more than two a day at most!) Coffee Bottled iced tea with sugar	WATER is #1! (Drink at least eight glasses a day!) Fruit juice Vegetable juice Herbal tea Green tea
Sugar	A factor in obesity, heart disease, diabetes, hypoglycemia Contributes to tooth decay Personality and behavior problems	Sugary soft drinks Candy, cake, cookies Ice cream Convenience foods (packaged meals or fast food may have lots of sugar)	Fruit Fresh foods that you prepare or that you get from a restaurant salad bar
Salt	Can be factor in high blood pressure Can increase miseries of PMS water retention	Canned soups and vegetables Frozen convenience foods Snacks such as potato and corn chips Fast food (even milkshakes have high salt content)	Lemon juice or herbal seasonings as salt substitute Fresh meals you make yourself or soups and frozen entrees that are low-sodium (check labels!)
Fat	Contributes to obesity, heart disease (which can start in adolescence!), and certain cancers	Fried foods Bacon, sausage, and spareribs Butter, margarine, fatty dressings Snacks such as donuts, chips, or rich nuts (such as macadamia nuts)	Lean meats and fish that are baked or broiled Low-fat or nonfat dairy products (including low-fat yogurt or nonfat sour cream as a potato topping) Low-fat or nonfat salad dressings

doing the planning, shopping and cooking, several days a week. You and your family will feel better—and you'll be establishing a healthy cooking and eating pattern for the rest of your life.

Making healthy food choices helps you look and feel better today—and establish good eating habits that will give you lifetime benefits. In these years, many of your long-term food habits and preferences are being formed. At age 30 or older, you may not be able to eat the way you do today without piling on weight. It may be much more difficult to change your eating habits—and, certainly, to lose weight—as you approach middle age. So start now! Even if healthy food tastes weird and lame, stick with it for a few weeks or months and you may be amazed to see how your tastes change. You may find that those old sugar- and fat-laden treats don't taste nearly as good as they used to.

Growing up with healthful eating habits—salads, vegetables, seafood, fish, turkey chicken, beans and tofu—will help you main-

GOOD FOOD ON THE RUN

Yes! It's possible to enjoy fast food with your friends
if you're savvy about substitutions!

Instead Of....	Try This!
High-fat burgers and sandwiches; potato salad, French fries, onion rings	Salad bars (greens, fruit, veggies; no creamy salads—e.g. potato, macaroni, ambrosia) with low-fat, nonfat, or minimum amount of dressing
Cheeseburger	Hamburger
Fried chicken or fish sandwich or chicken nuggets	Chicken breast sandwich or chicken fajita pita
Fried fish sticks	Seafood salad
Fried tacos and burritos	Soft tacos and burritos
Meat pizza	Vegetarian pizza
Milkshake	Plain or chocolate low-fat or nonfat milk
Cola	Water with lemon slices or iced tea (with no sugar)

tain your weight and your health now and throughout adulthood.

REACHING AND MAINTAINING YOUR BEST WEIGHT

If You Feel You're Underweight

I'm 14 and skinny and everyone teases me about it. Some of my friends are jealous because I eat whatever I want and never gain weight, but other people make fun of me. What can I do?

J.K.

While underweight teens may be the envy of their classmates, being skinny and unable to gain weight can be as serious and emotionally painful a problem for someone faced with this situation as being overweight may be to another teen.

What can you do? First, check with your physician to see if you are, in fact, underweight. If he or she agrees that you are:

- *Consider your age, state of physical development, and body type.* The growth spurt in early adolescence burns a lot of calories. As your growth rate slows down a bit, you may start to fill out. Some people, of course, have a naturally lean, angular (*ectomorphic*) body type. Many models and actresses fall into this category—which is why so many women who have different, more rounded body types, get so frustrated in their futile attempts to diet their way down to similar slenderness.

- *Work out with weights for greater muscle definition.* This can give a lean body a few more curves. Both men and women work out with weights in health clubs, at school, and at home these days—and this form of working out can help you look and feel stronger.

- *Keep a diary of everything you eat for at least a week.* Note your eating habits. Do you eat three well-balanced meals a day, or do you snack a little here and there and skip meals a lot? Do you have trouble eating when you're nervous or upset? Are you extremely active or so busy that you often find you don't have time to eat? Are you a nibbler who tastes food, but who never finishes anything? In your food diary, note how much (or how little) you actually eat. It could give you some important clues.

- *Change behavior that keeps you too skinny.* Never skip a meal, especially breakfast. Even if you're upset, try eating regular meals. Your body needs essential nutrients no matter what you're feeling. And a well nourished body can give you extra strength to deal with a crisis.

- *Eat more nutritious snacks.* Trying to gain weight on candy and other junk food does more harm than good. Instead, pamper your body with snacks such as granola, whole-grain bread and peanut butter, milk products, and fruits (fresh or dried), and vegetables.

- *If you're only a little underweight, consider counting your blessings.* A slender body that is nevertheless well-nourished can be a healthy, attractive one. Find a fashion style that works for you and dress to accentuate your best features. As time goes by and your calorie needs decrease, you may tend to put on weight anyway. You may want to start a little low and thus reach (and then maintain) the average weight for your height after your growing years are over.

- *If you're active, don't stop!* Regular exercise is a health must for everyone. If you're set on gaining weight, simply increase your calorie intake, but do keep exercising!

Diet Danger: Too Thin on Purpose

Some young people, usually girls, fit into a different category of underweight. These are teens who suffer from dieting-connected disorders, most notably anorexia nervosa and bulimia.

Because these disorders have psychological as well as biological aspects, we will be discussing them in greater detail in Chapter 9, "Mind over Body", but we'll mention both briefly here. Both disorders often begin when teens who are normal weight or slightly overweight start a diet regimen to become fashionably slender. Unlike many young people who go on and off diets regularly, these teens are unable to stop dieting and develop bizarre rituals to avoid gaining weight. A teenager with bulimia usually indulges in alternate binging and purging, eating too much and then getting rid of the food by vomiting and taking laxatives. She may also diet stringently between binges. Most bulimics don't get seriously underweight, but there are serious health risks associated with the binge-purge behavior characteristic of this disorder.

Teens with anorexia nervosa, however, diet and exercise compulsively, sometimes starving themselves down to skeletal proportions and risking a number of life-threatening complications.

Although these girls are often alarmingly thin—sometimes weighing only 50 or 60 pounds—they have a distorted body image, seeing their emaciated bodies as fat or just right, and so are very resistant to efforts to help them gain weight.

If You Feel You're Overweight

How can you tell if you're overweight? I feel fat even though my parents say I look fine. All of my friends are on diets even though some are much thinner than me. I'm into sports and am pretty health conscious. I don't want to be like a skinny model, but I want to be a healthy weight. How can I tell if I am?

Cherise A.

Whether a teen is normal weight, slightly overweight, or obese, weight is a major concern among teens—especially teen girls—today. Unfortunately, it's quite common for girls to be dissatisfied with their bodies—overweight or not—and to start dieting at a very young age. When scientists at the University of California at San Francisco studied dieting behavior in young girls, surveying 500 girls ages 9 to 18, they found that while 58 percent of the girls considered themselves too fat, only 15 percent were actually overweight. Nevertheless, some 50 percent of 9-year-olds, 80 percent of 11-to-12-year-olds, 70 percent of 12-to-16-year-olds, and 90 percent of 17-year-olds were dieting to lose weight. These findings and others like them, concern medical professionals for several reasons:

- *Low Calorie diets can interfere with adolescent growth and development.* You need 2,500 to 3,000 calories a day during the prime years of physical development in order to experience your full growth and development and to have healthy bones. Too few calories can stunt growth.

- *Early dieting* can put you on the road to a lifetime of yo-yo weight fluctuations. When you diet, you change your metabolism. Your body learns to get by on fewer calories and you gain weight more rapidly after you stop dieting. Trying to reach some impossible standard of thinness in your youth can set you up for a lifetime of struggling with your weight.

- *Intense focusing on body weight and dieting at a young age can* make you feel worse about yourself. When your body and your life are changing, it's quite common to feel insecure at times. But if you are constantly comparing yourself to famous models or actresses (whose body type may be genetically quite different from yours), you're setting up standards that may not be attainable for you. While you might like to look like a model, not looking like one doesn't mean that you're a failure, ugly, or without any redeeming value as a person. You have your own strengths and talents and unique beauty. Obsessing about what you aren't or can't be and dieting to reach a goal that might not be healthy or even attainable usually doesn't do much for your weight and it can do great harm emotionally to the special person you're struggling to become.

Before you compare yourself too much to others—models, actresses, or even your friends—there are several important facts you need to know:

1. *People have genetically determined body types. Ectomorphs* are thin and angular. Many models and actresses are born with such bodies. *Mesomorphs,* on the other hand, are muscular with broad shoulders and slim hips. *Endomorphs* tend to be rounder and have more body fat and softer curves. So if you're an endomorph, you may be at your ideal weight, yet look heavier than a friend of the same weight who has the ectomorph body type. Genes are important. You're not likely to be slender and willowy if you come from a family of short, stocky people. Studies of people who were adopted as children have found that their weight and body shape more closely matches those of their biological rather than their adoptive parents. This doesn't mean that if you have obese parents, you're doomed to a lifetime of obesity. It may mean that you have to watch what you eat and exercise regularly in order to maintain a healthy body weight.

   Certain ethnic groups may be more likely to have higher percentages of overweight people. This may be a combination of genetics, eating habits, and cultural preferences. (Not all cultures venerate thinness as the ultimate in beauty and virtue!) For example, in a study of percentages of overweight children and adolescents by ethnicity recently released by the Center for Disease Control, the percentage of overweight teenage males was 11.6 percent for whites, 12.5 percent for African Americans, and 15 percent for Latinos. Their overweight female counterparts comprised these percentages across ethnic lines: 9.6 percent for whites, 16.3 percent for African Americans and 14 percent for Latinos.

2. *Females quite normally have a higher percentage of body fat as they mature during puberty and, over a lifetime, more body fat than males.* As we saw in Chapter 2, adolescent girls need a certain percentage of body fat for the changes of puberty to even happen. And while both boys and girls gain weight during puberty, boys put on more muscle tissue while girls put on more fat—usually going from about 19 percent body fat in the pre-puberty years to 21 to 22 percent body fat after the changes of puberty. Striving for much less than that can be harmful. Unfortunately, the media ideal has been to keep women looking like pre-pubescent children. Think about the implications of that. At a time when you're struggling to assert your independence and become your own person, do you *really* want a childlike body?

3. *Before deciding that you're too fat, you need to understand what that means:*

   ✔ *Overweight* means that you weigh more than other people of your sex, height, and body build.
   ✔ *Obese* means that you carry too much fat on your body. It is usually used to describe someone who is more than 20 percent over his or her ideal weight.

   An athlete may be overweight, but not overfat, carrying that extra weight in muscle mass. On the other hand, a normal-weight couch potato may have too much body fat due to lack of physical exercise.

How can you tell if your weight may be a problem?

- *See if you can pinch an inch.* Pinch a fold of skin on one side of your waist or on your upper arm. If this fold measures an inch or more, you may have too much body fat.
- *Check your BMI. BMI* stands for *body mass index.* This is a ratio of height to weight. You can determine your BMI by dividing your weight (in pounds) by your height squared (in inches). Multiply the result by 705. Ideally, your BMI should be between 19 and 22 if you want to be healthy and avoid developing heart disease. Those whose BMIs are 25 have a 30 percent higher risk of heart disease, while those with BMI of 26 or higher have an 80 percent increased risk of heart disease as well as a higher risk of developing cancer than those with lower BMIs. Those with a BMI over 30 are at risk for much more immediate health problems.

    For example, a girl who is 5'4" (64 inches) would have a BMI of 20 at 116 pounds, 25 at 145 pounds and 30 at 174 pounds. If you want to calculate your own BMI but are feeling a bit mathematically challenged, consult the chart on page 82.
- *Consult your physician.* He or she can plot your weight to see if it's in line with your height, body build, and stage of development. If your doctor finds that you're just a little overweight—ten pounds or less—stepping up your activity level (maybe taking a walk after school instead of watching TV) or starting a new sport or an aerobic exercise program may be all you need to do.

SENSIBLE WEIGHT LOSS

It is better to make slight changes in your lifestyle and eating habits and to lose weight gradually than to go on and off strict diets, losing and regaining the same ten pounds over and over again. By taking your time, you'll have a better chance of reaching and maintaining your best weight.

Excess Weight Is A Serious Problem For Many Teens

The statistics are sobering. The obesity rate for teens has tripled over the past 25 years and, with it, there have been some alarming health trends. Type 2 Diabetes was once a disease of overweight, middle-aged adults, but it is increasingly common among teens today. It now accounts for 45 percent of newly diagnosed diabetes in children and adolescents. Experts observe teens who are diagnosed with Type 2 diabetes tend to experience a more rapid deterioration of their general health than newly diagnosed adults do. Many already have high blood pressure and the fear is that severe heart disease could become much more common in young adults.

Why are young people fatter today? Readily available fast foods and snacks are part of the problem. But calories can pile up not only with what you eat, but what you drink: not only sugary soft drinks, but also calorie dense lattes and smoothies. And a recent study found that those who drink as little as one can or bottle of soda a day—whether regular *or* Diet—are at increased risk of metabolic syndrome, which can lead to

FINDING YOUR BMI (BODY MASS INDEX)

Height						Body Weight							
4'10"	91	96	100	105	110	115	119	124	129	134	138	143	148
4'11"	94	99	104	109	114	119	124	128	133	138	143	148	153
5'0"	97	102	107	112	118	123	128	133	138	143	148	153	158
5'1"	100	106	111	116	122	127	132	137	143	148	153	158	164
5'2"	104	109	115	120	126	131	136	142	147	153	158	164	169
5'3"	107	113	118	124	130	135	141	146	152	158	163	169	175
5'4"	110	116	122	128	134	140	145	151	157	163	169	174	180
5'5"	114	120	126	132	138	144	150	156	162	168	174	180	186
5'6"	118	124	130	136	142	148	155	161	167	173	179	186	192
5'7"	121	127	134	140	146	153	159	166	172	178	185	191	197
5'8"	125	131	138	144	151	158	164	171	177	184	190	197	203
5'9"	128	135	142	149	155	162	169	176	182	189	196	203	209
5'10"	132	139	146	153	160	167	174	181	188	195	202	207	215
5'11"	136	143	150	157	165	172	179	186	193	200	208	215	222
6'0"	140	147	154	162	169	177	184	191	199	206	213	221	228
BMI	19	20	21	22	23	24	25	26	27	28	29	30	31

heart disease and diabetes. (Metabolic syndrome has a particular set of symptoms—excessive abdominal fat, high blood pressure, high blood glucose levels, high blood triglycerides and low levels of lipoprotein, better known as the good cholesterol.)

Besides having poor diets, young people today are less likely to be physically active than previous generations. Gym class has been elim-inated at some schools or is less frequent in others. And, in their free time, young people often spend hours at the computer or with video games or text-messaging instead of walking or biking over to a friend's house or playing sports.

We've had a number of questions lately from teens who have heard that overweight can be catching—and that having fat friends can make you fat, too. However, it's more likely that friends will share food preferences, sedentary activities and other lifestyle habits that can help pack on weight—whether these friends see each other on a daily basis or not. It's more likely to be shared habits than some kind of fat contagion that can result in friends gaining weight.

Many teens who *are* concerned about their weight, may make unhealthy choices—like skipping meals or smoking—to keep from overeating. And an estimated 5,000 teens chose liposuction surgery last year, according to the American Society of Plastic Surgeons.

There *has* to be a healthier, more effective way to manage your weight and live a healthy life—and there is. It isn't so much a matter of starving yourself as making better food choices and becoming more active.

If you and your doctor determine that you are overweight or obese, you need to take several steps:

Step One: Examine Your Eating Habits and Behavior

■ *I eat when I'm upset, angry, nervous, or bored or to reward myself.*

Action plan:
1. Find ways to deal with your feeling that do not involve food.
2. Make a list of healthy pleasurable activities you can engage in to reward or comfort yourself.
3. Find more constructive solutions to anger or stress—such as talking, meditating, or exercising.

■ *I skip meals (especially breakfast).* (Note: Meal skippers are, as a group, more likely to

be obese. This is *not* a good way to control your weight!)

Action Plan
1. Don't skip meals. Eating regular meals is a major step forward in controlling your weight because you never get starved and then lose control and load up on food (and calories) late in the day.
2. Always eat a nutritious breakfast. No time? Get up half an hour earlier. Or grab something portable, such as low-fat yogurt and a piece of fruit.
3. Try the following balance: hearty breakfast, reasonable lunch, and light, early dinner with no big evening snacks. Your weight-loss progress may surprise you

■ *I'm really busy and don't have time to fix fancy meals and my mom won't make special diet stuff for me. I usually grab…whatever.*

Action Plan
1. Eat what your family eats—only watch your portions. Drink a large glass of water half an hour before your meal: this will help you to eat less.
2. Read labels on convenience foods. Many are full of sodium, which doesn't exactly help your weight loss even if the food or low in fat or calories.
3. If you're eating on the run, carry healthy, portable meals and snacks: fresh fruit, raw vegetables, a piece of whole-grain bread, rice cakes, low-fat cheese, yogurt, or a healthy sandwich with vegetables and/or lean meat.

4. If you and your friends are into fast food, refer to Chart 9 to start making some calorie-saving, healthwise choices!

■ *My fat protects me from social situations I find scary.* (Note: Fat can be a protective shield against expressing your sexuality or dealing with pressures to be sexual or even to date another person. It's not uncommon for those with a history of sexual trauma to find solace in food rather than risking relationships.)

Action Plan

1. Explore and find ways to solve your fears—write in your journal. Talk with people you trust.
2. If you have trauma in your past, consider getting help from a professional psychotherapist to deal with these troubling feelings.
3. Understand that you can make active choices that protect you without using weight as a shield. You can stand up for yourself and still have friends. You can say no to sex and still have a social life. You can learn to handle pressure and stress. When you use fat to protect you from these, you may also miss a lot of fun.

■ *I watch TV a lot and never exercise.* (Note: if you want to control your weight and build a healthy lifestyle, you *must* exercise regularly.)

Action Plan

1. Start moving in small but significant ways: Walk instead of riding or driving whenever you can. Take stairs instead of elevators and escalators. Volunteer to walk the dog.

2. Rediscover old pleasures: Get that old bike out of the garage and ride it; swim laps; walk with friends or family or by yourself (this can be a time to think, plan and dream.)
3. Learn a new sport you enjoy—or find one you hate the least and give it a try. You may be pleasantly surprised.
4. Realize that even very moderate exercise can bring wonderful benefits. You don't have to jog five miles a day, seven days a week to improve your fitness (in fact, we'd advise against such a grueling regimen, especially for a beginner!). A half-hour walk three to five times a week will make a positive difference in your life and your health—especially if, until now, you've been immobilized in front of the television set most afternoons or evenings.

■ *I am rebelling against someone.* (Note: It's quite common for someone whose parents are really into thinness and/or popularity, looks, and so on to rebel by getting fat. A Harvard research project showed that the obese women studied tended to have mothers who pushed them to succeed at everything and who equated thinness as a moral virtue and being fat as the worst possible fate.)

Action Plan

1. There are other ways to be unique and to stand up to your parents. You don't have to fight them with your body—in a way that hurts you.
2. Work on asserting yourself more often. Tell your parents what you think and how you're feeling.

3. Express your uniqueness through conversation, creative hobbies, journal writing, or other activities you enjoy.

4. If your family conflicts feel impossible to resolve, ask your parents about the possibility of family therapy so that you all can learn to communicate better and work better together as a family.

Step Two: Be a Smart Diet Consumer!

Many people seek miracles to lose weight: magic pills, instant diets that let you eat all you want while the pounds melt off, and weight loss while you sleep. If it sounds too good to be true, it probably is. In search of weight-loss miracles, too many people endanger both their bank accounts and their health.

Learn to be skeptical of outrageous claims. Face it: You can't melt off body fat overnight or lose 20 pounds in 72 hours or have lasting weight loss with no effort on your part.

■ *Fact: There are no miracles.* Avoid quick fixes and magic pills. They don't work—and aren't good for you. Even approved over the counter diet aids like Alli have some undesirable side effects (loose stools and an oily anal discharge) and aren't meant for long-term use. Instead, a slow, steady weight loss—no more than two pounds per week—is best for your health, and the best way to achieve it is with a well-balanced diet and exercise plan.

■ *Fact: old-style diets don't work.* Dieting, especially dieting without exercise, doesn't help you lose weight and keep it off. You may lose weight initially, but are likely to regain it quickly. The deprivation of an old-style diet can trigger binge eating. The body will also adapt to lower calorie levels and begin to store fat and maintain weight at progressively lower calorie

GUIDELINES FOR HEALTHY WEIGHT LOSS

Courtesy of Dept. of Nutritional Services, Kaiser Permanente Medical Group, San Francisco

Food Group	Daily Servings	One-Serving Examples
Protein	2	2 eggs
		2–3 oz. poultry, fish, meat
		3–4 oz. tuna
		1 cup beans/lentils
		4 Tbsp. peanut butter
Milk products	4	1 cup yogurt
		2 cups cottage cheese
		1 cup milk
		2 slices cheese
Breads and starches	4	½ cup hot cereal
		¾ cup dry cereal
		1 slice bread
		1 tortilla
		½ hamburger bun
		½ cup rice, noodles, pasta
Fruits and vegetables	4	1 whole fruit
		½ cup fruit juice
		1 cup vegetables

intakes. Dieting keeps you on the lose-gain weight roller coaster.

- *Fact: Weight control takes effort and sensible action.*

1. Plan well-balanced food choices that do not eliminate any of the basic food groups.
2. Follow a regular exercise program.
3. Make the commitment to eat well and exercise and just hang in there long-term to see the positive results. (No instant magic, but lots of long-term rewards!)
4. Consult your physician for diet and exercise tips. You might also want to consider the plan shown in the "Guidelines for Healthy Weight Loss" from Kaiser Permanente chart in this chapter.

Step Three: If You Can't Do It Alone, Seek Help

You can get help from family, friends, or diet programs such as Weight Watchers, TOPS, or Shapedown. You can also get help from your physician. In fact, you need to consult with your doctor before you start any weight-loss program, especially if it will go on for an extended period of time. You and your physi-cian can determine together the best way for you to lose weight and the minimum number of calories your body needs to lose fat and still be well nourished. You man also find psycho-therapy useful if your eating patterns or weight gain have roots in psychological stressors or conflicts.

Step Four: Start Living a Full and Healthy Life Today

You don't have to wait until you're slim to do this. Living fully doesn't have to depend on the shape of your body. There is a lot more to look-ing good than having a certain body shape or wearing a specific dress or jeans size. And there is much more to value about yourself than your looks. Good health (the result, at least in part, of good nutrition and regular exercise), energy, and a positive outlook on life can make you wonderfully and uniquely attractive.

You *can* have a full and happy life—what-ever your weight, whatever your shape. Being enthusiastic is attractive. Being smart is attrac-tive. Being compassionate gives you a very special beauty. You can be the best possible you—starting today—no matter what your weight.

Making good health (rather than a certain weight) your top priority will help you build a rewarding new lifestyle—starting today!

EATING FOR GOOD HEALTH

✔ *There are seven steps to good health.* These include: eating a balanced, healthy diet; getting regular exercise; maintaining a healthy weight; not smoking or doing drugs; having regular medical and dental checkups; getting involved in work or activities you love; and developing strong friendships and love relationships.

✔ *There are some painless ways to improve your eating habits right away.* These include: drinking water or fruit juice instead of sodas; substituting herbal seasonings for salt; eating more fresh fruit and fewer processed sweets; eating chicken, fish and tofu instead of red meat; choosing fast-food salads, baked potatoes, and non-fried chicken sandwiches instead of burgers.

✔ *The best way to lose weight is slow and sensible.* Make slight changes in your lifestyle and lose weight gradually. That way, you have a better chance or reaching and maintaining your best weight. Strict diets and fad diets are out! They're nearly impossible to stick with for an extended time and they're especially unhealthy for growing teens.

CHAPTER SIX

Exercising For Good Health

I'm overweight and my doctor says I have to exercise as well as eat less to lose the weight. The problem is, I HATE exercise! Is it something I have to do?

Cory Y.

I used be active as a little kid, but the last few years I've been so busy with school, dates, and activities that I've stopped exercising much. What can I do that would help me get back in shape and yet not take a lot of time and money?

Megan M.

When you're busy, don't have a lot of money to spend, and/or are embarrassed about your body, it's hard to imagine even doing, let alone enjoying, exercise. If you're a couch potato, you're in the majority. Recent studies have found that preteens and teens today are less fit than ever before. Tightened school budgets that all too often eliminate daily physical education classes are a major factor. So, too, are some of the favorite pursuits of today's teens: watching TV, playing computer games, and surfing the Internet.

But if you're active, or open to the idea of becoming more active, you can reap enormous benefits that can far outweigh any investment of time or risk of initial embarrassment about your body or your beginner status in a sport. Exercise is important for everyone: young, old, overweight, underweight, and all those in between.

What's the best kind of exercise program?

YOUR BEST EXERCISE PLAN

1. *Aerobic exercise.* This strengthens your heart and lungs. It includes fast walking, biking, running, swimming, dancing, aerobic dancing, and rowing. You need to exercise for at least 30 minutes, five times per week. And that's a minimum. Aerobic exercise also helps build bones and aids digestion, helping you make the best

possible use of vitamins and minerals. It's essential to your good health!

2. *Strengthening exercise.* This helps build muscle and bone mass, and tones your muscles. It might include weight lifting, working out on gym equipment, or doing exercises at home such as pushups, abdominal crunches, situps, or leg lifts. You need to do strength exercises at least twice a week.

3. *Stretching exercise.* This might be yoga, ballet barre exercises, or simple stretches at home that help you be more flexible.

Exercise can have many addition benefits, beyond helping you lose weight and keep it off and being an important part of building a healthy, strong, flexible body that will serve you well for years to come.

- *Exercise can safeguard your mental health.* Studies show that being physically active increases your self-esteem, improves your body image, and decreases your risk of serious depression. Exercise also helps prevent or reduce anxiety. It can be a great stress reducer and mood enhancer.
- *Exercise can help to prevent catastrophic diseases.* It not only protects your heart and lungs, but also can be a factor in preventing certain forms of cancer. For example, studies have found that women who are physically active as teens and young adults significantly reduce their lifetime risk of breast cancer (as well as osteoporosis, the painful and debilitating loss of bone that cripples many women in their later years).

What are the best forms of aerobic exercise? It depends. To reap the benefits of such exercises, you must do them at least five times a week. Look at the following list of suggested aerobic activities and ask yourself which one(s) you would like best (or hate least) and would be likely to do on a regular basis. In building physical fitness, consistency is very important.

- *Brisk* walking.
- Jogging or running
- Cross-country skiing
- Bicycling—regular or stationary bicycle
- Lap swimming
- Racquetball, handball, squash—if played vigorously
- Jumping rope
- Dancing—including aerobic dance
- Ice skating or roller skating—if vigorous and continuous

Other factors besides immediate preferences may influence your choice of activity. For example:

- *If you're significantly overweight*: Jogging or running may not be a good idea until your weight is closer to normal. Instead, you might try sports such as walking, cycling, and/or swimming.
- *If you want to exercise in private*: Stationary bicycling, jumping rope, using one of the new stepping/climbing home exercisers, or exercising to any of a number of excellent aerobic tapes, CDs, or videotapes may be fun for you. Walking can also be a non-threatening form of public exercise.
- *If you have trouble with motivation*: Join an exercise class at your local Y or youth club, or

find a friend or family member with whom you can exercise regularly. A vigorous walk every day with a special friend or family member can be a great way to get fit and to share some special talking time together too!

- *If you're in very poor physical condition*: Stick to walking and swimming—at least at first.

FOR A SUCCESSFUL START TO YOUR ACTIVE NEW LIFE

- *Check with your physician.* This is especially important if you have an underlying medical problem, but can be helpful, too, in discovering the safest kind of exercise for you. A complete sports physical is especially important if you're going out for team sports, competitive sports such as gymnastics, or physically demanding activities such as cheerleading, serious ballet, or other dance training.

Why does this need to be a complete physical? Because where you are in your adolescent development can make a major difference in your bone and muscle growth. A physician needs to determine your physical readiness to take on such challenges and help you plan for an exercise training and nutritional regimen that will maximize your good heath and fitness and help you avoid serious injuries.

Your physician may not always tell you what you or your parents want most to hear. For example, if you're tall, but have not developed the muscle mass and strength to match, you may not be ready just yet to compete with more developed peers in a contact sport such as football. Taking time to let your strength build and your body develop may mean a better sports experience later on and a healthier, injury-free body throughout your participation in team sports.

Also, with a thorough sports physical, your physician may be able to spot potential problems and refer you to an orthopedic specialist or physical trainer before a little problem becomes a big one that may threaten your continuing with a sport or continuing to be healthy and fit.

Especially if you're active in a sport that has stringent weight demands—such as wrestling, running, gymnastics, ice skating or ballet—you need to get regular checkups and advice from your doctor on proper nutrition, eating habits, and health guidelines in general so that you will not lose your good health while pursuing your active interests.

Developing a cooperative relationship with your doctor can mean that you have a special advisor on your team! If injuries happen, it's important to seek medical care right away and to follow your doctor's guidelines for healing before returning to full participation in your sport. Though injury-caused waiting times can be frustrating, taking time to heal properly from a strain, sprain, fracture, or contusion can mean a longer and happier sports experience.

If you have a special medical condition such as diabetes, asthma, or epilepsy, it is very important that you check with your doctor before starting a new sport or stepping up your activity level. Chances are, your medical condition will not keep you from doing what you want to do. However, it's vital, for your maximum benefit, that your condition be well controlled. If you have diabetes, you and your

WARNING: BEFORE YOU REACH FOR THAT ENERGY DRINK . . .

Now that everyone seems to carry bottled water to the gym or the sidelines of a competitive sport, some teens are opting for energy drinks, something the American Academy of Pediatrics strongly discourages. And, in fact, some of the energy drinks say right on the label that these substances are not to be used by those under 18.

Among the dangers these pose for teens is that most energy drinks are loaded with caffeine and caffeine-like substances (such as guarana), as well as sugar. This can be a powerful combination, especially when mixed with alcohol—which is common among teens—and can lead to an increased risk of alcohol dependence as well as increased heart rate, heart rhythm problems and elevated blood pressure.

A recent Canadian study has linked energy drinks, especially when consumed with alcohol, with an increased risk of traumatic brain injury—most often among athletes. Teens who had a traumatic brain injury within the past year were found to be seven times more likely to have consumed at least five energy drinks in the past week than those without a history of traumatic brain injury. Those with brain injuries were also twice as likely to have mixed energy drinks with alcohol than teens without such injuries.

Researchers found, too, that teens who consumed energy drinks didn't recover as well from their brain injuries, possibly because the high caffeine levels changed the chemical state of the body. The researchers expressed concern about these teen brain injuries, particularly because the brain in adolescence is still developing.

In most instances, water is your best and healthiest drink if you're working out moderately to intensely. If your physical exercise level is intense, you may decide to add a substance like Gatorade, which replenishes carbohydrates and electrolytes lost when you're excising intensely. However, other drinks that contain large amounts of caffeine are not recommended, especially those also including ephedrine, which is the active ingredient in the FDA-banned substance ephedra. Ephreda was banned for a good reason: it was linked to a number of sudden deaths among young athletes.

Also not recommended: using decongestants as stimulants, diuretics and laxatives for sports where weight is a factor or over-the-counter products that claim to increase muscle mass.

It's important to avoid protein supplements, be it in the form of powder, shakes or bars. The most recent statistics show that as many as 40% of young athletes use these protein enhancements, but these can have harmful effects like weight gain, muscle cramps and high blood pressure. Overuse can cause blood acidity leading to decreasing bone strength and a higher risk of kidney stones.

Using these questionable substances in an effort to enhance performance, you may be putting your health at considerable risk—and missing the main benefit of living an active life.

HEALTHY EXERCISE

Exercise	Common Injuries	Prevention
Jogging	Shin splints, strain of Achilles tendon, foot and knee pain	Wear good running shoes with proper cushioning. Warm up and cool down. Run on softer surfaces such as soft track and asphalt rather than concrete. Use proper running technique—flat-foot or heel-toe rather than running on toes.
Walking	Plantar fascitis, blisters	Use proper warm-up and cool-down. Wear good walking shoes with proper cushioning and support. If previously inactive, don't try too far too soon.
Inline Skating	Wrist fractures, facial lacerations, elbow or lower leg fractures, wrist or ankle sprains	Wear protective padding every time! Learn proper techniques for stopping. Keep speed under control especially if you're a beginner.
Bicycling	Head injuries, knee injuries	Wear a protective helmet every time you ride. Change gears—and take stress off your knees.
Snowboarding	Wrist and ankle sprains and fractures, head injuries	GET INSTRUCTION before hitting the slope. Even one lesson will decrease chances of injury. Use proper equipment—helmet and wrist pads.
Skiing	Head injuries, broken bones	Use common sense–recklessness on the slope can be deadly. Get good training and be physically fit. If you're tired, stop skiing. Most injuries happen when the skier is fatigued.
Dance/ cheerleading	Knee, ankle, and back injuries	Do proper warm-up. Use correct technique. Wear correct, well-fitting shoes. Allow rehab/recovery for injuries before full activity again.
Surfing	Head and spine injuries for body surfers, various injuries from being hit by surfboard for board surfers	**BODY SURFERS:** Avoid crowded beaches. Do not surf unless waves are breaking in deep water. Arch body with head back while riding wave. When leaving wave, roll to one side—*do not somersault.* **BOARD SURFERS:** Surf with a companion and try to stay with your board. If you wipe out in deep water, try to fall behind the board, diving deep and staying under for a while. When you come to the surface, protect your head with your arms. For shallow water wipeout, try to fall flat, feet or buttocks first.

Exercise	Common Injuries	Prevention
Swimming	Middle ear infection if you swim with a cold, swimmer's ear.	Don't swim if you have a cold. Staying out for a few days is better than having to be dry-docked for six weeks with a painful ear infection. Keep your ears clean and dry. If your physician suggests it, use alcohol-based eardrops.
Tennis	Tennis elbow	Best prevention is playing well: power for swings should come from the shoulder, with the forearm used only for control. Try a two-handed backhand. Wear a band just below your elbow to keep the muscles of the forearm from squeezing bone ends.

doctor need to discuss what additional nutritional needs you may have when you increase your activity level. If you have asthma, a minor adjustment in medication may be necessary when you become more active. And if you have a seizure disorder, your physician will probably advise you against diving, equestrian, or rock-climbing activities (even if your seizures are well controlled by medication) while encouraging other sports activities.

■ *Start slow and set realistic goals:* If you've been sedentary for years, you won't become a marathon runner in a week. Instead, you might start your exercise training with brisk walking, followed by several weeks of walking and jogging before you try running full time. Remember: running isn't for everyone. Taking a 30-to-45-minute walk every day may be better for you. Do what you like most—but don't try too much, too soon. That's how injuries—and discouragement—happen.

■ *Don't torture yourself.* If you make your exercise regimen torture, you'll become a fitness dropout. Make it as easy as possible to do what you need to do. Exercise at a time of day when it is both convenient and comfortable. Avoid

the heat of the day and drink liquids as you need them. It's not only OK, but essential, to drink water while you exercise vigorously. And, while you need to engage in aerobic exercise five times a week to get maximum benefits, with strengthening exercise (working out with weights), you need 48 hours rest between workouts to avoid muscle damage.

■ *Try a fun exercise combination.* This is especially important if you're the type of person who, like many of us, needs to exercise every day in order to keep motivation high. Cut the risk of injury (and boredom) by alternating your activities. Three or four days a week, you might walk or swim or cycle. The other days, you might work out with weights—either with free weights or on a Universal machine or Nautilus equipment—to exercise a different group of muscles and build upper body strength. Or run or walk outside when the weather is nice and save your indoor cycling, rowing, climbing, or cross country simulation for days when the climate is less hospitable.

■ *Exercise vigorously enough to reach your target heart rate.* In order to realize the benefits

ANABOLIC STEROIDS
AND OTHER SPORTS SUPPLEMENTS

■ *Anabolic steroids are bad news.* Taking anabolic steroids to build muscle mass or, supposedly, strength, is dangerous—whether you're male or female. These synthetic hormones have not been shown to increase strength, though they may increase muscle bulk somewhat. But athletes who build muscles by taking such substances may pay a terrible price: serious liver damage or disease, jaundice, and/or cancer. These drugs can also adversely affect blood cholesterol level. In males, there may be some decrease in size of the testicles and possible infertility. In females, masculine body hair patterns, thinning of the hair on the head, deepening of the voice, and clitoral enlargement may be irreversible even after the use of steroids is discontinued. Also, for those who are still growing while they are taking anabolic steroids, there is the risk of permanent short stature as the hormones cause the long bones to fuse prematurely. Some synthetic hormones, popularly referred to as "brake drugs," have been used in some countries to delay growth and puberty in female gymnasts. Such drugs carry the same risks as other steroids and, furthermore, in closing off the long bones to prevent growth, cause some body distortion and spinal curvature as other parts of the body continue to grow.

■ *Don't take amphetamines to enhance sports performance.* Some athletes have used amphetamines to increase endurance, but these drugs, too, exact a price: They mask fatigue limits and may make you risk injury.

■ *Say "no" to creatine.* This popular sports nutrition supplement can cause muscle cramping and gastrointestinal problems. Since its long-term impact on athletes is not known at this time, it is best to avoid using this supplement until experts have a better idea of how it helps or hurts not only sports performance, but also long-term health.

■ *Be cautious about herbal supplements.* There has been some concern about herbal supplements such as ephedrine. Ephedrine is closely related to the stimulant methamphetamine and can lead to high blood pressure, heart attacks, seizures, and strokes in active young people trying to boost athletic performance. This substance may be found in such products as Herbal Ecstasy and Ripped Fuel.

In sum, these drugs are *never* advisable for athletes. Real strength, skill, and endurance are built only by hard work and commitment.

RX FOR SPORTS INJURIES: RICE

R = Rest! Stop what you're doing and rest the injured body part.

I = Ice. Apply ice immediately to reduce swelling and internal bleeding. Continue ice treatment for first 24 hours. Crushed ice in plastic bags works best.

C = Compression with an elastic bandage also helps reduce bleeding into the tissues.

E = Elevation. Keeping injured body part elevated may help to reduce swelling.

of aerobics, you must sustain the exercise for 20 to 30 minutes and your heart rate must go up to its target level.

How do you know what your target level is? Your target heart rate is 70 to 85 percent of your maximum suggested heart rate of 220 minus your age. Generally, someone under 20 years of age would have a heart rate range of 140 to 170. To test your heart rate, take your pulse at your wrist or at your neck for six seconds. Then multiply that number by 10. Ideally, your 6-second heart rate should be between 14 and 17. Multiplied by 10, this would put you between 140 to 170 heart-beats per minute—your target heart rate.

- *Remember the value of warm-ups and cool-downs.* You need to do stretching exercises before any kind of aerobic sport—including swimming or stationary bicycling or even walking. It's even more important to allow time to cool down gradually as well. Abrupt starts and stops can lead to injuries or dizziness and other negative feelings during or after exercise. If you warm up, exercise, and cool down properly, this activity should make you feel better and full of new energy instead of worse and more fatigued.

- *Do what you most enjoy (or hate the least!).* Going into a new exercise program with positive feelings is a must! If the activity is at least somewhat enjoyable, you're more likely to stick with it and make exercise an important part of your life.

EXERCISING FOR—AND IN—GOOD HEALTH

If you're a sports lover or an insecure beginner who has a penchant for getting hurt regularly, this may be a sign that you need to be careful. How can you boost your sports performance without injury?

- *Warm up properly—and every time!* Failure to warm up properly is a major cause of sports injuries.
- *Start slowly and build your strength.* Too much too soon causes injuries. Don't go for peak performance your first time out.
- *Know and admit when you've had enough.* Most sports injuries happen when people are tired and their reflexes, coordination, and judgment slack off.
- *If you're injured, rest and recover—don't quit!*

COMMON SPORTS INJURIES

Injury	What Is It?	Symptoms	Treatment
Strain	Injury to muscle or tendon	Mild aching, stiffness or pain and swelling	RICE
Sprain	Injury to ligaments	Pain, swelling, more pain on movement	RICE—but if severe, see a physician to make sure there is no fracture.
Muscle cramps	Cramping of muscle due to lack of potassium and insufficient warm-up	Pain in affected muscle	Moist heat, pressure and massage of affected area, then slow stretching.
Patellar tendinitis	Inflammation of the patellar (knee) tendon	Pain	As long as the pain is mild, you can keep exercising. If it gets worse, see a physician.
Tennis elbow	Tendinitis in the elbow	Pain	RICE—then see a sports trainer for tips on strengthening injured muscles. See your coach for improvement of technique.
Shin splints	Injured muscles as the result of muscle imbalance: calf muscle much stronger than shin muscle	Pain in front of lower leg	Strengthen shin muscles (running up stairs is a good exercise) and stretch calf muscles by leaning against a wall and stretching the muscles slowly (NO bouncing!).
Plantar fascitis	Tear of fascia covering muscles at bottom of foot	Pain just under heel bone or on bottom of foot	Rest. Then make sure your shoes have proper support.
Achilles tendinitis	Inflammation of Achilles tendon—caused by tight muscles	Pain in area of Achilles tendon (back of ankle/heel)	Stop exercising for several days until the pain stops. Then do slow, gentle stretches to help stretch out the muscles.
Blisters	Caused by friction of ill-fitting shoes	Pain and appearance of blister	Cover with sterile bandage. To prevent: make sure your shoes fit well and are specific to your sport. Also keep your feet dry with foot powder.
Stress fractures	Cracks on the surface area of bones	Pain—especially when you press on the injured area from above or below	Rest so the fracture can heal. Temporarily switch to a non-weight-bearing exercise such as swimming or cycling.

As you become more physically fit and expert in a sport or activity, you're less likely to be injured. Don't quit. Just rest and recover. Then work to strengthen the affected muscles as you ease back into full activity.

Remember that the better shape you're in, the less likely you will be to suffer injuries—and the more likely you'll be to stay healthy, active and attractive all your life!

QUICK SCAN ✓

EXERCISING FOR GOOD HEALTH

✔ *Establish a regular exercise schedule.* You need regular aerobic exercise at least three times a week for 30 minutes or longer.

✔ *Check with your doctor before starting an exercise regimen.* Regular sports physicals are especially important if you're in a highly demanding sport such as running, gymnastics, figure skating or ballet.

✔ *Remember the safeguards against sports injuries:* These include a good warm-up and cool-down; the proper equipment; good technique, and common sense.

✔ *Best advice if you're injured:* Rest and recover—but don't let an injury keep you sidelined for any longer than you need to heal.

CHAPTER
SEVEN
Good Health
and Good Looks

I feel ugly. I hate my zits. My nails break all the time and my hair is gross. I wear dorky glasses because my parents won't let me get contacts. I HATE HOW I LOOK!!!! Help!

Michelle A.

This girl at school won't go out with me because she only dates guys who are good-looking. I guess I'm pretty average-looking. How could I look my best so some girl (maybe not this one) will like me enough to hang around with me?

Austin H.

The secret to being attractive is to feel as good as possible about your strengths and all you have to offer as a person— right now. Then, because you deserve tender loving care, you need to take good care of your body. Good looks come from good health. Head-to-toe attractiveness starts out with a good diet and exercise program. Eating protein, for example, can help your skin stay smooth and your hair grow strong and shiny. Vitamin A, (acquired via diet, *not* extra supplements), is great for healthy skin, and the B vitamins help you have healthy hair.

Cleanliness is important, too. A daily bath or shower—plus extra face cleansings if you, like most young people, have oily skin—helps clear away dirt, oil, and dead cells, preventing the accumulation of bacteria on your skin that can cause body odor.

However, sometimes looking your best is a bit more of a challenge and takes a little more care than just the basics.

HEALTHY SKIN

Skin, not surprisingly, is a number-one concern among teens: acne is the most common skin problem that young people seem to have.

Acne

A recent survey on adolescents and acne that was commissioned by the American Medical Association found that most teens (83 percent of those surveyed) were very concerned about skin appearance and acne, with about a third of these teens saying that they thought zits were the first thing people noticed about them. Some 18 percent reported depression about acne. But only 16 percent had sought help from a doctor, with most (67 percent) using over-the-counter medications that weren't especially effective.

To find appropriate help—or to help yourself—you need to understand how acne happens, its stages, and the best treatments for each stage. You also need to know the truth behind common myths about acne, such as "You'll outgrow it," "Just give up chocolate," or "Just keep clean. Acne comes from dirt." The fact is, untreated severe acne can scar you for life, both physically and, perhaps, emotionally. There is no conclusive evidence that chocolate or any other foods trigger acne. And acne does not come from dirt, though a good cleansing routine can help keep excess oils from accumulating.

So why do some people have severe acne and others have little or none at all? Heredity, which determines your skin type along with other important characteristics, can have a lot to do with whether or not you have acne. The conditions of adolescence, however, seem to be a major factor, too. At this time, there are many changes going on in your body: growth spurts, physical maturation, and a surge—and possible imbalance—of hormones. These hormones— progesterone in girls and testosterone in guys— become part of your lifelong body chemistry. So acne can flare up at any time later in life, too. But it seems most common in adolescence. Acne may be a problem for you for a short time—a year or so—or for a number of years.

How do your hormones trigger acne? As hormone levels increase, the oil, or sebaceous, glands (which are quite numerous on your face, shoulders, chest, and back) become more active, producing a fatty substance called *sebum*. This sebum travels from the gland to the pore (opening of the skin) and produces the oily skin so common in teens. If this passageway becomes blocked with sebum, the first step of acne—blackheads—may develop. Blackheads are black, *not* from dirt, but from oxidation of sebum and skin pigments in the pore.

If these blackheads are not removed, the sebum continues to fill in the duct of the gland, pressure will build, and bacteria may invade the area. The resulting infection may cause red papules and pustules (filled with pus), which we most often call *zits* or *pimples*. In more serious cases of acne, these may progress to cysts and subsequent scarring.

Can washing your face and other affected areas help prevent acne progression? It certainly can. Removing oil from the skin surfaces and keeping pores open through cleansing with ordinary or antibacterial soap two or three times daily is the first step. Frequent shampoos—to keep oily, greasy hair from adding oil to the affected areas—may also be helpful. In mild cases of acne, some over-the-counter acne lotions and creams may aid in drying of the skin.

If you're female and wear makeup, be very careful about the makeup you use. Oil-based makeup will only clog your pores more. However, a non-oily and/or medicated makeup that may even have astringent qualities can be helpful.

If you're troubled by acne on your back, a

shower once or twice daily with antibacterial and abrasive soap, using a back brush to scrub the back thoroughly, may help, too.

If you have blackheads, a pulverized soap may help to remove the blackheads and open the pores, but do be careful! These soaps are abrasive to the skin, so don't use them more than once or twice a day. Wash your face in hot water and rinse with cold water to help close the pores again. You may even wish to swab your skin with an alcohol-soaked pad after washing to help remove the last trace of oil and dirt. Used in moderation, alcohol is a good astringent. If your skin starts to feel dry, however, you may be using too much, depleting your skin's natural oils.

Washing isn't always enough, however, since sebum and blackheads start below the skin surface. Blackheads may be removed with a device called *comedo extractor*. When used correctly, this device can be very effective in removing blackheads (also called *comedomes*). When applied over the blackhead, this device exerts uniform pressure, expelling the blackhead and thus removing the oil duct blockage. This extractor works well and does not leave scarring, which might happen if you pick at a blackhead with your fingers. Although the area around the blackhead may be a little red (from the pressure) right after removal, this will fade quickly.

Your physician may use a comedo extractor to remove blackheads for you, or you can learn to do it yourself. You can buy a comedo exactor at a surgical store (easy to find in most large cities) or, in some instances, at a drugstore or pharmacy.

We'd like to emphasize that a comedo extractor is useful for *blackheads only!* When the blackhead becomes infected and turns into the classic red bump we usually call a pimple, the comedo extractor will do more harm than good. At this stage, exerting pressure could damage the skin and cause scarring. So don't use this device for pimples *and* don't pick at or squeeze your pimples in any way!

Several conditions may aggravate acne. *Fluctuating hormone levels*, present just before a woman's menstrual period, cause increased oil production and the chance of an acne flare-up. *Stress*, which may be present before an important event, may also be a predisposing factor. While there is no absolute scientific proof that this is so, such ill-timed pimple attacks are seen by many doctors and suffered by many teens. While sunlight combined with dry heat may help to dry out oily skin, *hot, humid weather*—like that in Hawaii or Florida or in most of the United States during the summer—can aggravate acne. *Salt water* may also aggravate acne. If you're a beach lover, but find that you seem to break out more after a dip in the sea, try washing your face and showering with fresh water right after you finish swimming.

As you may have noticed from looking around at your friends as well as from your own experience, acne can range from mild to severe. Where are you in this scenario—and what can you do about it? The following chart may help.

As you can see from the chart, there are several ways your physician can work with you to control stubborn or severe acne. The following are among the most current treatments:

Prescription Gels and Lotions

These include a particularly effective benzoyl peroxide gel and various antibiotic lotions that combat acne by suppressing follicle

STAGES AND TREATMENT OF ACNE

Stage	Symptom	Recommended Treatment
One	Blackheads	• Wash once a day with pulverized soap. • Over-the-counter or prescription medications containing benzoyl peroxide 5–10% once a day. • Comedo extractor (buy from pharmacy). Use on blackheads only.
Two	Blackheads and pimples	• See your physician. • Use benzoyl peroxide 5 or 10% twice a day. • Prescription topical antibiotics twice a day. • Retin-A if your acne is severe or resistant.
Three	Pustules	• Benzoyl peroxide 10% twice a day OR benzoyl peroxide 10% in morning and Retin-A 0.05 at night (if physician recommends this regimen). • Birth control pills (females only; also only if not responsive to topical forms of treatment).
Four	Severe, cystic acne	• Try all of the above • Discuss use of Accutane and possible referral to a pediatric dermatologist with your physician. Please note: Accutane should only be taken when acne does not respond to any other form of treatment. If you take Accutane and are female, you must avoid pregnancy while taking this drug as it can cause severe birth defects.

bacteria. In the past, acne patients often took antibiotic pills (for example, tetracycline) to help clear up acne lesions. While many still do take oral medications, topical antibiotics, which penetrate to the follicles, have become quite popular in the past few years. The most widely used include clindamycin lotions (called Cleotin T) and an erythromycin lotion.

Retin-A, a vitamin A acid, has been used as an effective topical medication, but its use lately has become somewhat controversial since many physicians have found that it can cause a lot of skin irritation. If you use Retin-A, be sure to wash your face first with a very gentle cleanser, then wait about half an hour before you apply Retin-A. Spread it evenly over your face, avoiding areas right around the

eyes, nose, and corners of the mouth. *Don't* be tempted to spot-treat blemishes with it. Extra Retin-A won't make the zits go away sooner: it could simply irritate your skin. Be sure to pamper your skin during treatment, wearing a sunscreen and a moisturizer to protect your face from the elements. Retin-A is most effective when applied to your entire face just before bedtime.

Oral Medications

Tetracycline is the most common oral medication. This may be either plain tetracycline or doxycycline or sometime minocycline. Oral medications can be used alone or in combination with topical medications. However, because of possible side effects from oral medication, this is generally used only when a person's acne does not respond to treatment with topical antibiotics.

If you're female and your acne doesn't respond to any of the above treatments, your physician may prescribe birth control pills, which have been approved by the FDA to treat acne as well as to prevent pregnancy. Hormones, as we have seen, *do* exert a strong influence on acne. The hormone estrogen, which birth control pills have always contained, seems to suppress oil gland secretions and, in the process, may help to control acne.

For those with severe, cystic acne that has resisted other forms of treatment, there is an oral prescription drug called Accutane (13-*cis*-retinoic acid). This powerful drug should be used only in severe cases and then only under the direct supervision of a dermatologist.

Accutane treatment, which involves taking a pill daily, lasts eight weeks, followed by an eight-week rest period and then continuation of the drug another eight weeks, if necessary. Studies indicate that many patients continue to improve after the medication has been stopped.

The drug does have side effects—most commonly, severe drying and chapping of the lips. This occurred in most patients tested. A smaller number also experienced some rise in their cholesterol levels. And there have been some recent cases of teens on Accutane who have episodes of depression, psychosis, or suicidal behavior. (If you're taking this medication and begin to feel depressed, let your doctor know right away.) Significantly, medical experts say that the drug cannot be given to a woman who is pregnant or who has a possibility of becoming pregnant during

the treatment, since 13-*cis*-RA is in a class of chemicals known to cause quite devastating birth defects.

If you and your doctor feel that this drug treatment is your best alternative *and* you are sexually active, it is crucially important that you use TWO *very* reliable birth control methods during your course of treatment.

Eczema

I'm a 15-year-old girl who has bad eczema. I've had this for a long time. How can I get rid of it?

Desperate

Eczema is a chronic skin allergy and, like many allergies, there is no sure cure; however, there are ways to control it. Treatment with steroid creams to control the inflammation and itching may help a lot, but this is available by prescription only, so check with your physician.

Psoriasis

I have these awful patches that hurt and itch and have white scales on them. My mom thinks it's psoriasis and made a doctor's appointment for me. My friends think it's gross and won't be around me. How soon can I get rid of this?

Jessica S.

Psoriasis is a very common skin disorder that usually first appears between ages 15 and 35. It is caused by too-rapid skin cell growth. Cells build up on the skin surface with resulting swelling, redness, scaliness, and discomfort (either pain or itching). It's like having hyperactive skin! Parts of the body most likely to be affected are the hands, feet, knees, elbows and scalp.

Psoriasis is not contagious nor is it necessarily an inherited condition. While one in three people with psoriasis do have a family history of it, two of three do not. And while this condition is not curable, medication can control it and clear it up for varying amounts of time. Your physician will work with you to determine what treatment will be best for you. If you have just a few lesions, he or she might suggest using moisturizers and, possibly, a prescription topical medication, such as low- to medium-potency steroids for a short period of time. (Long-term use of steroids is not suggested due to possible side effects.) There are other types of topical prescription medications—such as vitamin D-3 (not the same as vitamin D sold over the counter), coal tar, or, in severe cases, anthralin.

Your physician may also suggest light treatments—from natural sunlight to ultraviolet light (UVB) treatments—which can bring some relief. In severe cases, a short treatment of UVB combined with an oral medication may be used.

The emotional impact of this disorder can be at least as painful as the lesions. You may feel very much alone at times. It's important to share your feelings with those who love you—and you may also find reassurance via a pen pal match with another teen with psoriasis. If you're interested in getting a pen pal (or special information about this disorder), write to the National Psoriasis Foundation, 6600 S.W. 92nd Ave., Suite 300, Portland, OR 97223-7195 or call (800) 723-9166.

Warts

What causes warts? Are they contagious? My boyfriend has a wart on his hand and I'm almost afraid to hold hands with him.

Shelly

I heard that putting duct tape on a wart can make it go away? Is that true??

Jake Y.

Warts are caused by a virus and come in many varieties. Some, like venereal warts, which occur around the genitals, are quite contagious. Others, such as those occurring on the arms, legs, hands, and feet, are usually not contagious. There is a great deal of speculation about how one gets these warts. We do know that warts are caused by a virus—not by frogs, as the old myth goes—but beyond that, we have very little conclusive evidence about what exactly causes this virus to happen in some people.

Some warts on the hand can be treated at home with topical application of an over-the-counter preparation such as Compound W. This type of treatment usually requires persistence and repeated applications, however, so don't get discouraged if your warts don't disappear on the first try.

There haven't been any studies yet on whether duct tape actually works in getting rid of warts. (In the one study on record, researchers used the wrong type of tape—clear stuff instead of the usual silver duct tape. The clear didn't help. The silver might.)

If your warts seem immune to nonprescription preparations, your physician may be able to help in several ways. He or she may remove the warts via electrocautery (burning off the warts with electrical heat), topical application of certain prescription medications, liquid nitrogen (which turns warts white, "freezing" them and causing them to die and eventually fall off), or even a systemic approach, using vaccines to remove and prevent recurrence of the warts.

Another kind of wart is something else altogether: the *plantar wart*. This type of wart, usually found on the sole of the foot, is not raised like most other warts, but burrows deep into the skin. This wart, which may be very painful, is also caused by a virus, which may be picked up by a minor break in the skin, in places like gym shower rooms.

Plantar warts should *not* be treated with home remedies. If the wart is not particularly painful and does not appear to be multiplying, some physicians prefer to leave it alone. These warts will often disappear in a month or so when the body begins to reject the wart. However, if the wart is painful and/or starts to multiply, the physician may remove it with liquid nitrogen or by treatment with an acid solution.

Moles

> I have several moles on my neck and chest. Are they dangerous in any way? Should I have them removed?
>
> Don R.

Moles, medically termed *nevi*, are very common in all age groups. Basically, a mole is an area of the skin where there is a heavy concentration of the skin pigment *melanin*. Generally, moles are harmless, though in some instances and locations, they may be cosmetically unappealing.

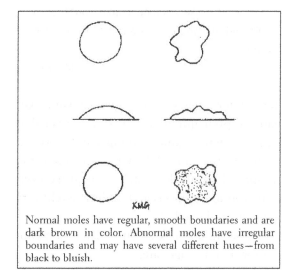

Normal moles have regular, smooth boundaries and are dark brown in color. Abnormal moles have irregular boundaries and may have several different hues—from black to bluish.

Moles—Normal and Abnormal

If you have a mole that begins to enlarge or change in color, however, this is a reason for concern. This could be a symptom of a rare but serious condition called *malignant melanoma*, a cancer that can kill young people as well as older ones—and can do so rather quickly without prompt treatment. So if you notice any changes in a mole, do see your doctor.

In examining your moles, use the ABCDE rule: look for *Asymmetry* (one side of the mole looks different from the other); an irregular *Border*; a change in *Color* (or sudden multiple colors); *Diameter* (an increase in size over a short time); *Evolution* (changes in A.B.C and D as well as bleeding, pain and/or itching. If you notice any of the above, see your doctor right away!

A Sun-Lover's Guide to Protecting Your Skin

> I practically live on the beach in the summer and love to get deep tans. I've read some stuff, though, about too much tanning making

you wrinkle like a prune before you're even old and that you might even get skin cancer. True—or not?

Mary B.

Yes—unfortunately, it *is* true that your skin can age prematurely or that you can get skin cancer, often at quite a young age, by overexposure to the sun. Malignant melanoma, the deadliest form of skin cancer, can strike even fairly young sun-lovers and, unless caught very early, it can be lethal.

Those most at risk for sun-related skin cancer (or skin damage) are:

- Those with fair skin and light hair and eye color.
- Those with a family history of melanoma.
- Those with unusual or changing moles on the skin.
- Those with painful or blistering sunburns in childhood or during adolescence.
- Those who spend their recreational time outdoors.

If you, like many young people, practically live outdoors in the summer, here are some common-sense tips that may help minimize skin damage from the sun:

- *Use a sunscreen.* This applies to everyone, especially to those with fair complexions. Use a sunscreen with the highest sun protection factor you can find. Look for a "broad spectrum" sunscreen that helps to block ultraviolet A and B (UVA and UVB) radiation. Apply your sunscreen before going outside. Once you are out, perspiration may dilute the sunscreen and prevent some of the sun-blocking ingredients from penetration your skin. Reapply the sunscreen occasionally while you are out.
- *Protect your lips.* Use a special lip sunscreen that applies like lipstick.
- *Realize that sunscreen can't do it all.* It offers protection, but it doesn't make you free to roast yourself for six hours in the midday sun in search of a perfect tan.
- *Shun the sun in high-intensity hours.* Avoid direct sunbathing or prolonged sun exposure between the hours of 10 A.M. and 2 P.M., when the sun's rays are most powerful and direct. If you must be in the sun at this time, wear sunscreen and protective clothing. Take refuge under a beach umbrella or in the shade of a tree.

  If you're swimming, remember that water is no protection. It admits the sun's rays, too. In fact, wet skin is more receptive to ultraviolet rays than dry skin, so apply a sunscreen before swimming and *after* you get out of the pool or the surf.
- *Take care to protect the most vulnerable parts of your body.* Your nose, ears, lips, knees, and shoulders are more exposed and will burn faster than other parts of your body, so give these extra protection. Be sure to apply sunscreen, too, to the areas often forgotten (until a painful sunburn reminds you!): your ankles, the tops of your feet, the tops of your ears, and the back of your neck.
- *Dress for maximum protection.* Don't use a sheer, gauzy cover-up when you're at the beach. Ultraviolet rays penetrate these fabrics easily. A long-sleeved, dark-colored shirt or coverup is better. Best of all would be clothing that is specifically made to block harmful rays: tightly woven fabrics

that have specific SPF ratings (and are sold in sporting-goods stores or in specialty catalogs). Also, wear a hat with a four-inch brim to give your nose (the most common site for skin cancer) some extra protection.

■ *Remember that weather is no protection.* You can burn as easily on a cloudy day as a sunny one, so use that sunscreen even when clouds or haze cover the beach!

■ *Your ethnicity doesn't make you immune to sun damage.* Black or other dark skin can burn, though not as easily as lighter skin. While whites have 20 times greater risk of getting skin cancer than do African Americans, everyone needs to be cautious and use sunscreen.

If all of this sounds more than a little sun-phobic, remember that we're talking to you from a health-oriented (rather than fun and fashion-oriented) point of view. However, protecting yourself doesn't mean that you have to become a creature of the night, forgoing any fun in the sun or any kind of cool clothing. Just be as careful as you can.

Why are we going on so about skin cancer? Because studies have found that malignant melanoma has its origins in these early years. What happens to your skin *now*, when you're in your teens, can have a major impact on your health in later years—or maybe even few years down the road. (Sandi, a close high school friend of Kathy's, was a blue-eyed, blond sun-lover who spent all her free time at the beach in search of the perfect tan. She was diagnosed with malignant melanoma when she was in her early twenties and died, despite extensive medical treatment.)

Other, less serious types of skin cancer can result from prolonged sun exposure over a lifetime. These are more easily treated than melanoma and have a lower fatality rate (1 percent compared to 25 percent among those with melanoma). But for optimal health and peace of mind, it simply makes sense to try avoiding such problems altogether.

Prolonged sun exposure can also make you look old long before your time. Damage to the elastic fibers of the skin by overexposure to the sun can cause wrinkles. These fibers, which keep the skin soft and elastic, cannot function well if damaged: this may lead to wrinkled, saggy, leathery skin at a fairly early age. You may find yourself at 35 looking like you're 70!

I'd like to get a sun lamp with a timer for safety. Could it still hurt my skin? I really would like to have a year-long tan.

Sunny

We do not recommend either sun lamps or tanning salons. The risks to your skin are simply too great. Tanned skin is, essentially, damaged skin and, as we pointed out earlier, can make you look old and leathery well before your time. In the more immediate future, sun lamps can give you a nasty burn if you spend too much time under them (usually by falling asleep and forgetting to set or not hearing the timer).

We recommend that, for your best healthy and lifetime good looks, you avoid tans both of the indoor and outdoor variety!

HEALTHY FEET, NAILS, AND HAIR
Feet

Some of the most common foot problems,

their causes and treatments are listed in the following chart.

TLC FOR COMMON FOOT PROBLEMS

Problem	Cause	TLC Solution
Blisters	Rubbing, friction	• Buy shoes that fit • Wear socks (preferably synthetics). • Put Vaseline or a sports lotion on area likely to rub or blister
Bunions	Ill-fitting shoes; can also be hereditary	• Buy shoes that fit comfortably. Avoid narrow, tapered styles. • Use orthotic inserts in your shoes. • If bunions are painful, use ice and elevation to alleviate pain and swelling.
Corns	Ill-fitting shoes; can also be hereditary	• Buy well-fitting, comfortable shoes. • Soak and moisturize your feet daily. • Use over-the-counter corn pads (such as Dr. Scholl's OneStep). • If you have diabetes, discuss foot care with your doctor before using any over-the-counter corn pads.
Fungus (athlete's foot)	Going barefoot in moist, warm environments such as gym showers or pool decks	• Avoid going barefoot in public showers and on poolsides. Use shower sandals or other shoes designed for use in water. • Treat with over-the-counter antifungal powder or cream. • See your doctor for prescription treatments if the above doesn't help.
Hammertoes	Hereditary; can also be caused by shoes that put pressure on toes (too small, very high heels, ballet toe shoes, etc.)	• Wear shoes that fit comfortably and do not put pressure on toes. • See your doctor about surgery if your case is severe.
Ingrown toenails	Too much clipping and/or tight shoes	• Soak and dry feet, use only toenail clippers, and file nails straight across. • Use antibacterial ointment to avoid nail fungus infection. • Wear sandals with open toes whenever you can. • See your doctor if the problem is severe
Toenail fungus	Injury to nail and/or too much clipping	• If over-the-counter antifungal medications don't work, see your physician for prescription oral medications.
Smelly feet	Heredity; wearing shoes without socks; wearing nylon stockings for long hours	• Wash and dry your feet thoroughly at least once a day. • Wear socks (preferably synthetic). • Use deodorant foot powder or cream or deodorant spray on feet. • Soak feet in warm tea.

Three Rules for Happy Feet

1. Wear shoes that fit your feet comfortably. Shop for shoes in the afternoon, when your feet tend to be bigger.
2. Bathe and powder your feet every day.
3. Use common sense. Avoid certain types of shoes: very high heels or platform shoes which can cause ankle-spraining (or ankle breaking) injuries; flats without adequate arch supports; and tight-fitting boots that may restrict blood circulation in your legs. Your best bet: comfortable, well-fitting shoes with a slight heel.

Nails

My fingernails are flaky and chip easily. Would drinking gelatin help? I want to have pretty nails like everyone else.

Bethany

If your nails are brittle and chip a lot, analyze your habits. Do you have nervous mannerisms, such as drumming them, or picking or biting them? All of these can retard nail growth and cause chips, spots, and pits in the nail. So can fungal infection or poor circulation. If there seems to be a skin infection involved, you may want to visit your doctor for treatment. If there is no infection involved, you might try soaking your nails in a combination of water and gelatin for temporary hardening—or use one of the nail hardeners-lacquers available at your local drug or department store.

I've been using artificial fingernails over my own nails, but I've noticed lately that my own nails are getting separated from the skin and really look gross. What's wrong?

Jill

You may have onycholysis, a condition usually caused by a fungal or bacterial infection or by an allergic reaction to the glue used on fingernails. Stop using the artificial nails (and the glue) immediately and see your doctor. Usually, removing the cause of infection will cure the problem and the nails will grow back.

Hair

I have oily hair and like to wash it every day. My mother objects because she thinks I'll lose my hair. I have acne, too, so feel it's especially important to keep my hair clean. Am I right?

Christy

It's a good idea to wash oily hair every day if desired, not only to keep from aggravating any acne that may be present on the face or back, but also to stimulate the scalp. This stimulation, in combination with a mild shampoo, may actually enhance hair growth by stimulating the hair follicles and the scalp's natural oils.

Recently when I shampoo my hair, I lose more hair than usual. Is something horrible wrong with me?

Worried

It's normal to lose some amount of hair every day. Hair follicles have distinct cycles, involving active growth of hair followed by shrinkage of the follicle, and then rest. After producing hair for several years, a follicle may shed its hair and rest for a few months. This is occurring on a constant basis with the countless hair follicles on your head.

Some factors can trigger some of the hair follicles to take an unscheduled rest and shed hair: bodily upsets such as stringent dieting (such as anorexia nervosa) or severe illness; certain anti-cancer drugs; infection of the scalp (which can be caused by allergies to a hair product such as shampoo, conditioner, or a hair-coloring agent); and hormonal changes brought about by thyroid abnormalities, some birth control pills, or pregnancy.

> My hair is dull and looks faded. How can I make it look shiny?
>
> Carla A.

There are a number of reasons for dull-looking hair. A buildup of dirt or hair products (like conditioner or hair spray) on the hair can make it look dull. So can a residue of shampoo if you don't rinse your hair thoroughly after washing it. Frequent shampoos—possibly with a protein shampoo product—may help make your hair shine.

As we have discussed, your diet is extremely important to your looks. Dull hair may be an indication that you lack vitamin B-12 and could use some more lean meats, fish, eggs, milk, and liver to start feeling—and looking—your best.

HEALTHY EYES

Your eyes, too, can be a reflection of your general health. A specially trained physician may be able to see symptoms of diabetes, liver disease, or high blood pressure—to name a few disorders—while examining your eyes. Your vision may also have a huge impact on how you do in school. If you suffer from headaches after reading or find it hard to keep your place while studying, you should get your eyes checked. But whether or not you experience any troublesome symptoms, periodic eye examinations are advisable.

Who are the professionals who do eye exams?
An *ophthalmologist* is an M.D.—a physician—whose specialty is diagnosing and treating diseases and defects of the eye. He or she performs surgery when necessary. An *optometrist* is not a physician, but has a Doctor of Optometry degree (O.D.) and is highly trained and licensed by the state to diagnose eye problems and diseases. He or she may prescribe glasses, contacts, or other optical aids. An *optician* is the technician who grinds lenses, fits them into frames, and then adjusts these frames to each individual.

If you go to an ophthalmologist, he or she may refer you to an optometrist or an optician for glasses or, if you desire, contact lenses.

Contacts

> I wear glasses now, but would really like contacts. My girlfriend says that they are great. I heard there are different kinds but don't know anything about them.
>
> Josh K., 17

Most contact lenses these days are soft lenses, made of watery, gel-like plastics. Usually, these are somewhat larger than the colored part of your eye (the iris). However, another type of lenses—oxygen permeable lenses—is made from more rigid plastic material and is smaller than the iris of the eye. A recent innovation—silicone hydrogel contact lenses—allow even more oxygen to pass through to the eye and aren't as likely to dry out.

In addition, contacts can be classified by how long you can keep them in continuously.

Daily wear contacts must be removed every night. Some of these are ones you cleanse and store for the next use. Others are disposables that you replace every day. *Extended wear* contacts are ones that can be worn continuously, including overnight, for a week. *Continuous wear* contact lenses can usually be worn for a month and then are replaced with a new pair.

Why are so many varieties of soft contacts disposable these days? Proteins and lipids build up in the lens, causing discomfort and possibly increasing the possibility of infection. Cleaning the lenses can help but buildup will still make replacement necessary over time. The disposables, some of which are replaced daily, take care of this problem with a minimum of inconvenience.

There are many different kinds of contacts that correct whatever vision problem you might have. In addition, there are some that can enhance or even change your eye color, or special effect lenses that can make your eyes look like a cat's or a zombie's or any variety of theatrical effects. (The latter would be used for special occasions and not for daily wear!)

There is no one kind of contact lens that is right for everyone. Check with your doctor to see which type may be right for you and your special vision problem.

My best friend and I both wear contacts. She

wets hers by putting them in her mouth. She says it's perfectly OK to do. But I heard it's not good. Who's right?

Amy L.

Amy is right. Placing your lenses in your mouth may spread infection. It is also not advisable to clean your lenses in tap water, according to a new warning from the American Academy of Ophthalmologists. Cleaning your lenses in tap water puts you at risk of getting an eye infection called acanthamoeba keratitis, which can cause blindness. Distilled water isn't completely sterile and shouldn't be used either. Clean your lenses in sterile saline solution *only*!

Other practices to be avoided: rubbing your eyes with contacts in; wearing them too long or; if you don't have extended wear lenses, sleeping with your contacts in place. If you're careless, your eyes could suffer serious irritations.

Eye Surgery

I've heard about an operation that stops nearsightedness and makes your vision normal without glasses or contacts. I'm really interested. Could you tell me more about this?

Brian K.

There are several laser surgeries including LASIK and PRK (Photo Refractive Keratotomy). Both treatments involve using a laser on the cornea to remove and then refold layers of corneal tissue to get the corrective angle.

However, these procedures are generally not recommended until early adulthood. The minimum age at which a physician will consider accepting a patient for this treatment is usually

21. These procedures are also quite expensive, running about $4,000 total for both eyes.

At this point, we would recommend putting up with your glasses or contacts for a few years more until you're 21 or until more is known about the long-term advantages or disadvantages of these procedures.

Caring For Your Eyes

I have normal, good eyesight, but my eyes get bloodshot and water sometimes. Why does this happen?

Alex G.

Bloodshot, tearing eyes can be the result of several possibilities—allergies, eye strain, and pollution being the most likely. Washing the eyes with water may help. If you have a chronic problem involving allergies, an eye preparation such as Visine may help. However, if the problem is severe or chronic, see a physician.

Is it true that you're not supposed to wash just under your eyes? Someone told me that and I just can't believe it. Why should that be true?

Brit W.

It's *half* true. The skin around the eye is very delicate, should not be scrubbed, and needs to be moisturized regularly. However, you can clean the area and remove eye makeup with remover made just for the delicate eye area.

For some time, the white parts of my eyes have had a slight yellowish color. Could this be serious?

Worried

A condition like this—called *icterus*—may or may not be serious, but it's certainly worth checking with your physician. Icterus may be a sign of a liver disease, such as infectious hepatitis. Then, too, it may mean nothing. There are some entirely healthy people who may have slightly icteric eyes. However, only your physician can tell whether this condition is normal for you or whether it is a symptom of a serious health problem.

HEALTHY TEETH AND GUMS

Help! I have bad breath and nothing, even mouthwash, does any good! What's the matter with me anyway?

Embarrassed

What causes bad breath? Persistent bad breath can be a symptom of indigestion or one of a number of diseases. However, it is often caused by decaying teeth and/or a gum problem.

Many people, young and old alike, worry about bad breath and the social problems it may cause, and try to mask the symptom rather than to cure the underlying causes by seeking dental help.

Your teeth and gums are an intrinsic part of your total health. Too many young people seem to be ignoring this fact. Among the statistics compiled by the American Dental Association, one in particular stands out: fifty percent of young people age 15 and younger have *never* been to a dentist.

Your dental health is an important part of your total health and can be an important barometer of your body's health—or lack of it. Decayed teeth and tender gums can serve as early warning signals that what you're doing—especially what you may be eating—is not good for your body. And dental problems are widespread among young people. The ages of 13 to 16 are particularly cavity-prone years.

Teens in this age group can be especially likely to get cavities because these are busy years: you may not be taking time to clean your teeth properly. Also, you may be eating a lot of junk food or convenience food that may be laced with sugar. Neglect plus sugar can equal a buildup of *plaque* on the teeth.

What *is* plaque? It is a film of harmful oral bacteria that forms on the teeth. Combined with sugar, certain bacteria in the plaque form acids that attack tooth enamel, leading to decay and, even worse, to gum disease. Although you can remove some of this plaque by brushing and flossing your teeth twice daily, regular visits to a dentist for a more thorough cleaning are essential to remove plaque from the hard-to-reach areas on your teeth. Too often, people put off going to a dentist until an emergency—such as a toothache—hits. But good preventive care can keep such painful emergencies from happening.

Although tooth decay is extremely common in young people (it is estimated that by 17, the average young American has nine decayed, filled, or missing teeth), the possibility of gum disease causes the most concern among dentists. Gum disease, also called *periodontal disease*, is what usually makes people lose their teeth later on in life. A third of all Americans have no natural teeth left at all by age 60. Sixty may seem a long way away, but the damage can start now.

The damage caused by gum disease may not be just to your teeth, but also to your health in general. Researchers have found a link between gum disease, heart valve damage, stroke and, in mothers who have gum disease, a greater possibility of giving birth to a premature baby.

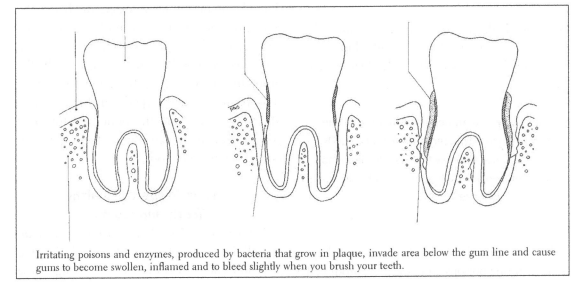

Irritating poisons and enzymes, produced by bacteria that grow in plaque, invade area below the gum line and cause gums to become swollen, inflamed and to bleed slightly when you brush your teeth.

Gingivitis

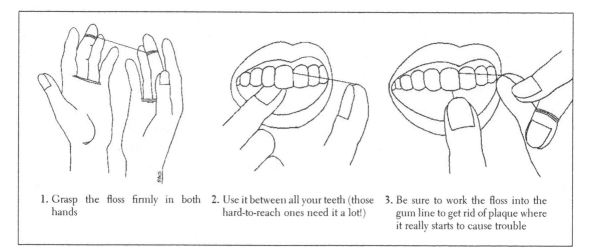

1. Grasp the floss firmly in both hands

2. Use it between all your teeth (those hard-to-reach ones need it a lot!)

3. Be sure to work the floss into the gum line to get rid of plaque where it really starts to cause trouble

Flossing Technique

Periodonal (Gum) Disease and Its Prevention

I have had a problem with my gums bleeding when I brush my teeth for a couple of months now. Is this serious or not? If it matters, I'm 14.

Allen

Periodontal disease—or advanced gum disease—is seen most often in adults, but teenagers can show signs of the early stage, called *gingivitis*.

During a visit to my dentist, I found out I had gum disease. My parents think that sounds strange, since they say that usually happens to older people. Can someone who is 15 have gum disease?

Lisa R.

What is gum disease and why does it happen? Irritating poisons and enzymes, produced by the bacteria that grow in plaque, invade the area below the gum line and can cause your gums to become inflamed and to bleed slightly during brushing. This "pink toothbrush" symptom is the most common sign of gingivitis. Other symptoms are gums that are swollen and inflamed.

What happens in more advanced gum disease?

The plaque on the teeth, extending below the gum line starts to harden, building up into a substance called *calculus*. This causes even more irritation of the gums, and eventually the gums begin to separate from the teeth. Bacteria begin to fill the spaces in between and attack the gums and the bone structure that supports the teeth, causing the teeth to loosen and, possibly, to be lost.

Four Steps to Healthy Teeth and Gums

1. *Visit your dentist at least once a year.* Twice a year for a professional cleaning and checkup is even better during these cavity-prone years.

2. *Brush your teeth at least twice a day.* Most dentists recommend brushing at least twice a day (and rinsing your mouth after eating in between). Use a soft-bristled toothbrush, and check it carefully for signs of wear. A toothbrush full of loose and bent bristles isn't going to do you much good. Plan to replace yours every one to three months.

In brushing your teeth, it's important to be thorough, covering the teeth and the gum line with a gentle, circular motion, and to follow up the brushing with dental floss, to reach the cavity-prone areas between the teeth where your toothbrush can't reach.

3. *Floss every day.* Flossing between your teeth is important, too. Lots of teens think that they don't have time to do this, but it's so easy. Just do it while you watch TV or listen to music. If you're not sure how to do it properly, just look at the following illustration. Note that flossing involves not only cleaning between your teeth, but also to the gum line. This removes food and plaque that may be forming at the base of your teeth.

4. *Eat a good, healthy diet.* That means lots of fruits and vegetables instead of sugary and sticky carbohydrate snacks. When you eat candy or granola or some other tooth-unfriendly snack, brush your teeth (or at least thoroughly rinse your mouth) as soon as possible. Better still, learn to like salads and raw vegetables. Carry strips of bell peppers, carrots, and celery sticks with you to school. You *can* acquire a taste for these (really!).

Bleaching, Bonding, Invisible Braces, and Other Dental Innovations

I'm real depressed. My dentist says I ought to have braces but I'm scared that this will interfere with my modeling career. I do modeling for a local department store several times a year and hope to get into some ads. I think braces would really hold me back. I heard about invisible braces and would like to know more about these. Are they for real?

Kerry A.

Advances in dentistry are giving hope to many people who have stained or chipped teeth or who can't face the idea of having metal braces. While some of these recent options aren't for everyone, they can be very helpful to many young people concerned about the appearance of their teeth.

My teeth are all stained because of tetracycline. Is there any way a dentist could make these stains less obvious or get rid of them completely? I heard about something called bleaching and wonder if that would work well for someone like me. What do you think?

Denise

I recently chipped my tooth playing football and it looks awful. My mom has been so mad because she thinks I'll need a crown or cap or something and that's real expensive. I haven't seen a dentist yet. Is there a way to fix my tooth that wouldn't cost so much?

Brad

- *Bleaching*. This dental treatment can remove or lighten a variety of stains on the teeth. It is particularly effective in removing stains from cigarettes, coffee, or excess drinking-water fluoride, but somewhat less so in improving the appearance of teeth stained by tetracycline, which causes stains to develop within the tooth rather than just on the surface. However, light tetracycline stains can be improved. Bleaching is a painless procedure that involves several visits to the dentist. First, the tooth is coated with hydrogen peroxide and another solution that aids penetration of the tooth by this bleach. Then a heating instrument starts the chemical reaction that penetrates and bleaches the tooth. The most dramatic improvement will probably be noticeable after the second treatment and the benefits of bleaching may last from one year to a lifetime. There are a number of dentists who point out that bleaching is not appropriate in every case of stained teeth: check with your dentist to review all the options available to you.

- *Bonding*. This treatment is also sometimes used instead of capping to improve the appearance of teeth that have been chipped or broken, are stained or cracked, or have gaps. This treatment is fast, requires no drilling or anesthetic, and is less expensive than crowns/caps. In this procedure, diluted phosphoric acid is applied to the tooth. This etches tiny pores into the tooth enamel. Then a sealer—a coat of liquid plastic—is applied. The next coat is a paste made up of plastic and very finely ground glass, silica, or quartz. This paste, which is tinted to match the natural color of the tooth, is put on in very thin layers and then molded to whatever shape is needed. Each layer is hardened and bonded by a 40-second exposure to visible or ultraviolet light waves: then, when all the layers have been applied and hardened, the newly constructed tooth is finely contoured and polished. The cosmetic results can be dramatic, but there are limitations. Bonding can't be used on the chewing surfaces of the back teeth and lasts only about half as long as conventional capping (about 5 to 10 years versus 10 to 20 years).

- *Invisible Braces*. Those who cringe at the thought of being called "Metal Mouth" may find some hope in recent advances that make braces more or less invisible. In one technique, clear plastic braces are bonded onto the surface of the teeth and held together with a single metal wire. To the casual observer, these braces are almost unnoticeable. There is also a new orthodontics technique pioneered by Dr. Craven Kurz in Beverly Hills, California. Here, braces are attached to the *backs* of the teeth and are unnoticeable to others. This new technique is becoming popular, especially among teens and adults, but there are drawbacks. These braces are more expensive that conventional braces and can cause speech difficulties and trouble chewing food until the tongue adjusts to their presence. Still, as more orthodontists offer this alternative, it could be a good option for many young people.

- *Implants*: We're mentioning these here only because dental implants are the best permanent replacements for missing teeth, and because we've had a number of questions from teens asking about them. While implants are a terrific advance in dentistry, you *will* need to wait until you are in your late teens or early twenties to have them. Why? Because implants are titanium screws that replace the lost tooth roots in the jawbone. Over time, they actually fuse with the bone, after which a crown is placed on top, making the implant look and function like a freestanding, natural tooth. The problem is that implants attach to your jaw in a different way from your natural teeth and aren't flexible, and are unable to adjust as your regular teeth do as your jawbone grows. So they can't be placed until your jaw and face complete their growth, and this doesn't happen until early adulthood. Your dentist will be able to work with you on an alternative until your jaw growth is complete and you can have an implant. It's well worth waiting for: a tooth replacement not only looks and functions like a real tooth; it keeps you from losing bone at the site of the missing tooth.

I'm 14 and hate going to the dentist because I have a lot of cavities. The shot of Novocain is just the worst and the drilling just makes me crazy! I hate it! What can I do? I don't want to have awful teeth, but I almost get sick from nervousness about going to the dentist. Help!

Pam A.

There is also hope for those who, like Pam, are upset by shots and dental drills. More dentists these days are using painless electronic anesthesia and lasers to reduce or eliminate that nerve-racking drilling! These techniques are expected to be the dentistry of the future in the next 10 to 20 years. In the meantime, some dentists are already using these new techniques.

Usually, with lasers, the work on the tooth is so quick that the pain doesn't have a chance to register so that Novocain is not necessary. Lasers are quickly replacing old dental equipment, including drills. However, currently lasers can be used to remove decay from a tooth, but have difficulty getting through the tough enamel outer layer of the tooth, so a little drilling may still be necessary for a while. (But it's definitely on its way out!)

Electronic anesthesia, which is painless and does not expose you to the risk of electric shock, happens when the dentist places two small electrodes, held in place by adhesive sponges in the patient's mouth. This slow electrical current blocks the brain's pain response and can be controlled by the patient during the dental procedure with the use of a hand-held device. There is no numbness later and this new anesthesia can be used by those allergic to conventional local anesthetics. However, it cannot be used by those with seizure disorders or who are pregnant.

SPECIAL HELP FOR GOOD LOOKS

Plastic Surgery

Cyber-savvy teens have their lives filled with a 24-hour parade of social media, pictures and videos, selfies, YouTube video stardom and, less happily, the threat of bullying, cyber and otherwise. Today's teens are even more conscious of how they look—and how they would like to look. There is more interest than ever in the possibilities of plastic surgery and cosmetics among self-critical and self-conscious teens. But it's important to know that, while plastic surgery can change certain physical features and cosmetics can enhance your looks, these can't necessarily cure a poor self-image.

Although a healthy, fit, well-nourished body is a great start to an attractive you, this may not feel like quite enough. What you may want most of all is to feel more attractive and more accepted by others. And you have this feeling that something physical is preventing you from looking your best.

You may have a feature that you feel keeps you from looking your best: a large nose; a receding chin; ears that stick out; or skin pitted with acne scars. You may be plagued with excess body or facial hair. You may wonder about the safety of ear piercing or the safety and effectiveness of cosmetics and beauty aids. You may be willing to settle for something less than stunning beauty. You may just want to look, essentially, like everyone else, minus an embarrassing flaw or two.

People see so-called flaws in a variety of ways. Many contend that flaws add to your character, your individuality. Many people aren't bothered at all by a prominent nose, for example. Others, plagued by self-consciousness and shame, find that for them a physical defect, however slight to others, is a major problem.

Help is available. Plastic surgery is the answer for some. Special cosmetics may be fine for others. However, it's important for all of us to realize the limitations of these beauty aids. They may help you look better, but how you feel about yourself and how you choose to

live your life go far beyond these procedures. Even though the results, in some cases, can look miraculous, it's important to realize two things about plastic surgery:

- *Plastic surgery can change a physical feature. That's all. It is* not *guaranteed to change your whole life for the better.* Plastic surgery to reduce the size and shape of your nose, for example, will do just that. It is not guaranteed to turn your life around, make you the most popular person in school, or drastically alter who you really are. It may help you feel better about your appearance, but it will not guarantee instant self-esteem or an immediate sense of self-worth.

- *Plastic surgery is* surgery, *not magic. It has its risks, discomforts and considerable costs. It is not a decision to be made lightly.* We're discussing it in this book *only* because we've had so many letters and questions about it and feel that we owe you some honest answers. And we honestly feel that plastic surgery has its limitations in terms of its ability to enhance your life and your own singular beauty.

The most beauty-enhancing quality one can have is self-acceptance. If you think that life is worthless unless you're a C cup or have a cute nose, instead of the smaller breasts or larger nose you were born with, then you need to do a lot of thinking and working on improving your feelings about yourself.

Think for a moment:

- Beyond the physical, what are your best qualities? Aren't these the qualities that make your best friends, the ones who really count in your life, like you?

■ What aspects of yourself make you feel glad to be you? Think about it. You're special and beautiful in your own way whether or not you decide to have cosmetic surgery. A surgeon's knife can make certain physical changes. But it can't change the person you've grown to become.

Special beauty help, combined with your growing sense of the worthwhile person you have always been, may add a great deal to the good feelings you already have.

Plastic surgery can be a great help to someone whose life has been adversely affected by a defect. It can also be a tragedy when practiced by an incompetent, inexperienced surgeon or when a patient is not given adequate screening to determine whether he or she will be able to have cosmetic surgery without undue physical or psychological side effects.

These two concerns often go together. The inexperienced surgeon, whose technique may be faulty, may *also* accept patients who have physical or emotional problems that preclude the possibility of successful cosmetic plastic surgery—patients that a more knowledgeable surgeon will advise *not* to have such surgery.

How can such incompetence happen? Any profession has its share of incompetent people, or course, but in the area of cosmetic plastic surgery, there is an added complication. The problem is that any licensed physician may do surgery, including plastic surgery, even if he or she has not had any specialty training.

Major surgery, of course, is usually done in a hospital, and hospitals generally don't grant surgical privileges to physicians without specialized surgical training beyond medical school. Therefore, it would be highly unlikely to find a physician without specialized training doing open-heart surgery.

Plastic surgery, however, is often done in an office or clinic setting. So physicians are not necessarily dependent upon hospital affiliation and may simply set up their own operating rooms in their own offices or clinics. (This is not to say, or course, that all plastic surgeons who do office or clinic surgery are incompetent. Many are well qualified and may also have hospital affiliations.)

If you're like most people, you probably want the best surgeon you can find. So how do you find a qualified, well-trained plastic surgeon?

1. Instead of looking for ads in the paper or in the Yellow Pages of your telephone directory, ask your family doctor for a recommendation or check with your county medical society.

2. Check the physician's credentials, making sure that he or she is a *board–certified plastic surgeon*. Most competent, experienced physicians who have specialties are board certified in that specialty. Make sure that the plastic surgeon you choose is board certified in *plastic surgery*. You can find out whether a surgeon is board certified by calling the American Board of Medical Specialties at (800)776-2378.

3. Choose a doctor who is affiliated with an accredited hospital. Even if the procedure that you're contemplating may not involve a hospital stay, it's important that your doctor have a hospital affiliation—both as a measure of competence and in case of an emergency.

COMMON PLASTIC SURGERY PROCEDURES TEENS SEEK

Procedure	What Happens	Discomfort Zone	Other
Rhinoplasty (Nose Job)	Doctor (in outpatient clinic or hospital) does surgery to change the shape and/or reduce size of nose. Local anesthetic is most often used.	Some pain, swelling, and discomfort (from surgical packing in the nose). Nose is splinted for several days. Eyes may be blackened for some days. Some swelling and bruising for 3–4 weeks. Complete healing may take six months.	Best age for this is 16–17 for girls and the later teens for boys. This is when nasal bone growth is complete and the face more adult.
Mammoplasty (Breast Enhancement)	Doctor makes incision just below each breast and inserts implant through incision to enlarge the size of the breasts.	Procedure done at clinic or hospital under general anesthesia. Some pain, swelling and discomfort after surgery. There are possible health risks involved in the use of silicone, as opposed to saline, implants.	We do not recommend this for teens, especially for those whose breasts are still developing. Breasts continue to grow through the adult years. Push-up bras work great, too!
Mammoplasty (Breast Reduction)	This is major surgery done under general anesthetic and usually only in cases of extreme physical discomfort due to very large breasts. Skin and excess breast tissue are removed. This usually involves several days in the hospital.	Considerable pain and discomfort. Sutures and bandages usually in place for several weeks. While general recovery is 3 weeks, women must be careful to wear a well-fitting bra for several months. There may be significant scarring on the underside of the breast.	This is major surgery that should only be done in cases of extreme necessity.
Liposuction	This is usually done in the "tumescent" form, which involves injecting a saline (salt water) solution mixed with lidocaine (a local anesthetic) and epinephrine (a drug that prevents blood loss) into the fat and then using a vacuum device inserted into small incisions to extract the fat.	Note: A newer procedure called lipolysis has yet to be approved by the Federal Drug Administration and some states are trying to ban this newer procedure Some countries like England and Canada have banned lipolysis altogether.	The "tumescent" pre-surgical injection speeds recovery and limits the amount of swelling and pain during that time. While this is usually done as an outpatient procedure, recovery isn't without discomfort. Patients usually "drain" saline solution from their incisions for a day or so. Support garments in affected areas must be worn for varying times: a chin strap (for double chin liposuction) for five days; a support girdle (for saddleback hips and thighs) for 2-3 weeks. If liposuction is in the

Procedure	What Happens	Discomfort Zone	Other
Liposuction (continued)			calves and ankles, support hose must be worn for 6 weeks. Swelling may last up to 3 months, with scars fading after a year or two. This is not magic solution to obesity. Only a small amount of fat can be removed at one time with relative safety. This is suitable mainly for stubborn fat deposits that have not responded to diet and exercise such as thighs with saddlebags, a double chin or fat deposits around the knees or ankles.
Tattoo Removal	Doctor uses laser to remove tattoo. This may require several sessions.	This procedure is painful and may need to be repeated several times.	Results vary: black ink is easy to remove, while green ink is difficult to remove. Homemade tattoos are often more difficult to remove than one done by a professional.

A competent, experienced plastic surgeon selects his or her patients with care. As we said earlier, some people are not good candidates for cosmetic plastic surgery. For some this may involve physical reasons: a tendency toward excessive bleeding or clotting difficulties, anemia, or diabetes. Those who suffer from asthmas or other respiratory disorders may be advised not to have surgery that may involve general anesthesia. For others, psychological factors may make the plastic surgeon hesitate or refuse to operate at all.

Even if cosmetic plastic surgery is not a miracle, it can help improve your appearance, sometimes dramatically. There are a number of different procedures. The ones that teens have asked us most about are rhinoplasty (nose surgery), mammoplasty (breast enlargement or reduction), liposuction, and tattoo removal. The chart above will give you an idea of what each of these procedures involves.

Cosmetics

I try all kinds of cosmetics, but it never looks as good on me as it does on the models. I feel cheated. I try to buy good stuff but can't afford really expensive makeup. Would it be worth it to save up my money and get the most expensive? Is the quality that much better?

Janine G.

Cosmetics play a big part in many of our lives. We spend billions of dollars each year on soaps, shampoos, deodorants, perfumes, aftershave lotions, makeup, and moisturizers—among many other items. All too often, these products disappoint us, failing to live up to the promises of the ads. They may even cause more problems for us, triggering allergic reactions, irritations or, in some cases, infections. They may also put a strain on our pocketbooks. As costs—and consumer expectations—rise, it's vital to choose cosmetics with care.

> I notice that ingredients are now listed on cosmetics. Why? Most of it doesn't mean that much to me and most things seem to have pretty much the same ingredients.
>
> Georgia B.

In an attempt to protect your health and your cash, the Food and Drug Administration (FDA) now requires cosmetics companies to list the ingredients on product labels in descending order, with the major ingredients at the top of the list. If you read labels carefully, you may find that there is little, if any, difference between a cheaper brand and a more expensive cosmetics line. In the latter case, you may be paying for a famous name and, perhaps, for more elaborate packaging.

The new labels can be health protectors, too, since if you do have an adverse reaction to a product, you and your doctor may be able to determine, possibly, which substances may be involved and which ones you might avoid in the future.

What are some of the ingredients you're likely to find on a cosmetics label?

- *Solvents*—primarily water and alcohol—are liquids in which solid substances are dissolved. Purified water may make up a large percentage of some cosmetics: generally, this is one of the cheapest and safest cosmetic ingredients. In fact, it may be better for your skin if you use a cosmetic with a high water content rather than one with a high oil content. This may be particularly true of makeup bases. In some cases, the cheaper brands, which tend to contain more water, may actually be better for you. Alcohol is a frequent ingredient in astringents, perfumes, and after shave lotions.
- *Emollients*—such as mineral oil, lanolin, and glycerin—make the skin feel smooth, either by preventing loss of moisture from the skin surface or by getting moisture from the air. These are particularly in moisturizers and hand and body lotions.
- *Emulsifiers*—such as sodium lauryl sulfate— are a component of lotions and keep water and oil ingredients from separating, and
- *Stabilizers*—such as sodium citrate—work with the emulsifiers.
- *Preservatives*—such as parabens—keep harmful bacteria from growing in cosmetics.

A number of teens claim to like the natural look in cosmetics and express desire to shun products with artificial preservatives. Most cosmetics, however, even those claiming to be "natural," contain preservatives. There is an important reason for this: growth of bacteria in cosmetics, particularly in eye makeup, may endanger your health.

> Is it possible to be allergic to makeup? I started using a new lipstick and got a blister on my lips. Could this be an allergy?
>
> Cecily J.

It could be an allergy or it could simply be a skin reaction, an irritation caused by a particular product. *Contact dermatitis*, as this is called, is usually confined to the site of contact: irritation, rather than allergies, account for most common adverse reactions to cosmetics. Such a reaction does not mean that you have to give up cosmetics. You may find that you can use another product that contains a different concentration of the irritating ingredients with no adverse reaction at all.

Identifying the source of irritation isn't always easy. Cosmetics may not be at fault, in some instances. You may, for example, have an adverse reaction to the metal in earrings or hairpins. However, some common ingredients are more likely than others to cause irritation. A study by the FDA found that the highest rate of adverse reactions was found in deodorants and antiperspirants, hair sprays, hair colorings, bubble bath, mascara, moisturizers, eye cream, and chemical hair removers. So if you suffer from an irritation and use one or several of these products, you might examine the possibility that this may be a likely source of your problem.

You may keep a troublesome irritation from happening on a large scale by trying a preliminary patch test, recommended particularly in the instructions for hair-coloring products, permanents, and chemical hair removers. If you're plagued with allergies, do a patch test on any product you're thinking of using, preferably before you buy it. Many stores have demonstrator samples available for such testing.

Are hypoallergenic cosmetics better than regular ones for any type of skin? Are they guaranteed not to cause problems? Just how good are they?

Pamela, 15

"Hypoallergenic" on the label of a particular cosmetic means that it is less likely to cause adverse reactions. The Food and Drug Administration now requires all cosmetics manufacturers using the term *hypoallergenic* to run numerous tests proving that these products really are less likely to cause allergic or irritation reactions than are competing products.

If you have a history of allergies or irritations, it's a good idea to pick a hypoallergenic product. These days, a number of choices are available in all price ranges. However, it's important to note that while hypoallergenic products may be less likely to irritate your skin, they will not clear up or cure existing skin problems such as acne.

I've heard that mascara may be dangerous. How come? Also, my girl friend says that you should never share eye makeup with anyone else. Is she right or is she just being selfish?

Sue Y.

It's true that mascara and other eye makeup have been under close scrutiny by the FDA. The problem is that possible contamination of the cosmetic through normal use may trigger physical symptoms—some serious—in the user.

While most eye makeup is pure at the time of purchase, skin bacteria can reach the makeup in a number of ways—for example, when you put your finger in any eye-shadow container or touch a mascara wand to your eyelid. This bacteria may grow in the cosmetic and become dangerous to the eye, causing red eyes, sties, inflamed lids, or, at worst, an eye infection that is unchecked may lead to blindness. This kind of infection might happen, for example, if your hand were to slip while you were applying mascara and the cornea of your eye were scratched by the contaminated mascara wand.

A number of reports of corneal infection and ulcerations due to use of contaminated cosmetics have reached the FDA, which is now strongly recommending that all manufacturers use special preservatives, particularly in eye makeup, to prevent the growth of such microorganisms.

There are several steps that you, too, can take to safeguard your eyes:

- Don't lend or borrow eye makeup.
- Be sure that the makeup you use contains a preservative (check the label!)
- Don't keep mascara too long. Preservatives may begin to lose their effectiveness after two or three months. Replace your mascara after that time, even if you have plenty still left.
- When you buy new mascara, *always* discard the old brush.
- Wash your hands before using cosmetics.
- Keep makeup containers tightly closed when not in use.
- Use Q-Tips—regular or new cosmetic-sized—to apply eye shadow.
- If a product needs water, use water, *not* saliva! Never lick an eyeliner brush or spit in any makeup.
- Don't leave cosmetics or a purse containing cosmetics in the sun. Intense heat may make the preservatives less effective.

Another safety tip that may apply to all cosmetic products is this: read directions carefully and use the product exactly as instructed! If the manufacturer suggests a patch test, do

it. Don't use a hair coloring product on your eyelashes. Don't put cosmetics on already irritated skin.

The more common sense you use and the more you know about what cosmetics can and can't do for you, the less likely you will be disappointed.

SPECIAL PROBLEMS

Ear and Body Piercing

I haven't read anything about this, but I wonder: Can you get AIDS from having your ears pierced? I know that people can share needles when taking drugs can get AIDS, but what about ear piercing? How can I make sure it will be safe?

Erin K.

Ear piercing has been a popular trend among teens, both male and female, for some years now. Done properly, under antiseptic conditions, piercing of the ear lobes can be quite safe. Piercing of the upper part of the ear, getting into slower-to-heal cartilage, may be more problematic, making you more vulnerable to infection. If you *do* decide to get your upper ear pierced, be sure to do the follow-up self-care on a daily basis in order to avoid infection.

How can I convince my parents that it's safe to get my tongue pierced? I REALLY, REALLY want to do it, but they are being totally stupid and say it's unhealthy. What should I do to convince them I know what I'm doing?

Austin S.

If you have a tendency to bleed heavily, have allergies to metals, are unusually susceptible to infections, or tend to form keloid scars, you may want to approach ear piercing with caution. Consult your physician first. In cases like this, it is especially important to have ear piercing done by a physician.

Some people try to go the do-it-yourself route and pierce their own ears—or have a friend do it. We don't advise this. Most of those we have seen with adverse side effects—such as infections—have been do-it-yourselfers. Infections like this may cause swelling around the ear puncture and, if unchecked, may lead to more serious health problems as well as scarring of the earlobes.

And while there have yet to be any reports of someone contracting AIDS through blood-contaminated ear-piercing apparatus, this could be a risk, especially if you try to do it yourself or with a friend and share a common needle or an unsterilized one.

The best way to avoid such risks and complications is to have your ears pierced by a physician with sterile equipment. The doctor will use a sterile stainless-steel needle or an instrument much like a stapler, which will insert a spring-loaded earring into your earlobe. Although the procedure is generally painless, the physician may use a topical local anesthetic on the earlobe to numb it.

Many department and jewelry stores have special technicians trained to pierce ears. Here, the ear is often pierced with the sterilized post of the earring itself. As long as your ear is sterilized with alcohol before and after the piercing and as long as the earring has been sterilized and has never been used by another person, such ear piercing is generally safe. But the training of technicians varies widely—as does the level of sterile precautions used.

After piercing, surgical-steel or 14-carat-gold studs are immediately inserted into the earlobe holes and must be worn continuously for about six weeks until the ears heal. Wearing post earrings for about six months before trying wires may also help your ears to continue to heal and may ensure that the holes in your earlobes will remain instead of shrinking down into mere slits.

Other after-care hints:

- As the ears heal, dab the lobes regularly with alcohol or mild soap to keep bacteria away.
- Always dip your earrings in alcohol before inserting them
- Be patient! Allow your ears to heal before removing or changing your earrings, or you may find that your earlobe holes will close up, making it painful (or impossible) to put the earrings back in.

In terms of piercing other body parts—such as the tongue, navel, lips, nipples, nose, and eyebrow—we don't advise it, no matter how fashionable it may be right now. This body piercing carries considerable risk of infection and can be quite painful. The risk of infection is especially great when it is done in the tongue, the lips, and the inside of the mouth. In addition, metal in the mouth can damage teeth: swelling of the pierced tongue can make breathing, speaking, eating—all those things we hold dear—much more difficult.

Given the risks involved, if you are still determined to do this, have the piercing done by a physician. It is much more likely that proper technique, sterile conditions, and good follow-up care will be part of your treatment package.

Even better, *don't do it!* There are less painful, less dangerous ways to look cool.

We would say the same thing for tattoos. Again, there can be danger of infection if a tattoo is applied under less than sterile conditions. And tattoos have a way of going from cool to burdensome very fast. Maybe you break up with "Amy" and no longer want her name immortalized on your arm (or your new girlfriend is less than excited about this part of your body art). Maybe you're trying to get a job and that serpent curling around your ankle isn't helping you make the impression you'd like. Or maybe you just get sick of a tattoo and decide you want a new look. It isn't as if you could just wash it off.

A better idea: Try temporary tattoos, especially the herbal variety that can be applied with a brush or plastic cone and last two to four weeks. Press-on tattoos and body painting kits can be fun, too. You can have all the fun of looking different—or like your friends—or shocking your parents or other adults without the painful removal part.

Excess Hair

> Help! I'm a 15-year-old girl who is HAIRY! I have hair on my chin and a few hairs around the nipples of my breasts. The hair on my chin really looks awful. What can I do about it? My mom says it runs in the family. Help!
>
> Maria G.

Excess hair growth, particularly on the face, can be an embarrassing problem. For many, the cause may be genetic. If your ethnic origin is Mediterranean (Italian, Spanish, Semitic, Greek, and so forth), you may have a greater-then-average tendency to have more body and facial hair than, say, someone of Scandinavian or Asian origin.

> I have excess hair on my upper lip and break out from using chemical hair removers. I've seen ads for do-it-yourself electrolysis devices. Would this be safe to try?
>
> Eileen S.

For a minority of young people, excess hair may signal a hormone imbalance or a gland problem. If you re well into adolescence—in your late teens—and suddenly develop excess hair you might want to consult your physician. For most, however, the cause is genetic rather than glandular.

What can you do about excess hair? Many women, of course, choose to shave leg and underarm hair (which is perfectly normal—and superfluous only because of fashion and grooming trends) or remove it with chemical removers called *depilatories*.

Depilatories dissolve hair on the skin surface, but do not remove hair permanently. They may also be somewhat irritating to the skin, so try them with caution (on a small area) first. If you have facial hair, use a depilatory designed for use on the face or a general one that is safe for facial use.

When a few hairs are involved on the chin or breasts, some women prefer to pluck the hair. This may be a bit painful and, again, does not remove the hair permanently.

Another effective, albeit temporary, treatment is the hot wax method. This can be done at home (following instructions from the hot wax hair removal kit *exactly*), but especially when a large area is involved, it is best done by a professional in a beauty salon or a special waxing salon. Here, hot wax is applied to the skin and then, after cooling, is pulled off, taking excess hair with it. One treatment does not remove hair permanently, but treatments over a period of time *may* retard hair growth. Waxing is not entirely painless and may cause an inflammatory reaction. Also, individual result very widely.

I have a lot of hair on my back. It looks weird. I'd like to have it removed. Obviously I can't shave it myself. Should I try something like electrolysis or waxing? I heard these are good ways to get rid of hair like this. I'm a 21-year-old male college student.

Mark M.

Someone like Mark, who has extensive hair on his back and limited funds, might try this method instead of the more expensive electrolysis. Electrolysis is a method of permanent hair removal. Here, a tiny electrode placed, via a needle, into the hair follicle discharges a high-speed electric current, destroying the hair root.

This method of hair removal usually works well, but there are some drawbacks. It is expensive and time-consuming, may be painful, and can produce scars, especially if it is done by an inexperienced technician. For this reason, we don't recommend homestyle electrolysis. You may not be able to locate each hair follicle exactly and, in addition, the do-it-yourself kits usually don't have automatic shutoff devices that stop the electric current after a few seconds to help prevent scarring.

Shop carefully for a qualified electrologist. Your search might begin with recommenda-

tions from your physician or your county medical association.

Many dermatologists today use a laser beam to remove excess hair. Although this method can be expensive, it can be quite effective when performed by a highly qualified physician or practitioner. Laser treatment is less painful than electrolysis and does not cause ingrown hairs. The best results are seen with fine dark hair and light skin.

For women whose excess hair is the result of hormone imbalance and who have large amount of such hair, there may be some hope via treatment with one of several prescription drugs. One of these drugs, cimetidine (Tagamet), has been used to treat ulcers in the past and was recently discovered to block the effects of male hormones on hair growth. The other drug, aldactone, is a blood pressure medication that also lowers male hormone levels. Since these drugs are not without risks and side effects, they should be taken only in instances of extreme *hirsutism* (excess hair) and then only under the close supervision of a physician.

Perspiration

I sweat a lot under my arms. By the way, I mean my shirts get armpit stains and big wet marks. I usually wear big, baggy sweatshirts so it won't leave a wet mark. Once in a while, I'll sneak on a short sleeve shirt. If I'm lucky, it'll last me about ten minutes before the wet marks appear. This has been going on for about a year and I use deodorant and stuff. My mom says I'll outgrow this, but I'm afraid I won't. Do you think I'll grow out of it soon?

J.C.

My armpits sweat and smell even though I wear deodorant. It usually happens when I'm around this guy I like. Never when I'm around my mom. It's very embarrassing to walk around like this. Help—and thank you verrrrrry much!

Christina P.

My hands used to sweat so bad that when I was doing my school work my paper would be soaked when I got done. My mom took me to the doctor and I got this wonderful stuff (my mom read about it and took the clipping to my doctor who hadn't heard of it but gave me a prescription to try). It's called Drysol. You put it on your hands before going to bed and put rubber or plastic gloves over it. You might have to do it one or two nights in a row at first but then all you do it is once every one or two weeks as needed. I've been using this for two years now and my sweaty hands are gone!

Amanda S.

As these letters show, excessive perspiration can be a huge embarrassment in the teen years. When your body is growing and changing in so many ways, the sweat glands are also developing fully and, at times, they may seem to be working overtime.

What can help?

- *Check with your physician if perspiration is persistent* despite use of antiperspirants, or if you have really sweaty hands. As Amanda's letter shows, there are special preparations he or she can suggest or prescribe.
- *Use antiperspirants exactly as instructed on*

the label. Some product labels advise you that, for maximum effectiveness, you should use the product at bedtime rather than first thing in the morning. Others may suggest, too, not to apply an antiperspirant right after emerging from a steaming shower: your perspiration from the shower may simply wash the antiperspirant away. Dry yourself thoroughly and let your body cool down a bit. Then apply the antiperspirant.

- *Keep learning to manage stress and overcome social fears.* As Christina's letter shows, being close to someone you like or feeling stressed out can work you into a sweat when you least want it. When you work on stress management (see Chapter 4), you may find, as an added bonus, that you're able to stay dry, too.

It's true, too, that time can help. We've seen a number of young adults who were plagued with perspiration problems as teenagers dry out remarkably when they hit their twenties. This may simply be an adjustment of the body to adult functioning, more expertise at dealing with stress, or perhaps a combination of the two.

Questionable Beauty Aids

I saw an ad for some device that would make me lose a lot of weight in an hour with no pills, no diet, and no exercise. Is this possible, do you think?

Sheila B.

Tell me the truth:
Do those bust developers that you see advertised in all the magazines REALLY work? Do

they increase your bust like they say? If not, how do they get away with such ads?

Mary Q.

Some beauty devices promise more than they could possibly give you: instant (and seemingly effortless) weight loss or a quickly blossoming bosom! Many people—especially the young—would like to believe such promises. Being a smart consumer, however, means using common sense and recognizing some basic facts:

1. True weight loss is never instant, nor does it happen without some sensible, moderate eating and regular exercise. Some "instant weight loss" devices come with diet recommendations and, in most cases, if you simply followed the diet itself, you would probably lose weight eventually. Keep in mind that there are no miracles or shortcuts to weight loss. It takes time and effort!

2. Creams can't really increase your bust size. Such creams usually contain hormones and may cause an inflammation of your breasts (which may be harmful), but will not bring about a true increase in the size of your breast.

3. Bust developers do not increase the size of your breasts. These devices, if used over a period of time, may increase your pectoral (chest) and back muscles. This will perhaps lead to an increase in our all-around bust measurement (as it is measured around your torso), but it will not increase your actual (cup) size.

A study by the Good Housekeeping Institute's Beauty Clinic confirmed that cup size was not increased at all by the use of several bust-developer devices.

Their conclusion: Eternal hope rather than effectiveness accounts for the sales success of such products.

Don't let money-back guarantees cloud your skepticism. In some cases, the money-back guarantee time limit expires before the product has a chance to show whether it will be effective. In many cases the manufacturer is betting that you will be too embarrassed, too lazy, or too eternally hopeful to return an ineffective device and demand your money back.

One fact to keep in mind as you scan the ads: If it sounds too good to be true, it probably *is* too good to be true!

It may be helpful, too, to keep all legitimate beauty aids—from cosmetics to plastic surgery—in perspective. These aids might help you to look more physically attractive—but that's all. Looking more attractive may help to improve the quality of your life, but it will not change your life or the person you are. The growth and development of the person you would like to be and the lifestyle you would like to have are very much up to *you*!

CREATING A BEAUTIFUL, HEALTHY FUTURE

When I look at my mom and some of her friends, who are all in their early forties, I see a big difference between those who look old and those who don't. It may seem strange to be worried about looking old when I'm only 17, but what can I do to make sure that I look good as long as possible?

Bree B.

We all would like to look good well into older age and to live long, healthy lives. Whether we can actually do this is, in part, out of our control. Our genes play a part in determining how we age, how healthy we are, and how long we live. However, lifestyle is also a major factor. And here you have choices. You *can* be in control!

Preventive medicine is an important aspect of medicine today. The purpose of this is to try to prevent as much as possible common killers such as heart disease, cancer, strokes, high blood pressure, and diabetes. Although the possibility of developing such disorders may seem remote to you right now, what you do or don't do now in your teens years may have a great impact on your health in later life. And the beginning of some of these common killers may be seen among teenagers! So what can you do right now to look and feel good now *and* later in life?

1. *Eat a healthy diet!* Do we sound like an endless recording on this? The reasons: it's so important to your health and it's so within your control. Eat more vegetables and fruit. Cut way down on fatty meats that contribute to high cholesterol.

   If you think you have to wait years to see the impact of too many cheeseburgers, think again. A survey sponsored by the American Health Foundation and *Current Science* magazine examined the health habits and food preferences of almost 22,000 teenagers in 46 states. Researchers concluded that many of those in their early teens are already in trouble. The survey revealed that *as many as 30 percent of the 11- to 14-year-olds surveyed already have high cholesterol levels.* High cholesterol, which can stem from a diet high in animal

fat and cholesterol, is related to atherosclerosis, or hardening of the arteries, and may lead to heart disease and strokes later in life.

The study also revealed an alarmingly high salt intake among American teens. So what? Too much salt in your diet (translate that to mean salt on your food and salty snacks) can lead to hypertension (high blood pressure), a widespread health problem among Americans that may lead to life-threatening crises such as heart attacks, strokes, and kidney failure, as well as serious vision problems.

2. *Don't smoke.* Nearly 10 percent of the younger teens surveyed smoke cigarettes: it is estimated that up to 40 percent of them (more girls than boys) will be smokers by high school graduation.

   Don't smoke! Smoking not only exposes you to health risks, but also makes you wrinkle sooner and more severely than you might otherwise. Smoking also is a factor in cancer of the lungs, bladder, lips, mouth, and esophagus. Chewing tobacco, popular among teens, has been known to cause cancer of the mouth.

3. *Don't drink—especially when you drive.* Alcohol, which high numbers of teens (11- to 13-year-olds included) drink in some form, can have a number of tragic consequences if abused. Shattered lives, fatal liver damage, and possible cancer are longer term future possibilities for young alcoholics.

   Tragedy, however, can happen much faster than that. The most common cause of death in teenagers is accidents—usually car or motorcycle accidents—and about 42 percent of these are alcohol related.

Don't drink and drive. Don't ride with a driver who has been drinking or taking drugs. Alcohol has also been implicated in skateboard, cycling, and boating accidents, among others. Not abusing alcohol or hanging out with others who do will do more to protect your health and your life right now than *any other single lifestyle choice or change.*

4. *Exercise.* Lack of exercise can be a killer—eventually. American teens, especially girls, do not get enough exercise. Only 58 percent of the girls surveyed were getting *any* form of strenuous exercise!

Get regular exercise. This can help your heart to become more efficient, your bones to grow stronger, and your weight to stay at its best. Especially for girls, getting lots of exercise and eating calcium-rich food is important in the teen years—when the bones are still adding mass—in order to prevent osteoporosis, a crippling disorder linked with loss of bone mass in middle and old age.

Lack of exercise can lead to obesity, which carries with it a greater risk of developing diabetes, high blood pressure, strokes, atherosclerosis, and heart attacks later on. Even if you don't become obese via sedentary existence, you are at a greater risk of having a heart attack or stroke if you continue to avoid regular exercise.

Right now, exercise can make you feel good and look great! You just need to take that first step.

5. *Keep your weight down close to what you and your doctor determine is your ideal weight.* Don't be a yo-yo dieter. It's too hard on the body. And obesity ages you inside—as well as making you look old before your time!

6. *Safeguard your skin.* Use sunscreen whenever you are outdoors (even in cloudy or hazy weather).

7. *Don't use and abuse drugs—legal or illegal.* This goes for prescription as well as street drugs. All can take a toll—as we will see in the next chapter.

8. *Don't take chances with sex.* These days, sad but true, sex can be hazardous to your health and your future fertility—and may even ultimately endanger your life. If this sounds impossibly melodramatic, turn quickly to Chapter 12 to read about how sexually transmitted diseases can threaten your health and fertility. Abstinence is the only way to be completely safe from these diseases. The next best choice is to be in a monogamous (faithful) relationship with someone who has never had another sex partner. Beyond this, safe-sex practices may decrease your risks.

9. *Learn healthy stress management.* Learn to deal with stress in constructive, healthy ways. Talk with people you trust. Write in your diary or journal. Take a walk. Listen to some of your favorite music. See a counselor or therapist if there are things in your life that you can't handle. Use relaxation techniques or exercise when you're feeling tense and stressed out. Act in ways that make you proud of yourself. Building good self-esteem is a major part of lifelong health and well-being!

10. *See your doctor and dentist for regular checkups.* Seeing your doctor and dentist at least once a year for checkups can help

with early detection of problems before they become major, as well as helping you take advantage of preventive medicine and dental care. These visits also give you a chance to ask questions and get information that will help you take better care of yourself for now and for a lifetime.

These are the basic health maintenance rules. And they're important to remember and follow *now!* It's important that you work to maintain your good health while you're young and healthy and while whatever damage there may be is reversible and/or not extensive. While it's impossible to predict how long you will live or to say, "If you do this and this, you will never have a major health problem," it *is* possible for you to be healthy—and happy—for many years to come. But whether or not you will be is very much up to *you*.

QUICK SCAN

GOOD HEALTH AND GOOD LOOKS

✔ *There IS help for acne!* If you have acne, even a mild case that doesn't respond to over-the-counter treatments, see your doctor. There are prescription medications that *will* help.

✔ *Good dental health is vital to your overall health.* Brush and floss your teeth several times a day. See your dentist twice a year for checkups and cleanings.

✔ *Plastic surgery isn't magic.* Plastic surgery can change a feature—such as your nose—but it doesn't necessarily change your life. And it is real surgery—with pain and discomfort, some scars and necessary healing time.

✔ *Pierce with caution.* Piercing your earlobes can be safe if done under sterile conditions. But piercing other parts of your body, especially your tongue, can be hazardous to your health.

✔ *Remember the following when you see an ad for instant weight loss, perfect skin, larger breasts, smaller thighs or any other instant beauty claim:* If a beauty aid seems too good to be true, it probably *is* too good to be true!

CHAPTER EIGHT

Safeguarding Your Health with Wise Choices

MAKING WISE CHOICES

Me and my friends are really sick of all the stuff we get from our parents and at school about not drinking or smoking or doing drugs. It isn't like we're addicts. We like to party. It's our choice, right? All the bad things happen when you're old anyway and we can always quit before then. So what's the big deal now?

Adam N.

We're all for parties and fun. But there are many different ways to enjoy yourself—and some of them, unfortunately, are quite hazardous to your health and your future. It's true that how you have fun and what you put into your body is *your* choice. But it's important to know what you're choosing.

CHOICES ABOUT BEHAVIOR

There are a lot of things that influence your behavior in your teens.

Your friends make a difference for sure. Statistics show that teen drivers take many more risks and are much more likely to have an accident when one or more of their friends are riding in the car with them. This may have to do, in part, with distraction and in part with friends urging you to take a risk you probably wouldn't take if you were alone—everything from speeding to not wearing a seatbelt.

You may be tempted to try a weird or risky behavior out of curiosity simply because your friends or people at school have been talking about it. For example, some teens have been trying "iDosing", downloading digital "drugs" in the form of repetitive, atonal tracks that can put one in an altered state of consciousness.

Though this is harmless for most teens, it isn't a good idea to try this if you have neurological conditions such as epilepsy. Some experts fear that, because some iDoser tracks—like the Recreational Simulations pack that purports to re-create the sensations of cocaine, marijuana, peyote and opium—could be a "gateway" habit that prompts some teens to experiment with the real stuff.

A trend that is even more concerning is the popularity of The Choking Game, a dangerous practice using strangulation (by a friend or a belt or rope around the neck, compressing the internal carotid artery) or hyperventilation. Both can cause fainting and an altered state of consciousness. But this practice is very dangerous, all too often leading to accidental death (especially if you try this alone) that may look like suicide, or permanent disability as a result of falling and hitting one's head. Even if the worst doesn't happen, depriving the brain of oxygen can impair neurological function, making it harder to concentrate or damaging short term memory.

Sometimes teens are tempted to take a risk, not because of their friends, but simply out of curiosity. It just seems like a good idea at the time.

But why do intelligent teens make choices that can turn out to be misguided, even lethal?

Parents, experts and teens themselves have wondered about this for years, and now researchers are making some break-through discoveries about the adolescent brain: essentially, it's still a work in progress.

Even though you may be a math whiz or a champion debater or otherwise intellectually awesome, the frontal lobes of your brain—the areas responsible for planning and judgment—are not fully developed until you're in your twenties, maybe even your early thirties. So, as your frontal lobes are still maturing, you may be more likely to make impulsive rather than rational decisions, underestimating the risk of a certain behavior or substance. The impact of alcohol and certain substances may also be greater when your frontal lobes are still a work in progress.

Of course, that doesn't mean that impulsive behavior is a given when you're a teen. Most teens *do* stop, think and make rational decisions, helped by parents or teachers, responsible friends and their own innate common sense.

And it does make sense to choose to behave in ways that are health-enhancing rather than health- or life-threatening. You have the power to choose what to put into your mouth, what (if anything) to drink or smoke. You have the power to choose safety when you drive by observing speed limits, not texting ever when driving and talking as little as possible on the phone when you're the driver. Even with hands-off Bluetooth devices, conversations can be a distraction, particularly if you're an inexperienced driver. You have the choice to buckle up for safety. You have the choice to wear a bike helmet. You have a choice to pass on trying a new trend like iDosing or The Choking Game. You *always* have a choice.

You also have a choice about whether to drink or not. Or drinking and driving…or riding with someone who has been drinking. Alcohol-related car accidents are a leading cause of death for teens and young adults. Alcohol can also be a factor in other accidental deaths.

Researchers have discovered that addiction to alcohol or drugs can happen more quickly in teens and in young adults—in part because young people tend to consume in greater quantities. Binge drinking is increasingly common among high school and college students and is responsible for a number of deaths.

You have a choice about whether or not to smoke—and more teens are choosing not to these days. It's important to know when making this choice that studies have shown that cigarette smoking damages lung development in teens—particularly in girls—and that most lifelong smokers report having started the habit by age 14.

The choice to say no to harmful substances is a health-affirming one in many ways. Today's illicit drugs are more dangerous than ever, with marijuana, for example, generally stronger and quite different from the typical joint of the sixties or seventies. The substances most often abused—the ones we too often don't take seriously—can be the most hazardous to your health. Alcohol, a factor in a rising number of fatal accidents that take young lives each year, kills more teens than any other drug. And although the harmful effects of smoking tend to be more long-term, more and more is being discovered each year about this habit's awesome potential for harm, not only to the smoker, but also to those around him or her and even to that person's future children.

To begin to make your own healthy choices, you may need to begin to think in a whole new way about your life and the role substance abuse may play in it. If you do use or abuse substances—or are tempted to do so—this does not make you a bad person. Most people begin ultimately harmful habits because they want to feel better. They want to feel less shy, less awkward, less lonely, less depressed. They want to belong and be part of a group of accepting and caring friends. Wanting and needing to belong is something that we all feel. All of us have coped—with varying degrees of distress and eventual success—with shyness and social awkwardness. Doing this is part of growing up and part of simply being human. This fact of life can't be changed or alleviated in the long run by any chemical substance.

You also need to know and accept the fact that the dangers of drugs, alcohol, and nicotine are real. Bad things *can* happen to you if you take drugs, drink (especially if you drink and drive or ride with a drinking driver), or smoke. These dangers aren't scare tactics dreamed up by fun-shunning 40-year-olds. These are facts. You need to get past the "It can't happen to me!" mindset and look at the facts in a new way. Developing a realistic attitude about the risks and the possibilities you face will help you make choices that are best for you. This may be the beginning of a new balance of healthy habits *and* all the fun that is part of being young.

What Does All This Mean for You?

If you're like a lot of people, you've seen all the facts, scary statistics, horror stories, and maybe even a few real-life examples of the impact substance abuse can have on young lives—such as people you know in your school or community who have been killed in grad-night or prom-night car crashes or a classmate who disappeared into a questionable future. And yet it may all seem pretty irrelevant to your own life:

Maybe you smoke a little—but feel you can stop whenever you want.

Maybe you drink more than a little—but it doesn't feel like a real problem to you.

Maybe you've used drugs now and again or even pretty regularly—and nothing horrible has happened: in fact, you like the way you felt.

Before you can begin to sort out your healthy choices from the less healthy ones, you need to ask yourself some direct questions about how what you're choosing right now is affecting your life. You don't have to write to us with the answers. You don't have to tell your parents or even your best friend. You just need to be honest with yourself as you consider the following questions:

1. Have you lost time from school or work due to drinking or drug use?

2. Has drinking or drug use made it difficult for you to get along with your family?

3. Do you drink because you're usually shy—and can only relax and open up when you've got a buzz on? Do you use drugs or smoke when you're feeling tense? Are you finding that's you really *need* substances in order not to feel shy or tense or depressed?

4. Has drinking, drug use, or smoking affected your reputation? Have you lost longtime friends because of this? Has your circle of friends changed to a faster-moving crowd (and sometimes it's a little scary or exhausting or just a pain to keep up with them)?

5. Have you ever felt unhappy after drinking or drug use? (This can be unhappy with how you acted when under the influence or just depressed in general.)

6. Do you crave a cigarette, a drink, or your drug of choice at a certain time every day or in specific situations?

7. Do you ever want a drink the morning after (even if you're feeling fairly hung over)?

8. Is your drinking or drug use making it difficult to do well in school? Have your grades (not to mention your motivation) dropped since you began using?

9. Have you ever had a loss of memory after drinking or drug use?

10. Do you ever drink or use alone?

11. Do you ever drink, use drugs, or even smoke to build up your self-confidence? Do you find it difficult, if not impossible, to get through school or a social event without this confidence crutch?

12. If you smoke, have you been having more colds lately? Has anyone told you that you have bad breath and/or refused to kiss you? Have you been burning holes in clothes due to dropped cigarettes or ashes? Do you find yourself on the outside looking in—standing outside of food places while friends or family enjoy themselves inside—because you have to have a cigarette? Has your smoking caused conflicts between you and people who really matter to you?

13. Has your habit—drinking, drug use, or smoking—caused you to break a law?

14. Have you ever been sent to a hospital or jail as a result of drinking?

15. Have you ever stopped caring about how you look?

16. Do you eat irregularly while drinking or using drugs? Or do you smoke a cigarette instead of eating a meal?

17. Do you stay drunk or stoned for long periods (such as several days)?

18. Are you noticing any physical symptoms that you didn't have before, such as fatigue, frequent colds or other illnesses, or feeling hung over in the morning? Or do you just not feel quite as well as you used to feel physically (except when you're using)?

19. If you're an athlete, have you noticed your performance slipping or becoming harder to maintain?

20. If you're taking anabolic steroids, have you noticed any physical symptoms such

as an increase in acne or, if you're a girl, a deeper voice, increased body and facial hair, or thinning hair on your head? Have you noticed that you're getting into fights or flying off the handle at other people over stuff that didn't bother you as much before?

If you could honestly answer yes to any of these questions, your substance use is a problem. Even if you answered no to all and are still using, your choices could bring problems in the future.

MAKING CHOICES ABOUT SUBSTANCE USE

People use drugs, alcohol, and cigarettes for a variety of reasons: to cope with shyness, nervousness, loneliness, anger, or social awkwardness, among many other problem feelings: to appear sophisticated and with it, to be part of the group—and share the group's experiences. Or, some just want to escape reality. The problem is that these substances are artificial means of coping. They don't really make you courageous or socially adept. If you take substances instead of learning to cope with the pressures and important lessons you face during these growing years, your social and emotional skills will lag behind your physical development well into adulthood—and maybe even forever. Letting substances mask your feelings, letting substances mask your feelings and substitute for vital learning experiences, will only perpetuate shyness, discomfort, loneliness, alienation, and depression.

In short, substances will only add to your problems instead of solving them. Why make adolescence any tougher than it already is?

KNOWING WHAT YOU'RE CHOOSING

Smoking
What is it?
Teens who smoke may smoke cigarettes, cigars, pipes, or a combination of all of these.

So what's the problem?
- *Smoking can shorten your life significantly.* A habitual smoker may be giving up six to nine years of life! You're at higher risk for several kinds of cancer (lung cancer as well as cancers of the lips, mouth, pancreas, esophagus, bladder, and uterus). Smokers have a two or three times greater chance of dying from a heart attack than nonsmokers. They also have many more strokes than nonsmokers and are nineteen times more likely to become victims of emphysema, a crippling respiratory disorder that destroys the lung's elasticity and leaves the victim gasping for breath.
- *Smoking can make you a lot less attractive.* As well as bad breath, smelly clothes, and stained fingers now, smokers get wrinkles sooner than their non-smoking friends. Medical studies have found that the level of wrinkling in women who smoked heavily was equivalent to that of women *20 years older*! This wrinkling pattern may be due to the fact that smoking cause constriction of blood vessels and may make the skin more susceptible to wrinkles.

- *Your secondhand smoke can hurt those you love.* Recent studies have found that women who smoke during pregnancy are almost *twice* as likely to miscarry or spontaneously abort. They are more likely to have a stillborn baby or to give birth to a smaller-than-normal child. Studies indicate that children of smokers are also more vulnerable to SIDS (Sudden Infant Death Syndrome) and respiratory problems. Also, children of mothers who smoke more than ten cigarettes a day have a 50 percent higher risk of developing childhood cancers. They may also have lower IQ scores, have difficulty reading and adjusting socially, and be significantly shorter than children of non-smokers.

- *If you smoke, you have a greater risk of dying in a smoking-related accident.* More than 25 percent of all fires are caused by smokers, and so many car accidents are smoking-related (caused by a smoker taking his or her eyes off the road or hands off the wheel to light up or to retrieve a dropped cigarette) that some auto insurance companies offer discount rates to nonsmokers.

- *All smoking injures you to some extent.* If you're lucky, you may simply experience more than your share of illnesses every year, missing more work or school than a nonsmoker.

Smokeless Tobacco
What Is It?

Called *dip* or *snuff*, this is tobacco that is placed between the lip and the gum. A number of teens, especially those involved in team sports such as baseball and who feel that smoking is unhealthy but that smokeless tobacco is a less harmful substitute, are taking up this habit.

So what's the problem?

Unfortunately, this habit is terribly unhealthy in its own way, putting users at considerable risk of developing oral cancer. Teens as young as 15 have suffered—and died—from this disfiguring cancer.

E-Cigarettes
What is it?

E-cigarettes are hand-held, battery operated devices that are used like cigarettes but do not involve smoke or tobacco. Instead, they vaporize a liquid nicotine solution, giving the user a slower dose of nicotine. These were developed in an effort to help smokers to break their addiction to tobacco over time. The success of this method has yet to be proven scientifically. But what has captured the attention of researchers is the sudden popularity of e-cigarettes among teens.

While fewer than 10 percent of teens smoke regular cigarettes these days, more and more are embracing e-cigarettes. E-cigarette use increased 200% between 2011 and 2013 and, in just one year—between 2013 and 2014—e-cigarette use tripled among U.S. teens, with 13.4% now using e-cigarettes on a regular basis.

So What's the Problem?

There are several concerns that medical experts have about teens and e-cigarettes:

- *Despite claims to the contrary by manufacturers, e-cigarettes are being marketed aggressively to youth.* There are flavors like bubble-gum and cotton candy. The mechanism of the smoking behavior is similar to tobacco, and some fear it could set the stage for making traditional cigarette use cool again among youth. Not everyone agrees, of course. "Are you kidding?" one teen laughed when we asked her about e-cigarette use among her friends. "Holding this plastic tube between your fingers is really NOT cool at all! Never will be!" That may well be true, but some experts fear that in search of a cooler alternative, today's teens may rediscover traditional cigarette smoking. And it isn't just the cool factor that makes this a danger.

- *Nicotine, a major ingredient of the e-cigarette liquid and vapor, is highly addictive and can be detrimental to brain development in adolescents.* Experts fear that, as e-cigarette users become more tolerant of the side effects of nicotine, they will turn to traditional cigarette smoking.

- *Some teens are finding ways to vape marijuana.* Teens combining e-cigarette and marijuana use—in a small but growing trend—has researchers concerned.

Alcohol
What is it?

Alcohol is a drug that is being abused more and more by teenagers and young adults—and this fact is causing widespread concern. Nearly half of male high school seniors and one-fourth of female seniors who drink are problem drinkers. (This means that they get drunk six or more times a year or have problems in three or more areas of their lives because of drinking.) Of particular concern are drinking behaviors such as funneling (putting a funnel in the mouth and pouring beer or another alcoholic substance down the throat, enabling a teen to drink much more at a faster rate) and binge drinking, which is defined as having five drinks or more at one sitting.

So what's the problem?

- *Funneling and binge drinking can kill.* As a number of well-publicized college campus tragedies have shown, alcohol ingested in this manner can kill in a number of hours. (Teens who die may do so because of alcohol poisoning or by choking on their own vomit.)

- *Alcohol-related auto accidents (as well as drownings, suicides and homicides) kill a shocking number of teens each year.* Drinking and driving—whether it is a car, motorcycle, bicycle, boat, JetSki, or other recreational vehicle—can be deadly, even if you don't feel drunk.

- *Regular use of alcohol in the teens can put one at risk for alcoholism.* As we saw in the statistics at the beginning of this chapter, teen drinkers are at high risk for becoming problem drinkers or alcoholics later on. Those from families with a history of alcoholism or other substance abuse are at highest risk.

- *Alcohol is hazardous to your health—especially if you're a female.* Alcohol can affect women faster, more seriously, and in a shorter time because they have more body fat and less body water than men, and this causes the alcohol to enter their bloodstream in a less diluted form. Women tend to develop health-threatening complications from alcohol in less time than men and by drinking less alcohol.

Overall, teens who drink are likely to have poor eating habits, more respiratory problems, general fatigue, and sleep disorders. Long-term health risks of alcohol abuse are much more serious, including severe liver damage that, in some instances, can kill while a person is still in young adulthood.

- *Alcohol can have a devastating impact on the life and health of a female drinker's unborn baby.* Fetal alcohol syndrome (FAS) in newborn babies is a tragic disorder that has been linked to drinking during pregnancy. These babies may be mentally retarded and have heart, facial, and body defects. A study at Boston City Hospital found that 74 percent of infants born to women who had ten to fifteen drinks a day suffered one or more symptoms of FAS. Scientists in Seattle discovered something even more alarming: in a group of 164 women who drank two ounces of whiskey a day during pregnancy, 9 had infants with FAS.

Subsequent studies have found that even a can of beer, a glass of wine, or a cocktail twice a week is enough to increase by 30 percent a woman's chance of either miscarrying or having a brain-damaged baby. And recent research from the University of Washington and the University of Michigan has revealed that heavy drinking (two drinks daily or at least five in one sitting) on the part of a baby's *father* during the month before conception can significantly lower the birth weight of the baby. (Low-birth-weight infants are more likely to die during their first year and are more likely to have birth defects or respiratory problems.)

The National Council on Alcoholism recommends that pregnant women stay away from liquor altogether during pregnancy. Men who also have the potential to—or are trying to—father children would also do well to abstain from alcohol.

Prescription And Over-The-Counter Drugs
What is it?

Non-medical use or abuse of prescription drugs that may well not have been prescribed for you is what we're talking about when we include prescription drug use and abuse into our discussion of substance abuse. The fact is, while illicit drug use is declining, use of prescription drugs remains high.

Some of the most frequently misused prescription drugs among high school students: the painkillers OxyContin and Vicodin and over the counter medications such as cold or cough medicines with dextromethorphan (DXM). Stimulants such as drugs commonly prescribed for ADHD (attention-deficit hyperactivity disorder) are also commonly abused.

So what's the problem?

There is great potential for harm when prescription drugs are taken without a physician's supervision and/or when over-the-counter medications are taken for a high—in a higher than recommended dosage—rather than for quieting a cough.

- Barbiturates like Nembutal, Seconal, Phenobarbital can cause lowered inhibitions, slowed pulse and breathing, lowered blood pressure, poor concentration and confusion, respiratory depression or arrest (you stop breathing!), depression, impaired memory and judgment, and addiction.
- Opioids like codeine, fentanyl and drugs like OxyContin, Percodan, Percocet, Vicodin, Lorcet, Darvon and Darvocet can cause

drowsiness, respiratory depression or arrest, unconsciousness, coma and addiction.

- Stimulants like amphetamines and Ritalin, misused, can lead to increased heart rate and blood pressure, irregular heart beat and heart failure.

Club Drugs
What is it?

These are drugs commonly used at clubs, raves and concerts. Club drugs in general can affect your brain and result in impairment of your judgment, memory and coordination.

All of these drugs are illegal and include Ecstasy, GHB and Rohypnol, among a number of others. The drug of choice changes with the club scene and, because these drugs are often produced in home or otherwise makeshift labs, it's impossible to know exactly the strength of the drug you may be taking.

So what's the problem?

- Ecstasy and other stimulants can increase heart rate and blood pressure, sometimes leading to heart and/or kidney failure.
- GHB and Rohypnol are common "date rape" drugs, so called because they have a powerful sedative effect that can cause you to lose consciousness—and control of your situation. Furthermore, Rohypnol causes amnesia so you have no memory of what happened while you were under the influence of the drug.
- Mixing club drugs and alcohol is very dangerous and can even be lethal.
- Even without alcohol, club drugs can kill. High doses of certain club drugs can cause you to have breathing problems, go into a coma and perhaps even die.

Marijuana
What is it?

The substance most used by teens (after alcohol and tobacco), marijuana is made from the hemp plant and is usually smoked in a *joint* or with a pipe or *bong* (though it can be ingested as an ingredient in cookies or brownies). It causes a sense of euphoria and relaxation as well as increased appetite. On a positive note, it has been used by cancer patients to help decrease pain and nausea after chemotherapy.

So what's the problem?

- *Marijuana can have some undesirable short-term side effects.* These include lethargy, lack of motivation, bloodshot eyes, and dry mouth. Some report paranoia and impaired memory or reflexes.
- *Marijuana can come laced with other drugs—and give you a nasty surprise.* Some teens have the misfortune to smoke a joint laced with PCP ("angel dust") and suffer violent hallucinations, impaired judgment and muscle coordination, and at times aggressive, even violent behavior.
- *Smoking marijuana may even be more damaging to your lungs than smoking cigarettes.* An increasing number of medical studies are finding links between smoking marijuana and conditions such as chronic bronchitis, coughing, wheezing, frequent respiratory infections, and a greater risk of lung cancer, especially in people who also smoke tobacco. Researchers estimate that smoking three or four joints a day does as much damage to the lungs as smoking a pack of cigarettes! Joints are unfiltered and

thus deposit four times more tar on the lungs than cigarettes. Also, people smoke marijuana differently: it tends to be more deeply inhaled and held in the lungs and airways longer.

- *Marijuana can impair the immune system.* Researchers at the University of Illinois at Chicago have found that THC, the active ingredient in marijuana, may disrupt the complex chemistry of the immune system, diminishing the body's ability to fight off disease-causing viruses and bacteria.

- *Marijuana can cause your brain to age faster.* A study at Wake Forest University's Bowman Gray School of Medicine reports that laboratory animals exposed to THC five times a week for a period of eight months showed a significant decrease in nerve cells in the vital part of the brain that plays a role in emotional behavior. This decrease in nerve cells seems to mimic the aging process. Thus, someone who smokes marijuana regularly and loses 30 percent of brain nerve-cell density at a young age may not notice the effects immediately. However, the normal aging process may account for another 30 percent loss over time. Reaching old age with as 60 percent loss of brain density could seriously affect one's quality of life.

- *Marijuana can affect your future fertility.* Heavy use of marijuana can disrupt hormone production in both males and females, cutting down the level of testosterone and sperm cells in men and interfering with menstrual cycles and ovulation in women. There is no proof, as yet, for pot-induced infertility (thus marijuana should never be considered as a contraceptive!).

However, in pregnant women, THC can cross the placenta and cause damage to the developing fetus.

- *Marijuana can linger in your body and impair performance in a number of ways.* Unlike other drugs, which are fairly quickly processed out of the body, THC lingers in the body for four or five days. If a teen smokes marijuana even once or twice a week, this means that he or she may have a constant level of the drug in the body. THC tends to accumulate in the reproductive organs and in the brain. The results may be difficulty concentrating; impaired reflexes, depth perception, and sense of time, sleep disorders, and personality changes. The habitual marijuana smoker may be just as unsafe a driver as a teen with a drinking problem.

- *Second-hand marijuana smoke can pack a punch.* This is important to know if you are tested for drugs at school or work or for a sports team. Hanging out with marijuana-smoking friends and inhaling second-hand smoke from their joints can affect you more than you realize. According to a recent study at the National Institute of Drug Abuse's Addition Research Center, being exposed to the equivalent of only four joints in an hour can make you come out positive on a drug test!

Inhalants
What is it?

Inhalant abuse—often called *huffing*—is a growing practice among young preteens and teenagers who inhale solvents, typewriter correction fluid, Scotchgard, and other household products. (One manufacturer—3M—has been so concerned about this that they have sponsored a rock video warning teens of the dangers of huffing).

So what's the problem?

These toxic fumes affect the nervous system and can cause paralysis and also sudden death by cardiac arrhythmia. These health- and life-threatening events could happen the first time you try huffing or the 100th time you try it—or maybe nothing terrible will happen. But why take the chance?

Stimulants
What is it?

Stimulants include such popular teen drugs as crystal methamphetamine (crystal meth) and Ecstasy, as well as herbal Ecstasy. Cocaine and crack also fall into this category. Crystal meth, crack, and cocaine are usually snorted or smoked. Ecstasy and herbal Ecstasy are taken orally. These drugs can give a quick and intense high. While crack and cocaine highs are short, the high from crystal meth lingers for hours (but can be followed by a depression that lasts for days!). Ecstasy-induced euphoria and energy can also last for several hours.

So what's the problem?

- *Some stimulants are highly addictive.* Among these are crystal meth, crack, and cocaine. Crystal meth, in fact, is so highly addictive that some experts feel that to use it even once—if you inject it—is to become addicted. Those who smoke crystal meth may take a little longer to become addicted, but most do and go on to inject it as their needs for ever higher levels increase. With increasing amounts of this drug, the risks to health and life become higher.

- *Stimulants are unpredictable.* You may get a pleasurable high—or you may get a medical emergency. Crystal meth, for example, in addition to the previously mentioned depression, can cause increased blood pressure, rapid heartbeat, high fever, and nausea. Some users have suffered strokes, lapsed into comas, and died. Crack and cocaine can cause fatal seizures or heart attacks. Ecstasy and its herbal cousin can also cause high blood pressure, seizures, high fever (even heat stroke), heart attacks, and sudden death.

  If you think heart attack and stroke can happen only to some aging baby boomer tottering around snorting cocaine, think again. In studies of cocaine-related heart attacks, researchers have found that in most cases, these were healthy young people who had taken relatively small doses of cocaine. Many were not chronic users.

- *Abuse of some stimulants can damage your central nervous system.* Studies have shown that habitual use of stimulants, especially cocaine, can also cause a younger person to develop Parkinson's disease, a disabling, progressive disorder of the central nervous system. This apparently happens when cocaine upsets the balance of essential brain chemicals and at the same time destroys vital brain cells connected with motor skills. While Parkinson's disease—characterized by tremors, rigidity of muscles, and progressive crippling—occurs most commonly in the elderly, some cocaine users may develop this disorder some 20 years sooner than susceptible individuals in the general population.

- *There are uncomfortable side effects between amphetamine highs.* Snorted amphetamines can cause ulcers inside the nose: all amphetamine use can result in insomnia, anxiety, and paranoia.

- *Habitual use of some stimulants, especially crystal meth, can make you look HORRIBLE!* While some people try crystal meth as a weight loss aid, they soon find that, though they may lose weight, that is off-set by terrible changes in physical appearance: rotten and lost teeth, highly visible and unattractive skin blemishes, sunken eyes with purple or dark circles, and accelerated aging. You can look like a toothless, wasted hag in very little time if you use crystal meth. The before and after photos of users are dramatic—and heartbreaking. Don't throw away your youthful good looks—and your life—using this drug!!

LSD
What is it?

LSD is a hallucinogenic drug. It can be licked off a postage stamp; ingested in sugar cubes, pills or liquid; or eaten off one's clothing. Under the best of circumstances, it can cause a euphoric "trip" that can bring pleasant hallucinations; and go on for hours.

So what's the problem?

LSD is highly unpredictable. LSD trips tend to be highly individual—some are reported to be pleasant, some nightmares—and it's impossible to tell when a bad trip or "bummer" will happen. Dilations of pupils, flushing, occasional chills, and increased pulse and respiratory rates are some of the minor side effects. Paranoia and hallucinations are common major side effects, often lasting for the twelve to eighteen hours that LSD usually remains active in the body. For some, however, these effects can linger—or come back—for weeks, months, and even years. Long after taking the drug, a user may be confused and paranoid and have flashbacks of the LSD experience.

Heroin
What is it?

Heroin is a highly addictive narcotic drug. It can be smoked, snorted, or injected. Most teen users these days tend to buy heroin in antihistamine capsules that are broken open and snorted. Heroin causes a euphoric high that can last for several hours.

So what's the problem?

It's easy for teens to overdose on heroin—and the consequences can be deadly. This drug can cause the lungs to fill with liquid. It can also cause convulsions, coma, and death. Users who inject heroin into their veins with needles face another risk—AIDS—if they use or share needles contaminated with blood that has the AIDS virus present.

Anabolic–Androgenic Steriods
What is it?

These synthetic derivatives of testosterone, the male sex hormone, are used by many athletes to build muscle mass and strength in a relatively short time. Unfortunately, use is not uncommon among high school athletes and enthusiastic teen weight lifters and body builders. As noted earlier, an increasing number of teen girls are using steroids, often in an attempt to build leaner bodies.

So what's the problem?

Using this drug can be a shortcut to a lot of trouble. As well as triggering aggressive, violent behavior, anabolic steroids can lead to the following:

- *In males*: a decreased level of male reproductive hormones, shrunken testicles and reduced sperm count, permanent short stature, breast enlargement, high blood pressure, liver damage, and perhaps some forms of cancer.
- *In females*: an increased level of male hormones, resulting in shrinking breasts, male-style hair growth (on the face and body), male pattern baldness on the head, a deepening of the voice, enlargement of the clitoris, and menstrual problems. Some of these side effects are permanent. Long-term problems include cardiovascular disease, liver damage, and reproductive illnesses.

It's possible to excel in sports and to build a lean, strong body the healthy way: with good nutrition, responsible training, and the patience to let the body grow and develop in its own way.

MAKING A DECISION ABOUT DRUGS, DRINKING AND SMOKING

Everyone in the world keeps saying "Just say no" but I don't think adults realize how hard it is. If I said no all the time, I wouldn't have any friends and everyone would make fun of me. Do you know what it would be like to be going through high school with everyone hating you?

Talia C.

I've been smoking since I was 13—so it has been three years. Sometimes I think about quitting, but it's SO hard! I can't begin to explain it to someone who has never smoked. They think it's so easy, just a matter of stopping one day. But it's not like that. I get really nervous and jittery and feel awful when I go without cigarettes. And, also, I'm scared of gaining a lot of weight if I stop smoking. I'd rather take my chances on some health risks later on than be fat now (and besides, being fat is a health risk, too, isn't it?), if I'm going to risk my health, I'd rather risk it looking good!

Marti Y.

Saying no to alcohol, drugs, and/or smoking is much easier said than done. And we never said that stopping a habit like smoking was easy. But it's possible to do both—and live a happy, healthy life.

Saying No From The Beginning

While it's easier to never start smoking or drinking or taking drugs than to stop a substance use or abuse habit, it isn't always easy to say no. Some of the most common obstacles to saying no include the following:

- *"I don't want to be considered 'out of it'"* You will not be out of it if you pass up drugs, alcohol, or smoking. When you look at the statistics, *most* people, including teens, don't use these substances. It is becoming more and more acceptable and is considered quite sophisticated among adults and older teens *not* to smoke, drink, or use drugs.
- *"I'm afraid of losing my friends. They'll think I'm a prude or a baby."* Some of the people

you know may think that. But having your own point of view and your own strong feelings about what's right for you is a sign of *maturity*. Also, a friend worth having and keeping will respect your choices, even when these differ from his or hers. A real friend respects you as a distinct individual and wants the best for you. A friend who doesn't feel that way would probably be simply a temporary friend anyway. So when you lost a friendship like that, you're not losing as much as you're gaining good health, self-esteem and the respect of people who really care about you.

■ *"I'm going through a tough time right now and I need something to make me feel better."* Feeling hurt by a special problem such as a romantic breakup, the death of someone dear to you, a parental divorce, an alcoholic or abusive parent, or a major disappointment can make you want to grasp onto anything that will ease your pain, if only for a little while. Feeling frustrated by school problems or lonely due to a family move, a change of schools, or feeling intrinsically different from your classmates can also make you want to escape your problems.

Using alcohol or drugs to escape, or smoking to mask your social shyness and awkwardness, are only temporary measures. They don't do anything to solve your very real and painful problems. There *are* other, more constructive ways to cope: if you think about it, you can probably come up with some that sound possible to you.

✔ Talk with someone: a special friend or relative, an empathetic teacher, a school counselor, a hotline listener, or even a professional therapist or clergyperson.

✔ Listen to music that makes you feel better. (Studies show that this is what a *lot* of teens do when they're feeling depressed and down.)

✔ Exercise your anger, anxiety, or depression away. Regular exercise can release natural body substances called *endorphins*, which can make you feel better emotionally as well as physically.

✔ If you're facing a difficult situation at school or at home, consider your alternatives, by yourself or with the help of someone else. What can you do to change this problem situation to minimize or eliminate what is causing you pain? If nothing can be done right now, or the loss has happened and is final, take a deep breath and *feel* your pain, crying if you need to. Crying and grieving over a major loss are important steps toward healing and resolving your pain.

All of these alternatives can help you to grow, to cope more readily and constructively next time. All are far superior to postponing your resolving and healing with artificial substances.

Saying "No Thanks" Without Becoming An Outcast

■ *Say no and move on—without making a scene.* You don't have to rant, rave, and give long impassioned explanations. A simple "No, thanks" or a short reason will do.

The following are some reasons we've heard from teens who have said these in a number of situations without any major problems from friends or acquaintances:

"I'd rather not."

"I tried it and didn't care for it."

"I get sick when I drink."

"One of us has to be sober to drive, and I've decided to be the driver."

"I'm allergic to it."

"I have a physical condition that makes it dangerous to do that."

"I feel better when I don't (drink, do drugs, smoke) and I want to make the most of this time with you"

- *Seek help and ideas from others you respect.* Talk with older teens and adults who have said no successfully. They can help you feel good about your own choices and give you some ideas that have worked for them.

Helping A Friend

Your ability to help a friend may depend on your friend's ability to hear your concern and his or her own motivation to stop using whatever harmful substance is involved here. Your friend may need to stop using in his own way and in his own time, but that doesn't mean you shouldn't try to express your caring and concern. You never know when a friend may be needing just the sup-

port you're giving and ready to make some changes.

Stopping A Harmful Habit

Stopping a habit, especially one you've had for a while, isn't easy. It takes effort. It takes time. It takes patience with yourself. If you try and fail today to give up smoking or drinking or a drug, don't give up. Just try again. And don't be embarrassed to ask for help. If you have a serious drinking or drug problem, you may well need outside help to get you through, at least at the beginning.

Where can you get help?

- *Check with your physician.* If you want to stop smoking, your physician may be able to help you or to refer you to a stop-smoking program. Some of these treatment plans include not only support during the difficult time when you're trying to stop, but also medical help such as a prescription-only nicotine patch (doctors report that teens tend to prefer the patch over nicotine gum). This can help ease the difficulty of withdrawal from nicotine, one of the most addictive substances known and a major reason why people find it so hard to quit smoking. Such programs will also help you develop other behaviors to replace the soothing impact smoking has had in your life.

  Your physician will also be able to refer you to appropriate inpatient (in the hospital) or outpatient (you go to the hospital at certain times for treatment but don't stay overnight) treatment for drug or alcohol abuse treatment.
- *Make use of self-help support groups.* This can include so-called 12-step groups

founded on the model of Alcoholics Anonymous. There are 12-step programs for many different addictions, including drug abuse (Narcotics Anonymous). You can find listings for these organizations in the white pages of your phone book. Members get together—on a first-name only basis—and work through the steps of the program. Quite often, participation in a 12-step or similar group support program is a mandatory part of drug or alcohol rehab. But even if you aren't in a formal program or don't feel your addiction is quite so bad, participation in one of these programs can help you to sort out your choices and priorities. Some offer groups for young people so that you will have the support of peers as you go about the difficult task of overcoming your addiction and building a new life for yourself.

Many people have a lot of resistance to joining a group or getting professional help to overcome a habit or addiction. "I can do it on my own anytime I want!" you may be saying. Really? Think about it. If you could have done it on your own, you would have done it already. While it's true that some people can stop smoking or drinking on their own, it's best to have medical supervision when stopping a serious drug or alcohol habit. And many people find that they need extra support in stopping smoking, too.

Remember: knowing and accepting the fact that you can't conquer a harmful habit alone is a sign of strength—and the first step toward recovery.

You can help yourself in many ways—

whether you're going it alone or in a treatment program. Here are some suggestions:

- *Stop your habit "just for today".* Don't tell yourself that you will never, ever have another cigarette (or drink, or joint, and so on). Tell yourself, instead, "Just for today, I will not smoke (or drink, or use drugs)." Stopping a habit forever is too formidable a task. Just do it day by day. You will feel your strength, your resolve, and your self esteem grow over time as one daily success follows another.

- *Take responsibility for your choices.* No one forced you to smoke, use drugs, or drink—really. You chose to do this. So you can choose to change the habit. Knowing that you have power over your life—and your habit—can help a lot!

- *Don't put yourself in situations where the pressure is greatest.* If there is a particular crowd whose major activity seems to be drinking or taking drugs, stay away from that crowd, even if you like certain individuals in it. (It's easier to say no to one or two people you see individually than to a crowd.) Avoid unsupervised parties. When someone whose parents are gone for the weekend is throwing a party, you know going in that there is likely to be more pressure of all kinds: to drink, to use drugs, to engage in sexual activity. If your have doubts, don't go. It's better to miss a party than to get talked into doing things you don't really want to do. Don't get into a car with people who are stoned, drinking, or drunk—even if it means calling your parents to pick you up.

- *Learn from the pressure.* Remember that

peer pressure and taunts can be a learning experience. It's all part of learning to think for yourself. If you can withstand the pressure and make your own decisions, you'll have a good head start toward healthy adulthood.

- *Announce your new intention to family and friends who care.* Those who love you most are most likely to help and cheer you on. They also have great memories for this kind of thing, and, if your resolve is wavering, will be quick to remind you of your good intentions.

- *Seek the best way of stopping—for you.* Some people do better in a group—for example, a stop-smoking clinic sponsored by the American Cancer Society, or similar services for others with substance abuse problems. Others can do it on their own. Those with certain drug problems—such as addiction to prescription drugs—may need to cut down gradually, under medical supervision, to minimize the danger of serious withdrawal symptoms. Others, particularly smokers, may do best if they simply stop "cold turkey." (Some medical studies have found that smokers who cut down to a few cigarettes a day were inhaling so deeply that they were really minimizing the benefits of cutting down.) If you're stopping smoking or another substance habit, keep in mind that the first day is the hardest and that the urge to indulge will usually go away after a few minutes. Tough it out. You can do it.

- *Seek healthy alternatives.* If you're dying for a cigarette, a drink, or a drug, ask yourself what else you can do to ease whatever feelings or situation is contributing to your longing for this substance.

1. Find new ways to feel less awkward socially—such as easing your expectations for yourself (you don't have to be witty and brilliant or the life of the party to have a good time and be liked by others) or learning social skills in stages (for example, focus on saying hello to and talking with one person at a party, in the school lunchroom, or wherever you feel awkward before you contemplate mixing in a crowd).

2. Explore alternatives for dealing with loneliness, depression, or tension. Talk to a friend or relative. Take a walk. Listen to music. Read a book. Answer a letter. Plan for the future. Make a list of things you like about yourself—or of five people you can really count on. There are many alternatives you can pursue—if you choose.

- *Be patient with yourself.* If you slip and have a cigarette, a drink, or a drug, don't consider the battle lost or label yourself as a hopeless addict. You're just human. You had a slip. Admit it and limit it to that one instance rather than using it as an excuse for a binge of substance use. Decide what you can learn from it—such as how to overcome the temptation better next time. What feelings, situations, or people were connected with your slip? How can you cope better in the future?

You can do it! In saying no to drugs, alcohol, and smoking, you're making a positive choice: You're saying yes to personal growth, self-discovery, and a healthier, happier life!

QUICK SCAN ✓

DRUGS, DRINKING AND SMOKING

✔ *Early use can get you hooked for life.* Alcohol and tobacco are the substances teens use and abuse most often. Studies show that the earlier you start drinking or smoking, the more likely you are to become addicted. One study found that 43% of teens who began drinking by 14 developed alcoholism. And most lifelong smokers report having started the habit by age 14.

✔ *Prescription drug abuse is a new health threat among teens.* While use of illicit drugs has dropped in the past few years, according to some studies, abuse or prescription drugs and over-the-counter medications has increased. Teens need to remember: when prescription drugs are taken without a doctor's supervision or over-the-counter medications are not taken according to directions, there are significant health risks, including potentially fatal side effects.

✔ *Marijuana isn't as harmless as it seems.* Studies have shown that smoking marijuana can be even more harmful to the lungs than smoking tobacco. And second-hand smoke from marijuana may cause you to test positive on a drug test—even if you never use this drug yourself!

✔ *Girls pay a particular price for bad habits.* Smoking cuts down much more dramatically on teen girls' lung capacity. And anabolic steroids can have a devastating and permanent physical impact—balding, deepening of voice, growth of body hair, shrinkage of breasts, and enlargement of the clitoris.

✔ *Boys pay a price, too.* Boys who use and abuse anabolic steroids can end up with shrunken testicles, reduced sperm count, permanent short stature and breast enlargement—among many other undesirable side effects.

✔ *Crystal meth is total bad news!* It is so highly addictive that some experts feel that to use it only once (particularly if you inject it) is to become addicted. Not only can this addiction be life-threatening, it also can make you *seriously* ugly incredibly fast. So unless bad skin, rotten teeth, dark circles under your eyes and accelerated aging sound good to you, don't touch crystal meth!

✔ *You can say no to drinking, drugs and smoking without being a friendless outcast.* Say "No, thanks" without making a scene or lecturing others about it. Find other ways to ease tension, stress and social discomfort in your life. You can have friends, fun and all the advantages of being young without harming your health.

✔ *If you want to stop a harmful habit, see your doctor.* If you have a serious drug or alcohol problem or have been taking too many prescription medications, it's important to have medical supervision and support as you begin to withdraw from your substance of choice and begin your journey to sobriety. Even if you're a smoker looking to quit, medical help can make a difference. Many teens have found the nicotine patch (prescription only) helpful whether they're trying to stop smoking on their own or in a special program.

Mind Over Body

Have you ever heard of people getting the runs because they're nervous about an exam? I do that during finals every semester and it's really bad. Once I had to leave the room DURING a final. I get stomachaches a lot, too, when I have to give a report in class. My folks put a lot of pressure on me to make good grades, but that's something I want, too. It isn't just them. What can I do about my stomach problems?

Jeremy L.

When I get stressed out, I eat a lot of stuff I shouldn't. I know better than to eat cookies and candy like I do, but when I'm feeling stressed, I do it anyway. How can I start dealing with stress in a way that doesn't make me gain weight? (I'm not fat, but I gain and lose the same five pounds like every few weeks!)

Amy J.

Mind and body are inseparable. What affects one will affect the other. So some physical diseases such as mononucleosis can bring about depression. And stress and depression can give you headaches, stomachaches, and a variety of other ills. Although the mind-body connection is one of the hot medical topics of the millennium, and more people are understanding the mind-body connection both in terms of diseases and in terms of healing, disorders with a psychological component are all too often misunderstood:

"It's all in your head."

"It's just nerves."

"Forget it. It'll go away."

Too often, people dismiss disorders that we call *psychosomatic* (caused, at least in part, by emotional factors) as imaginary and unimportant. Contrary to popular notions, the pains and other symptoms of psychosomatic disorders are connected with the mind and the emotions, but are not imaginary.

THE STRESS CONNECTION

How does the mind enter into these problems? Feelings, especially emotional responses to stress, may help trigger or aggravate certain physical conditions. It's virtually impossible to separate your body and your mind.

Stress, anxiety, depression and trauma not only affect the way you feel emotionally, but also trigger changes in hormones that can promote inflammation in the body and lead to a wide range of health concerns—from diarrhea, to headaches, to lowered resistance to colds and flu. Long-term stress and trauma in childhood and adolescence can make you vulnerable to serious health conditions later in life, according to research by Dr. Victor J. Felitti of Kaiser Permanente Medical Center in San Diego. He was joined in further research by Dr. Anda of the Centers for Disease Control in examining adult patients who reported suffering from a wide range of stressors in childhood and adolescence, including parental divorce, marital fighting, emotional or physical abuse from a parent, or sexual abuse. A significant number of those reporting trauma or ongoing stress when younger exhibited a range of medical conditions, such as autoimmune diseases, heart disease, migraine headaches, bowel disorders, heightened anxiety and depression more frequently than those without a stressful history.

While the doctors supposed that some of these troubling symptoms were the result of stress-related behaviors, like overeating or smoking or drinking too much, many of the patients had practiced none of these and still had symptoms suggesting that stress hormones (and the resulting physical inflammation) were the primary cause of the link between stress and illness.

While you may have little to no control over the life choices your parents make, it can help to be aware of the health conditions and risks that are linked to stress and what you can do right now to help yourself feel better in the present and enjoy a healthier future.

What are some of the feelings that can give us physical symptoms? Anxiety, tension, and depression—to name only three—are some of these and may all be related to stress. And no one is immune to stress. It's an inescapable fact of all our lives. We can see—and even expect—stress as we cope with exams, the breakup of an important relationship, the death of someone close, or an increase in fights and tensions at home.

But stress can come from positive events, too. Winning an award, graduating from high school, going away to college for the first time, getting married and/or moving into an apartment of your own, getting your first full-time job, having a baby—all of these positive life changes bring stress along with the challenges and the joy.

Dr. Thomas H Holmes III, professor of psychiatry at the University of Washington, studied the relationship between illness and the stresses that change may bring. His 43-item stress-rating scale covers everything from the death of a spouse (100 points) or a close family member (63 points) to marriage (50 points), pregnancy (40), outstanding personal achievement (28), starting or leaving school (26), change in schools (20), a vacation (13), and minor violations of the law (11). Dr. Holmes found that if a person scores 300 change points in a year, he or she has an 80 percent chance of experiencing a change of health as well.

Your body may react to stress by becoming

more prone to illness (such as colds), or you may develop one of the more common health problems that may be rooted, at least in part, in stress—and in how you handle this stress. Migraine and tension headaches, gastrointestinal problems such as irritable bowel syndrome and ulcerative colitis, bulimia (overeating or binge eating) can bring you very real pain, both mentally and physically.

HEADACHES

There are many types of headaches: not all of them are tied in with emotions. Some, for example, may result from illness: colds, flu, a sinus infection, a dental problem. Others may come from allergies, eye strain, or high blood pressure. Still others may result from something you do—such as eating big bites of ice cream too fast, skipping a meal, drinking or smoking too much, or becoming fatigued. Only in rare instances does a headache signal a brain tumor, although this is a possibility that occurs to anyone who gets headaches regularly.

If you are plagued with regular headaches, however, it's important to see a physician. He or she may help you identify the type of headache you're having and its possible causes. If you're like most chronic headache sufferers, your physician's examination and tests are likely to reveal that there is nothing organically wrong with you.

What can cause chronic headaches? A variety of physical and psychological factors can combine to bring pain and suffering via tension headaches (caused by muscular contraction), psychogenic (depression) headaches, or migraine

headaches. Tension and depression headaches are, of course, rooted in the emotions and in muscular responses to these feelings.

Tension Headaches

Tension headaches are most often felt at the front and/or the sides of your head or at the base of your skull. These headaches are often caused by stress-induced anxiety, which also causes muscular tension and tightness in your shoulders and neck. Aspirin or other analgesics and rest are the best way to deal with tension headaches.

Depression Headaches

Depression headaches, stemming from depression and anxiety, may involve tense muscles in the face, head, neck, and/or a pattern of pain that may feel like a band circling the head. These headaches are more likely to strike early in the morning or in the evening and on weekends. They're the result of longstanding depression. Other signs of depression may be present.

Sleep patterns, researchers have found, can help one tell the difference between tension and depression headaches. A person with tension may have trouble getting to sleep at night. A depressed person, on the other hand, may fall asleep readily, but his or her sleep pattern may be fitful—with awakening during the night or early in the morning.

Pain relievers are only part of the answer in combating a depression headache. It's also important to deal with the feelings behind the physical pain. You may do this with the help of a professional or maybe combine professional help with support from family and friends.

With tension and depression headaches, it's vital to attack the source of your pain, not just the symptoms.

Migraine Headaches

Migraine headaches are something else again. They can be extremely painful, with severe, sometimes throbbing pain, usually on one side of the head. There may be nausea, blurring of vision, sensitivity to light and noise, and dizziness.

There are several different types of migraine headaches, but all are classified as *vascular* headaches. That is, they are triggered not by muscular tension, but by changes in blood vessels that are not in the brain, but *around* the brain.

What happens when a migraine strikes? For reasons as yet unknown, there is a change in the concentration of a substance called *serotonin*. This causes the blood vessels in and around the brain to experience changes, too. In some people who suffer from migraines, these blood vessels will *constrict* first, causing a phenomenon known as an *aura*. This is characteristic of the *classic migraine*. The person may see flashing lights or colors, spots before the eyes, or blind spots, or may experience extreme sensitivity to light and visual distortions—with people or objects growing smaller or larger. (It is said that Lewis Carroll wrote much of *Alice in Wonderland* while under the influence of migraine headaches.) Mood changes may accompany the aura, or may occur even without an aura. The migraine victim may feel giddy and euphoric. Then the pain hits. The pain of the migraine headache, which comes when the blood vessels *dilate* (swell), can be intense.

What causes migraine headaches? Heredity can be a factor in migraines. If both of your parents suffer from migraines, you have about a 70 percent chance of doing so. If one parent had these headaches, your chance of having them is about 45 to 50 percent. Of all migraine sufferers, 65 to 80 percent have a family history of these headaches. Some researchers theorize that there may be a migraine-prone gene at work here, giving you a physical, genetic predisposition. Others contend that migraines may be learned or acquired from your environment. You may imitate your parents or experience migraines as a reaction to an atmosphere of tension and high expectations. Whatever the reasons behind the phenomenon, migraines can, indeed, run in families.

Stress can also figure prominently in migraine attacks. The headaches may come in times of stress or in the letdown period after a stressful time (the weekend after final exams, for example, or on the first day of a long-awaited vacation).

Hormones may also influence your headaches. Some women experience migraines just before or during menstruation or in response to the synthetic hormones in birth control pills. For this reason, women who begin to suffer migraine-type headaches while taking birth control pills should consult their physician and, possibly, switch to another brand of pill or another form of birth control.

Certain emotions—such as anger and frustration (particularly if these feelings are repressed)—may be a factor in migraines.

What you eat may also bring on a headache. The chemical *tyramine*, which is found in most cheeses, many citrus fruits, freshly baked bread, lima and navy beans, pork, vinegar (except wine vinegar), onions, and nuts, has been pinpointed as a possible migraine trigger. Chinese food continuing the food additive MSG, chocolate, and, in some instances, the artificial sweetener aspartame (NutraSweet) can also cause problems. Some feel that alcohol may also stimulate the blood vessels and should be avoided if you suffer from chronic migraines.

What treatments are available? Some prescription drugs can prevent or interrupt a developing migraine. Some of the newest of these include Amerge and Zomig, medications in pill form that alleviate migraine symptoms. Also quite promising are the nasal sprays Imitrex (it gives relief in a matter of minutes, but can leave a temporary, unpleasant taste in the mouth) and Migranal (which can offer relief in 30 to 60 minutes along with a temporary stuffy nose). Maxalt, a quick-dissolving wafer, is currently being tested and has been found to ease migraine pain within half an hour.

Some people find that nonprescription drugs such as aspirin and ibuprofen may help during the painful part of the migraine. There is a fairly new product called Excedrin Migraine (which contains caffeine as well as aspirin) that a number of people have found helpful.

There are also some alternative-medicine migraine prevention measures, which we will discuss in more detain in the "Alternative Medicine" section of this chapter. These include the herb *feverfew*, as well as biofeedback and acupuncture.

STRESS AND YOUR STOMACH

The gastrointestinal tract—most notably the stomach and intestines—may also be affected by stress. Some of us, in fact, are so good at burying our feelings that it may take a stomachache, diarrhea, or more alarming symptoms to tell us just how tense, frightened, or angry we feel. Often only a physician can tell the serious from the minor, so if you do experience frequent gastrointestinal problems, it's a good idea to consult your physician.

The following descriptions are included not so that you can diagnose and self-medicate your condition, but simply to give you an idea how stress can affect your stomach—and how important it is to seek help and treatment early.

Many young people suffer from stomach pains. A recent study at the University of Connecticut evaluated 507 junior high and high school students and found that 75 percent of them reported abdominal pain from time to time. About 15 percent reported stomach pain on a weekly basis. And 8 percent of the junior high school students and 17 percent of the high school students reported symptoms of irritable bowel syndrome.

Irritable Bowel Syndrome

Irritable bowel syndrome (IBS) is one of the most common gastrointestinal problems in teens. Symptoms include abdominal pain and bloating, alternating bouts of diarrhea and constipation (or just diarrhea), nausea, and a feeling of faintness. Many teens with this condition also report feelings of anxiety and depression.

With IBS, it is important to avoid spicy foods, as well as alcohol, coffee or tea, and some diary products. Dietary fiber may lessen IBS symptoms in some cases. Good sources of fiber include whole grain breads, fruits, and vegetables.

Learning to manage stress and your feelings in general—whether these are fear (before exams, a special date or any other event in your life), anger, or general anxiety—is probably one of the most effective ways to combat this stress-related intestinal ill.

Some young people suffering from irritable bowel syndrome may need professional help to deal with the troubled feelings that can be linked to this problem. A study at the University of North Carolina found that more that half of 206 young women patients with irritable bowel syndrome had a history of physical and/or sexual abuse. If that describes your situation, you may need some psychotherapy or other counseling that may be comfortable for you before your physical condition begins to improve.

STRESS AND EATING DISORDERS

Stress and pressure to meet our society's unrealistic standards of model-thinness puts many adolescent girls at risk of developing eating disorders. A relatively small number of males develop eating disorders, too, usually because they are engaged in sports such as gymnastics or wrestling that tend to have strict weight requirements.

What are the most common eating disorders and who is at risk? Fear-of obesity syndrome, anorexia nervosa, bulimia, and compulsive overeating are the eating disorders most likely to afflict teens—and we'll be describing these in detail in a moment. But since the risk factors for developing an eating disorder are quite similar, let's take a look at those first.

Who is most at risk of developing an eating disorder?

- *An adolescent girl.* This may be due to the fact that women in our society are more

likely to be judged by how they look. And female standards of beauty are more geared to the media ideal of model thinness than are male standards of attractiveness.
- *A person with a perfectionistic personality.* These are often excellent students, well-behaved and intent on doing everything just right—including pursuing the elusive ideal of svelte perfection.
- *A person from a family where weight is an issue.* Parents may put a great value on slimness: the teen may either try to please parents by becoming perfectly slim or rebel by overeating and becoming obese.
- *A person who has had early sexual trauma.* Studies show that those who have had sexual trauma (abuse or molestation) may unconsciously try to protect themselves by making their bodies sexually unattractive and by focusing their attention on something safe—such as food—rather than dangerous—such as human contact and sexual relationships.
- *A girl who reaches physical maturity earlier than her peers.* Early-maturing girls, who experience the normal puberty weight gain while their classmates still have the slim, straight shapes of preadolescence, may be incorrectly identified as overweight by peers, parents, and themselves. Studies show that these girls are particularly likely to have poor body images.
- *Girls with authoritarian parents.* Those raised by strict, authoritative parents or who feel compelled to please their parents may see control of their weight and body shape as their only means of independent choice and expression.
- *Teens growing up with a substance-abusing parent or in an otherwise dysfunctional fam-*

ily. Having an alcohol- or drug-abusing parent can create a lot of stress. So can being in a family where expressing feelings, especially angry feelings, is taboo. Some teens may eat compulsively when they have these unexpressed feelings or when they're feeling depressed or lonely. Others may react to this stress by compulsively dieting, or binging and purging.

- *Teens who are depressed and/or have low self-esteem.* These young people may be especially sensitive to critical remarks and suggestions that they may be overweight—whether or not this is really the case.

Fear-Of-Obesity Syndrome
What It Is
Fear-of-obesity syndrome is characterized by self-induced malnutrition due to an exaggerated fear of becoming fat. It differs from anorexia nervosa in its intensity and the fact that teens with this syndrome do not exhibit some of the emotional problems common in those with anorexia nervosa. However, some of the behavior patterns are the same.

Symptoms
Food avoidance, stringent dieting, and body image distortion (thinking you're fat when you're really not).

Special Characteristics
These teens have an exaggerated concern with obesity, regardless of actual body weight.

Dangers
Fear-of-obesity syndrome can evolve into an eating disorder such as anorexia nervosa or bulimia. In the meantime, it can also interfere with a girl's growth and development, since this self-induced malnutrition comes at a time when the body needs nutrients and a certain level of body fat to complete the growth and maturation process. It can be hazardous to self-esteem as well, since model-thinness is often an elusive goal.

Treatment
Fear-of-obesity syndrome can be treated with nutritional and behavioral counseling. Check with your physician for help.

Anorexia Nervosa
What It Is
This disorder is a serious psychosomatic disorder. Characterized by compulsive dieting and self-starvation, anorexia nervosa may have some contributing physical as well as emotional factors. A recent study at the National Institute of Mental Health found that a group of women with anorexia had unusual brain secretions of a hormone called *vasopressin*, which regulates the body's water balance. The effects of this hormone on behavior are not yet known, but researchers theorize that this unusual hormonal response could be a factor in tipping the balance between an ordinary diet and compulsive starvation.

Other researchers at the University of Pittsburgh did studies comparing brain function in women who have suffered from anorexia with the brain function of healthy women. What they found was that those with a history of anorexia do not distinguish between positive and negative feedback. The main researcher, Walter Kaye, who is Director of the Eating Disorder research program, observed in a summary of his findings that anorexics are preoccupied with fear of making mistakes and have difficulty experiencing immediate pleasures.

Recently, Dr. Joanna Steinglass and her research colleagues at Columbia University Medical Center/New York State Psychiatric Institute suggested that, in cases of women suffering from anorexia nervosa, the severe dieting associated with the disorder may have become a well-entrenched habit, one that is inflexible and slow to change. This study may help our understanding of this serious disorder and why it is so difficult to treat.

Symptoms

Food avoidance, compulsive exercise, intense fear of fat, distorted body image (feeling fat even when emaciated), refusal to maintain a body weight at or over the minimum normal weight for age and height, amenorrhea (cessation of menstrual periods), heavy use of laxatives, and occasional binges punctuated by self-induced vomiting.

Dangers

The dangers of anorexia nervosa are well documented medically. Even when not fatal—as it is in 5 to 15 percent of cases—anorexia can cause severe malnutrition, very low blood pressure, cardiac arrhythmia (irregular heartbeat), bone weakness, and general poor health.

Treatment

Prompt medical help—preferably early, before a dangerous amount of weight has been lost—is vital. Treatment is often multifaceted, with medical treatment—sometimes inpatient hospitalization—used in conjunction with individual and family therapy. In this era of

managed care, it can be difficult for a family to get either sufficient coverage or sufficient inpatient treatment in some instances. This phase of treatment, however, can be crucial: it's important to work with your physician and your insurance company to get as comprehensive a program as possible. In addition to medical care, family therapy is especially effective since anorexia nervosa can be a symptom of family and parent-child relationship problems.

There is increasing interest these days in drug treatment for anorexia, with research being done with a class of drugs called opioid inhibitors. These drugs block the action of pleasure-causing brain opioids and help to break an anorectic person's addiction to dieting. The results of treatment with the drug in several studies have been promising, with 75 percent of patients treated with the drug Naltrexone gaining a healthy amount of weight.

Bulimia
What it Is

Bulimia is a common eating disorder affecting 4 out of every 100 women between the ages of 17 and 25 (while anorexia affects about 1 in every 100 girls). The major characteristics of this disorder are binge eating followed by purging via self-induced vomiting and laxative use.

Both psychological and physical factors can be involved in developing bulimia. Some studies show that as many as 75 percent of bulimics experience major depression: other studies link bulimia with both major and manic depression, anxiety disorders and substance abuse. Other medical experts believe that bulimia and some forms of depression may be caused by the same underlying chemical imbalance involving lower than normal levels of the neurotransmitters that facilitate commands between nerve cells in the brain.

Symptoms

A person with bulimia alternately binges on food, sometimes consuming thousands of calories an hour, and then purges via self-induced vomiting, enemas, and laxative abuse. Unlike people with anorexia, those with bulimia tend to be within their normal weight range, so the disorder can remain undetected for years. However, some signs that may appear over time include severe tooth decay (from stomach acids eating away tooth enamel during purging), swollen salivary glands, and irritated mouth tissues.

Dangers

Like anorexia, bulimia can be fatal, with most deaths occurring as the result of rupture of the esophagus from vomiting or from ipecac poisoning or cardiac arrest, the latter most common in women who abuse laxatives or diuretics or who are also alcoholics. A person with bulimia may also suffer from ulcers, hernia, and dangerous body chemistry imbalances that can lead to kidney and heart failure.

Treatment

Bulimia is usually treated with a combination of medical care and psychotherapy. A number of anti-depressant drugs relieve symptoms of bulimia. In recent years, Prozac has become, perhaps, the most frequently prescribed medication for bulimia. Like other serotonin reuptake inhibitors, Prozac's side effects are few and patients may actually lose some weight on the medication.

Many experts feel that though drug therapy can be helpful for some people with bulimia, there is no substitute for psychotherapy in helping a patient overcome this disorder.

Binge Eating Disorder
What It Is

Binge Eating Disorder was recently recognized as a new category of eating disorder and included in the DSM-5, a diagnostic manual that medical professionals use to diagnose mental health problems in patients. People with this disorder eat significantly more food in a shorter period of time than most people would eat under similar circumstances. They feel out of control, eating quickly and when not hungry.

Symptoms

People with Binge Eating Disorder not only eat a lot of food quickly and feel out of control. They also frequently have feelings of disgust, guilt and embarrassment about their eating behavior, going to great lengths to hide the evidence of their eating. This disorder is associated with great distress. Binge eating episodes happen, on average, at least once a week over a three-month period.

Dangers

The majority (an estimated two-thirds) of those with Binge Eating Disorder are obese and face the health risks of obesity—developing conditions like diabetes, high blood pressure, and cardiac problems. People with Binge Eating Disorder tend to have higher levels of anxiety and major depression than normal weight people or obese people who do not suffer from Binge Eating Disorder.

Treatment

There are medications that can be helpful in reducing binge eating, such as SSRI anti-depressants and certain anticonvulsants such as topiramate. Since all medications do have risks and side effects, your doctor will weigh the risks of the disorder against the risks and benefits of the medications.

Psychotherapy can also be help in managing some of the emotional symptoms of Binge Eating Disorder. Cognitive Behavioral Therapy (CBT), which focuses more on what you can do to change your thoughts and behavior (rather than delving into your past), has been found to be particularly helpful to those with this disorder.

Compulsive Overeating
What it is

This eating disorder is characterized by a large intake of food, more often than not as a result of emotional factors rather than physical hunger. Since this binge behavior takes place without purging, the compulsive overeater's weight may range from slightly to significantly overweight or obese.

What's the difference between Compulsive Overeating and Binge Eating Disorder? It is, to a large extent, a matter of degree: the symptoms in Binge Eating Disorder are much more severe, both in terms of the amount of overeating and the feelings that come before and after the eating behavior. The person with Binge Eating Disorder has more significant psychological and physical problems.

Symptoms

Eating large quantities of food, often in secret, without the purging behavior characteristic of anorexia or bulimia. Compulsive overeaters may eat normally at mealtimes, but eat large quantities of food secretly between meals. The often eat in response to emotional rather than physical cues, binging when angry, sad, nervous, or depressed or even when excited or happy about something. Food is often used as a stress reliever or a way to silence angry, hostile feelings the person feels he or she can't express.

Dangers

An obese teenager's greatest dangers are social: he or she tends to be ridiculed and excluded, facing discrimination not only from peers but also from employers and, in some instances, from college admission officials. There are some long-term physical dangers, however, since an estimated 80 percent of obese teenagers become obese adults at risk for life-threatening cardiovascular disease, adult-onset diabetes, and some forms of cancer.

Treatment

A well-balanced eating plan that can be maintained long-term (rather than relying on stringent diets, liquid meals, or prepackaged-food diet programs), combined with regular physical exercise, is the best way to overcome the physical results of compulsive overeating. A doctor- or nutritionist-supervised regimen of participation in programs such as Shapedown or Weight Watchers, which also feature behavior modification help, are commonsense alternatives.

However, as well as treating the symptoms, the underlying pain of this eating disorder needs to be addressed in individual or family therapy for best long-term results.

Body Dysmorphic Disorder

What It Is

Body Dysmorphic Disorder (BDD) is an obsessive dissatisfaction and preoccupation with one's body, seeing all manner of defects when none exist. While some with BDD may focus on weight, most worry about one or more aspects of their appearance, feeling they look ugly and defective. Researchers believe that the majority of BDD cases begin before 18 and the disorder tends to affect men more often than women—who are more likely to suffer from anorexia. However, some 30 percent of those with one disorder may be diagnosed with the other as well. BDD is classified as a psychosomatic disorder. The distress is very real, but the key characteristic of this disorder is constant preoccupation with a physical defect or series of defects in a person who appears completely normal to others.

The causes of BDD are not yet well understood, but some researchers believe that it is caused by chemical imbalances in the brain. Others feel that there may be some abnormality in how the brains of those with BDD interpret what is seen. In a recent study at UCLA, it was found that there were noticeable differences in the way those with BDD and those without the disorder viewed the same series of pictures that included an untouched photo, a blurred photo and a line drawing of the same face. Performing brain scans on their subjects as they viewed the pictures, researchers found that healthy people used the left, analytical, side of the brain only when viewing fine details while those with BDD had a left brain focus the entire time they were studying the images—which meant that their minds were searching for tiny details that really didn't exist.

Symptoms

People who suffer from BDD obsess about physical defects, most of which don't exist, and see themselves as ugly despite all efforts to correct their imagined physical problems. They tend to spend a lot of time in front of mirrors, studying themselves critically and engaging in constant and repetitive grooming activity. This goes far beyond a more typical adolescent embarrassment about pimples or a few extra pounds or a larger than average nose. For someone with BDD, this preoccupation can be life-limiting, with some not wanting to leave home or to go to school.

Dangers

Some of those suffering from BDD become so distraught over their imagined defects that they withdraw socially, even dropping out of school or work and becoming reclusive. Some become plastic surgery addicts, but are never pleased with the results. Some even consider suicide.

Treatment

This is a treatable disorder, usually with a combination of medication (anti-depressant/anti-anxiety drugs tend to work best) and cognitive-behavioral therapy. The latter is a very specific form of treatment that focuses not on revisiting your past but on finding and changing negative, erroneous beliefs the person may have about himself or herself. Cognitive behavioral therapy can also help vulnerable people learn to handle stress in more effective ways and take steps to change the obsessive habits that are part of a compulsive behavior.

Many of these disorders we've been discussing are part of the Obsessive-Compulsive Spectrum. One person may have an eating disorder. Another may feel compelled to wash her hands until they're bleeding and raw. Another may need to check and re-check certain things before leaving the house. Yet others may have repetitive thoughts they just can't get rid of.

If you find yourself showing symptoms of the disorders we have just described or having thoughts that keep turning around and around in your head, whether you want to concentrate on these or not, or when you do something over and over that makes no sense, but you can't seem to stop doing it, it's time to see your doctor. He or she can refer you to a mental health professional who can help you with therapy and medication. This doesn't mean you're crazy. It just means—as we've seen from some of the research—that your brain may work differently, yet respond well to medication and therapy focused on changing problematic thoughts and behavior.

A Note About Sleep Problems and Your Weight

There has been a lot in the news lately about lack of sleep making people gain weight. Is there anything to that?

Yes, researchers are finding some interesting links between young people in high school and college who stay up late and gain weight. There are a number of theories about why this happens.

In a study looking at freshmen at Brown University not long ago, researchers found that half of the students studied (who kept sleep diaries for nine weeks) had gained an average of six pounds during that time. The findings?

When teens are sleep deprived, they're more likely to reach for sugar-filled snacks like candy for quick energy. Another finding was that the greatest weight gain was associated with sleep variability, or the extent to which a student's bedtime and waking up times varied on a daily basis. This variability causes the body's metabolism rates to adjust and then readjust with the students feeling tired, and feeling less inclined to exercise and more inclined to eat sweets.

Another study, this one at UC Berkeley, has found that weight gain is correlated to lost sleep, particularly later than usual bedtimes. The study found that students who go to bed earlier "will set their weight on a healthier course as they emerge into adulthood."

PANIC DISORDER

What is it?

Panic disorder combines intense fear—the feeling that something really horrible is happening or about to happen to you—with a lot of physical symptoms that occur for no obvious reason. You might be doing something very ordinary: sitting in class or shopping at the mall with friends or driving. Then, all of a sudden, you're on high alert, as if your life were in danger.

Some people might have only one or a few panic attacks, sometimes during times of stress due to loss or a significant life change or after drinking too many caffeinated drinks. Panic attacks can be so intense and so unpredictable, however, that a person who has even one or a few may live in fear of having another. And, for some people, panic attacks become a chronic condition called panic disorder.

Symptoms

In addition to suffering from an intense fear that their lives are in danger, that something terrible is about to happen, those having a panic attack or suffering from panic disorder have a distressing array of physical symptoms: a racing, pounding heart and possible chest pain; sweating, nausea, shortness of breath and dizziness. Some fear they are having a heart attack. Others fear going crazy or totally losing it in a public place. Some feel certain they're about to die.

While a panic attack is self-limiting, the aftereffects can linger: the fear of having another one and trying to avoid situations that a person feels might trigger another attack can be seriously life-limiting.

Dangers

Panic attacks can become chronic, effectively disabling a previously healthy person who now finds himself or herself unable to go to work or to school or engage in other normal, everyday life activities. Some have difficulty leaving their homes—a condition called agoraphobia. Some of those with panic disorder also suffer from depression. A number of studies have found that this combination can make a person more likely to engage in drug abuse or to have suicidal thoughts and tendencies.

Treatment

Panic disorder can be treated by a combination approach of drug therapy (tricyclic anti-depressants or high potency benzodiazephines) along with cognitive behavioral therapy to change some of the thought patterns that lead to a panic, anxiety and depression. Group therapy, sometimes involving whole families, can also be helpful in diminishing a patient's isolation and increasing the family's understanding of this sometimes alarming disorder.

POST TRAUMATIC STRESS DISORDER

Post-traumatic stress disorder (PTSD) is a condition that can occur after you have experienced or have witnessed life threatening events such as car crashes, seeing someone killed or being threatened with death or severe injury yourself, rape, childhood physical, sexual or emotional abuse, natural disasters like being caught in a tornado or severe earthquake or fire, or experiencing combat during wartime. What happens here is that you re-experience the memories and the feelings of the original event over and over through constant flashbacks or debilitating nightmares.

While most people who live through a traumatic event will show some signs of PTSD initially, only a small percentage will go on to develop lasting PTSD. Researchers theorize that those who experience trauma at an earlier age, those who may have a genetic predisposition to mental disorders, those who felt the most helpless or horrified by the events and those who lacked a supportive environment and instead were made to feel ashamed or responsible for their trauma tend to be more likely to have symptoms of PTSD linger, sometimes for a lifetime.

Symptoms

Symptoms of PTSD include: feeling that the trauma is happening all over again—either in flashbacks or in nightmares; feeling that life is out of control, that one is helpless; a feeling of unreality; difficulty sleeping; irritability; difficulty concentrating; and extreme vigilance as you anticipate further trauma.

Dangers

PTSD on its own can be a disabling condition, interfering with every aspect of one's life. However, many people with PTSD try to block out these disturbing feelings with drugs or alcohol. Others experience serious depression and have a greater risk of suicidal feelings and behaviors.

Treatment

A combination of medication (like anti-depressants) with intense therapy can be most helpful to those with PTSD. Ideally, a therapist working with someone with PTSD might use a variety of techniques, from cognitive behavioral therapy which can help the person deal more effectively with stress and anxiety as well as any residual anger about what happened, to re-experiencing the trauma in the safe, supportive environment of therapy. Sometimes, a therapist may use Eye Movement Desensitization and Reprocessing (EMDR) when doing therapy that revisits the original trauma. Group therapy can be helpful as well because it can be immensely comforting to know that others have experienced and survived similar traumas. It makes one feel much less alone and can help the healing process immensely.

SELF-INJURY (CUTTING)

What Is It?

Self-injury, often in the form of cutting, is a behavior that often occurs when some-

one is feeling overwhelmed by painful feelings. It can be a way of gaining control in a world where a young person may feel very little control over what happens. It can be a distraction from these feelings or a way of feeling *something* when the distress has had a numbing effect on one's emotions. Some people who cut do so because they feel bad about themselves while others are experiencing significant depression. Some of those who self-injure report that this activity brings feelings of relief from pain, possibly from the release of endorphins in the brain. Whatever function cutting plays in a teen's life, it can become an addictive behavior.

Self-injury can be triggered by chronic feelings of depression, isolation and/or low self-esteem. It can happen in the wake of a major loss, family problems, difficulties at school, physical, sexual or emotional abuse. It's a way of dealing with feelings that have built up and threaten to get out of control.

Symptoms

Self-injury most often seems to take the form of cutting—cutting oneself with a knife, a razor or any sharp object that's handy. But some of those who engage in self-injury may pick at their skin until it bleeds. They may pull and even pull out clumps of hair—or their eyebrows. They may hit themselves until they're bruised or burn themselves with cigarettes or matches.

Dangers

Self-injury is a stop-gap measure to deal with overwhelming feelings. You may feel better for a time, but it doesn't really do anything to resolve your feelings. You risk not only lasting physical scars and injury from cutting behavior, but also the possibility that those overwhelming feelings will become severe depression or anxiety.

Treatment

Depending on the severity of this behavior, there are several possibilities. A logical step is therapy that can help you to explore the feelings that are consuming you and causing you to self-injure. But just talking with friends or family about this problem can be a big relief, a way of blowing off steam and keeping your emotions from building to the point that self-injury seems your only alternative. Many people who self-injure feel a lot of shame and isolation. Telling someone who will be supportive of you can be an important first step toward healthy coping with the stressors in your life.

HYPERTENSION (HIGH BLOOD PRESSURE)

Hypertension, or high blood pressure, can strike at any age, including childhood, adolescence, and young adulthood. High blood pressure means increased stress on the walls of the blood vessels. This can be serious if the pressure becomes so great that it actually causes a break in the vessel wall and bleeding into surrounding tissues. If this occurs in the brain, it is called a *stroke,* and can be most serious. Bleeding into the delicate tissues of the brain can result in paralysis and even death. The higher one's blood pressure, the higher the risk of stroke.

Some people are more likely to develop hypertension than others. For reasons not fully understood, African Americans suffer a much higher incidence of high blood pressure. So do people who are obese and those with serious ailments such as kidney disease. High blood pressure may occur for a number of physical reasons: stress and anxiety may also be major factors influencing your blood pressure.

The blood vessels are regulated by the nervous system. Given the body's "fight or flight" response to severe stress, tension, and anxiety, these blood vessels may constrict and high blood pressure results, especially in someone who may already have a pre-existing tendency toward hypertension.

How do you know if you have high blood pressure? You probably won't know unless you have your blood pressure checked. Many victims of hypertension have no symptoms. Others experience dizziness, headaches, and nervousness, symptoms often associated with high blood pressure. But it is possible to have one or all of these and not have high blood pressure.

Two readings—*systolic* and *diastolic*—are taken in a blood pressure examination. In a blood pressure reading of 120/80 (considered normal for young adults), 120 is the systolic. This is the higher pressure achieved each time the heart pumps, and may be affected by tension and anxiety. (If you had a bad day, for example, your systolic might be 150.) The diastolic reading is the low pressure as the heart is filling up once again with blood. This is usually considered the more significant reading.

Although the blood pressure reading for those in their mid-twenties or younger should not, as a rule, be higher than 120/80, there are significant variations of normal. Athletes, for example, have wide pulse pressure with a strong cardiac output. Wide pulse means that the person has an efficient cardiac output, requiring fewer heartbeats to circulate the blood. Consequently, an athlete's blood pressure might be 110/50. Children and very young teenagers whose vessels have not aged may have a 90/60 reading.

When does a reading cause concern? Generally, a flag goes up if you have a diastolic of 90 or greater as well as a systolic of 140 or above. If you have high blood pressure, your physician will investigate possible causes. If you show no evidence of a disease that might be a factor, your doctor may advise you to cut your salt intake, avoid taking birth control pills (which may elevate blood pressure) and, possibly, take diuretics. A diuretic will cause you to urinate more frequently and thus help to remove salt and fluid from your body. If you're overweight, this, too, may be contributing to your hypertension. Losing weight may also mean a drop in your blood pressure.

A *point to remember*: If you do have high blood pressure, you *must* be under the care of a physician. But you can care for yourself in important ways, too, since hypertension can be tied to stress. Taking time out from your hectic daily schedule just for you—to listen to music, just stare at the ceiling, write in your diary, or take a walk—can help alleviate some of the stress you may be feeling every day. Learning to say no when you want to and taking care not to overload your already busy schedule are important preventive measures. You need time to just *be*.

ALTERNATIVE MEDICINE: NEW/OLD WAYS OF HEALING

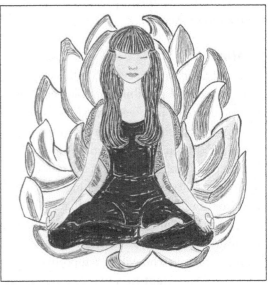

Yoga Lotus

Especially when it comes to mind-body concerns, alternative medicine offers relief and new hope to many. Even though some people see these techniques as quite new, many are rooted in folk medicine—from Asian, Native American, and African healing methods. Some techniques, too, are products of modern technology, but enable you to use the power of your mind to help ease your physical symptoms.

Chiropractors, who treat pain and injuries via manipulation of the spine, are probably the most common and familiar "alternative medicine" practitioners now being recognized by tradition medicine—with many more insurance companies and HMOs covering expenses for such treatments. Other somewhat less familiar forms of alternative medicine include the following:

- *Biofeedback.* Biofeedback is one of the most common nondrug treatments used for treatment of migraine headaches. Here the patient, hooked up to the electrodes of a biofeedback machine, learns to relax by listening to the sounds emitted by tensing and relaxing muscles, and learning to control other functions at will. Many migraine victims learn, via biofeedback, to concentrate on raising the temperature in their hands. Some feel that warm hands mean relaxation, while cold hands mean you're tense. Concentrating on warming your hands, then, may also cause you to relax. It may also mean sending more blood to your hands—and away from your head. When the patient learns how to control body responses like this, he or she can do it anywhere, any time, without having to be hooked up to a feedback machine.

- *Herbal Remedies.* Some folk remedies have become positively mainstream as people become dissatisfied with rational medicine. Ginger is being rediscovered as a remedy for upset stomachs—from stress to motion sickness to morning sickness. Feverfew can help to prevent migraine headaches. And some neurologists now recommend riboflavin (400 mg/day) for those who suffer from migraines. St. John's wort is newly popular as a mild anti-depressant. Chamomile (most often ingested as tea) can help gastrointestinal ills and menstrual cramps.

Caution:

1. Don't overdo it with herbs. Take only the dosage recommended by your physician or other licensed medical practioner. Don't mix a lot of different herbs.

2. If you have a pre-existing condition, such as diabetes or epilepsy, it's important to check with your physician before taking any herbal medicine. One teen patient we saw recently had a seizure while taking St. John's wort. It appeared that this teen, who had a seizure disorder that had been well-controlled by medication, had her seizure threshold lowered by the addition of the St. John's wort. If you have a similar condition or are taking regular medication of any kind, check with your doctor first before even trying an herbal medicine.

3. If your physician or pharmacist isn't knowledgeable about herbs, check with a licensed naturopath. (To find one, call the American Association of Naturopathic Physicians at [206] 323-7610.) Or you might look for a doctor of Oriental medicine (or a licensed acupuncturist who has received special training in Oriental medicine) if you're interested specifically in Chinese herbs.

- *Guided imagery and music therapy.* Guided imagery and music therapy have been around for years. You can find many different relaxation CDs using this technique. Also, many psychotherapists use this tool to help clients deal with stress and anxiety. A combined technique, using soothing music while a patient imagines a tranquil scene, has been found useful in the treatment and prevention of migraine headaches.

- *Hypnosis.* Far from being the strange stage trick where a hypnotist gets people to cluck like chickens and otherwise make total fools of themselves seemingly against their wills, hypnosis, when it is used by a licensed medical or mental health professional, can be very therapeutic. It is often used to help patients deal with stress and anxiety or a specific phobia—such as fear of dentists or of a specific medical procedure. Many reputable professionals these days are trained in hypnosis. All of them would tell you that it is impossible to make you do anything against your will. Hypnosis may be quite useful in getting past a feeling or fear that has been an obstacle for you. Hypnosis can also be useful in stress management, anxiety, and phobias and is sometimes used as an adjunct treatment for compulsive overeaters.

Caution: We highly recommend that, if you are interested in hypnosis for a specific problem, you go to a licensed physician or a psychotherapist who is trained in hypnosis rather than someone who is listed as a certified hypnotherapist (CHT). Although there are undoubtedly some capable, highly professional CHTs, many, unfortunately, are very poorly trained, with only a weekend course in hypnosis and little if any knowledge of medicine or psychology or any legal obligation to observe specific professional ethics. Since hypnosis is most often used as an addition to medical or psychotherapeutic treatment, it is better to see a licensed professional in either field who can offer you a full array of treatment.

- *Acupuncture.* This ancient Chinese healing remedy uses fine needles at very specific points in the body (depending on the ailment). It has received increasing acceptance by Western medicine in recent years and has been found useful for treating many different kinds of pain, perhaps by triggering pain-blocking endorphins. Although there are licensed acupuncturists (in some states that require it) and many others who are certified by the National Certification Commission for Acupuncture and Oriental Medicine (call (703)548-9004 for a referral to one in your area), it's also important to know that many traditional physicians are trained in acupuncture. If your doctor doesn't have this training, you can find one who does by calling the American Academy of Medical Acupuncture at (800)521-2262.

- *Meditation:* There are a number of ways to meditate. Some people do it on their own, finding a quiet place and imagining a peaceful scene; others practice religious meditation. Some find peace in mindfulness: in being fully in the moment, letting all the senses savor the sights and sounds, smells and sensations around one. There is a new meditation technique called mindfulness-based stress reduction that has been found to be especially helpful to those feeling pain and stress over life events. It is a fascinating combination of mindfulness meditation, mindful movement and yoga. The best way to do this, at least initially, is to take an MBSR class. Many of these are now available at yoga studios, hospitals and community centers. Meditation can be especially effective in managing stress, alleviating anxiety, high blood pressure and other physical problems related to stress.

- *Moving Meditation:* Tai Chi, widely available at community centers, hospitals and some gyms, is a series of slow movements that are called "moving meditation." Even some teens who were initially skeptical of this have reported to us that they feel much calmer after a session.

- *Diet, nutrition, and lifestyle changes.* In their landmark 2014 study, "Stress in America," researchers for the American Psychological Association found that teens often reacted to stress with unhealthy habits like overeating or eating unhealthy foods (26 percent of those surveyed), skipping meals (23 percent) or lying awake at night (35 percent). Stressed out teens also spent significantly more time online or watching television than teens who reported low levels of stress. Moreover, teens who got regular exercise—at least once a week or more—had significantly lower stress levels as did those who got at least eight hours of sleep each night.

As we noted in Chapters 5, 6, and 7, choices you make about what you eat, how you exercise, and how you take care of your body can have a huge impact on your continuing wellness. Medical science is recognizing that exercise can help you manage stress: this, in turn, can help prevent some stress-related physical illnesses. In the same way, watching what you eat can alleviate the symptoms of conditions such as irritable bowel syndrome, migraine headaches, and high blood pressure. In a growing number of medical centers, nutritionists and exercise physiologists are becoming valued members of preventive-medicine teams.

This approach also gives you more power in your own health maintenance. Instead of expecting a doctor or a pill to fix a condition, you can prevent it or control it by wise and healthful lifestyle choices.

MAKING SENSE OF THE MIND-BODY CONNECTION

It's important to see your health in a holistic sense with emotional health, stress management, and good self-care (in all ways) just as important as good nutrition, regular exercises, good health habits (such as brushing and flossing your teeth), and regular checkups are to your overall good health. With all the stresses in your life—because you're a busy teen who is juggling school, work, friends, and family as well as dealing with a body that is constantly changing—it's not surprising that stress-related physical ailments happen. It's important to understand your psychological needs as well as your physical needs and ask for help when you need it. It may be easier when you see counseling as necessary for healthy, strong people who want to grow.

Growing may mean accepting responsibility for your health: asking for help when you need it and helping yourself when you can. It may help a great deal to realize that feelings must be expressed in some way. If you can't express your feelings in a way of your choosing—talking or writing, for example—these feelings will choose their own way to come out. If you let anger build up, for example, it may burst out in a temper tantrum, a throbbing headache, or stomach cramps—or even trip you up in an accident! In the long run, then, it may be much less painful to say "I feel angry" than to find yourself yelling "Ouch!" or moaning "Oh, my aching head!"

It's important, too, not to put yourself down for feelings or characteristics that you consider negative. We *all* have flaws and failings. Having compassion for your faults and accepting feelings such as anger as normal may reduce stress in your life considerably.

A certain amount of stress, however, is inevitable. So it's important that your body be ready for it. Regular exercise, for example, will not only help you work off some of your tension and frustration, but it will also increase your body's capacity to handle stress when it does come. A physically fit body and the knowledge that a rich assortment of professional help—from traditional medicine to alternative medicine—is available when you need it can be reassuring as you face the rigors of daily life. Even more important, however, is the conviction that *you* have the power—if you use it—to keep a healthy balance in your life and to prevent many feelings from hurting you physically. If you know where to turn for help and how to manage stress, you will be well equipped to handle those stresses that are simply part of being alive and a part of the world of the 21st century.

QUICK SCAN

MIND OVER BODY

✔ *Mind and body are inseparable.* Many disorders that affect your body can also cause emotional symptoms. And some emotional states—such as depression—can cause physical symptoms such as psychogenic headaches.

✔ *Some of the most common teen physical disorders can have an emotional component.* These include tension and depression headaches, migraine headaches, stomachaches, irritable bowel syndrome, eating disorders, and hypertension.

✔ *There are traditional and alternative ways to treat mind-body ills.* Traditional medicine has a number of remedies, but alternative medicine can help, too. Meditation, yoga, tai chi, biofeedback, acupuncture, guided imagery and herbal remedies, to name a few, can be helpful.

✔ *You have the power to keep balance in your life, by taking responsibility for your own health and well-being.* This is accomplished primarily by living a healthy lifestyle and learning to manage the stress that is inevitable in all our lives.

CHAPTER TEN

Your Special Medical Needs

I have diabetes and I'm really sick of it. Everything in my life is so complicated. I hate the insulin shots and having to test my blood all the time. And it's so hard sometimes to do things with my friends when I have to be so careful about when I eat and stuff like that. Sometimes I feel on the edge of giving up. Will it always be this way for me?

Tonia P.

Special medical needs can have a considerable impact on your life. Any kind of illness or physical problem can be especially hard on you during the teen years. You're so conscious of and concerned about your body. When something goes wrong, it's easy to get scared—and to feel very much alone. If you're like most people, you want to be active and may resent any illness that you feel keeps you from doing what you want to do, either temporarily or permanently. You may also feel that a special medical need is keeping you more dependent than you would like to be on your parents, and your parents may—even with the best intentions—tend to foster such dependence.

You may hate feeling different, yet when you have special medical needs, you may be intrinsically different. You may have to take medications and be on a special diet. There may be certain procedures you have to follow that make it necessary to have detailed plans for simple things that other teens take for granted, such as slumber parties and field trips, which point up the fact of your difference even more.

Maybe you don't have a special medical need yourself, but you know someone who does: a college roommate with eczema (a skin disease), a cousin who has asthma, the girl next door who has scoliosis (curvature of the spine), or a boyfriend with diabetes. If someone you know and love has a special medical problem, it's natural to be concerned. We have received a number of letters from teens asking questions such as the following:

"My boyfriend is diabetic. Is it true that he'll die young?"

"My sister has asthma really bad. Can she ever get better?"

"A friend of mine at school has epilepsy. If she would have a seizure at school, how could we help her?"

So this chapter is for everyone—for those who may have either temporary of chronic medical problems and for those who know and love someone who does. We hope we can help you to better understand some of the common medical problems that adolescents can have and, more important, to learn how to *live* with these special medical needs.

We are focusing on medical problems that are most likely to be part of your life, either directly or indirectly. Some are temporary. Others may be chronic. Some of the problems may be relatively minor. Others can have serious consequences. All may cause pain, upset or a feeling of being different, and may impinge on your life in a number of ways.

What problems are we talking about? All kinds, including mononucleosis, urinary tract infections, bed wetting (nocturnal enuresis), allergies, asthma, anemia (iron-deficiency and sickly-cell), ADHD (attention-deficit hyperactivity disorder), diabetes, scoliosis, Osgood-Schlatter disease, and epilepsy.

We hope that this information will give you new insights into special medical needs, whether they are your own or those of someone close to you.

ATTENTION-DEFICIT DISORDER (ADHD)

I've always had trouble keeping my mind on my work, especially in class, and I just don't

remember things the way other people do. I've always thought it was because I wasn't smart, but my doctor thinks I may have ADHD. My younger brother has that and he runs around the classroom and makes a fool of himself. I don't do that at all. I just can't keep my mind on the teacher or on my schoolwork. Could I really have ADHD? Is eating too much sugar making me this way? Does this mean I have to take pills forever? Also, does it mean I really am stupid?

Emma Kate, 13

ADHD has nothing to do with lack of intelligence. It's a real medical condition!

What causes it: ADHD often runs in families and is caused by changes in how the brain works. Two chemicals, dopamine and norepinephrine, send messages between brain nerve cells, especially those in parts of the brain that control attention and activity level. It is one of the most common chronic medical conditions of children and adolescents, affecting four to twelve percent of school-aged children. Boys are three times more likely than girls to be diagnosed. (But many girls, like Emma, may have the attention problems without the agitated behavior and may not be diagnosed as promptly or as often as more hyperactive boys, who can disrupt a whole classroom with their behavior.)

Some people with ADHD were born prematurely or exposed to alcohol during the mother's pregnancy. However, sugar, immunizations and food allergies have not been found to cause ADHD.

How do you know if you have it? ADHD is most often diagnosed on the basis of behavioral problems and difficulties in school. People with ADHD:

- Show inattention—including frequent day-dreaming, having trouble listening or concentrating, making careless mistakes in schoolwork, having difficulty finishing tasks, and having more than a slight tendency to be disorganized and forgetful. Girls with ADHD most often have an attention deficit without the hyperactivity.
- May have problems with hyperactivity. This is most often seen in boys. This is the person who is in constant motion, can't sit still, runs and climbs when and where this is not permitted, can't ever seem to be quiet, engages in constant fidgeting, and talks all the time.
- May show significant impulsivity. This means the person can't wait his or her turn, interrupts others, acts (or speaks) without thinking, dashes into the street without checking for traffic or takes other risks that most people his or her age wouldn't.

While there isn't a definitive test for ADHD, the physician will usually make the diagnosis after taking a look at the problem behavior and how long this has been going on and how significantly it has impaired the child's or teen's ability to function.

The physician will also do a complete physical and history to rule out other possibilities including vision or hearing problems, learning disabilities, depression, seizure disorders, emotional problems (depression or a reaction to abuse) or a sleep disorder.

How is ADHD treated? Medication and behavioral therapy have been the most effective treatments over time for controlling symptoms and allowing those with ADHD to concentrate and perform better in school and on the job. Usually, people with ADHD are not intellectually impaired. Some have very high intelligence. And medication can help all of these achieve their potential—instead of continuing to struggle in school.

There are a number of commonly used medications, most often stimulants (perhaps the best known of which is Ritalin) that help relieve ADHD symptoms. Sometimes these are combined with behavior therapy to bring about positive changes.

How can you help yourself? Self care doesn't replace medication, but it can help your life—both at school and at home—run more smoothly. Some things that have worked for a lot of teens with ADHD:

- Set a specific time to do homework or chores—so it's harder to forget.
- Organize your stuff—homework, clothes, your smartphone or tablet—so that you can grab it quickly when you need it and are less likely to misplace it or forget it.
- Make "To Do" lists and keep them in a specific place
- Use a daily planner for school assignments, doctor's appointments, meetings at school and with friends—all the details of your life
- Be aware that ADHD can put you at risk—either because you can forget (unless you build these precautions into your routine) to use precautions like seatbelts or protective sports gear like a helmet when you ride a bike or because you are more likely to act impulsively and take chances others wouldn't.
- Also be aware that those with ADHD are more at risk of tobacco and alcohol abuse than their peers without ADHD. So it's even

more important for you not to experiment with these substances.

- Make positive use of your extra energy by going out for sports, dance, drama or debate.

- Be aware that those with ADHD are at greater risk that their peers for mood disorders like depression or bi-polar depression or anxiety disorders. If you find yourself feeling depressed or anxious or having troubling mood fluctuations, talk with your parents and others you trust. Check with your physician. Talk with a counselor. There are many people ready to help—and that can make a huge difference!

ALLERGIES

Since coming to college in the Midwest this fall (I'm from California) I feel like I've got a cold all the time! I'm beginning to think I might have an allergy. But I've never had any problems with allergies before. What could be causing this?

Puzzled

Allergies afflict people of all ages, causing a variety of uncomfortable symptoms including nasal congestion, sneezing, nasal dripping with throat discomfort, redness and watering of the eyes, itching, hives or skin rashes, nausea, diarrhea, and, in some serious types of allergies such as asthma (which we'll discuss in detail a little later on), respiratory disorders and difficulty in breathing.

What exactly is an allergy? It is a reaction by the body against a substance that it recognizes as foreign. Such a substance is called an *allergen*. In response to an allergen, the body forms antibodies and releases certain chemicals that, in turn, cause the allergy symptoms. While many people are able to adapt to allergens, many remain sensitive to common substances that may be completely harmless to those without allergies.

Allergies may run in families. If both parents have allergies, you have an 80 percent chance of being allergic, too. Even if only one parent is allergic, you still have a 50 percent chance of developing allergies.

There are many different kinds of allergies:

- *Environmental allergies* mean that you're allergic to certain pollens, plants, flowers, weeds, grasses, molds, dusts, or tobacco smoke.
- *Food allergies* are quite common. The allergens may be common foods such as chocolate or eggs, milk, or more unusual foods such as macadamia nuts or shrimp. Reactions may include bronchial congestion, trouble breathing, skin rashes, and diarrhea.
- *Drug allergies* happen when people are extremely sensitive to certain drugs—often aspirin, sulfa drugs, or penicillin. Reactions range from mild itching to severe hives and shock.
- *Cosmetic allergies* are triggered by substances ranging from eye makeup to shampoo. People are often allergic to the oils in some of these products and may suffer reactions such as rashes after using the product.
- *Animal Allergies* are also fairly common.

Here people may be unusually sensitive to the dander (skin and hair) of dogs, cats, or horses. While a clean, brushed animal may trigger fewer allergic reactions, some people cannot be around animals at all.

- *Contact allergies* are an unusual sensitivity to certain metals such as nickel, gold or silver. You may experience redness or itching of the skin when you make contact with the metal in a piece of jewelry.
- *Hives*, incidentally, may be classified as a sign of an allergy, but, especially in teens and young adults, may be a sign of extreme stress and nervousness as well.

How do you know if you have an allergy and what the allergen might be in your case? The answer is not clear-cut. Like "Puzzled," you may suffer what you think of initially as prolonged cold symptoms after moving to another area of the country. It may be helpful to know that certain geographic areas have different allergens. So if you grew up in the East and go off to college on the West Coast, you may find yourself with a long-lasting "cold" that may prove to be an allergy. Some people find that a stressful situation, illness, or injury may lower the body's resistance to allergies. Other people have very mild or seasonal allergies that are often mistaken for colds.

However, if you have more than an occasional problem—if your symptoms are chronic and stressful—you are probably fairly sure *already* that you have allergies. You just might not know what may be triggering these reactions.

By going to a physician who specializes in allergies or to an allergy clinic, you can get skin tests to help determine your specific allergy or allergies. Here, prepared solutions of common allergens are injected under the skin at different sites to see if any reaction occurs. In this way, your specific allergy may be determined.

However, if you have only an occasional problem or already know what your specific allergen is, it may not be necessary to go to the expense and time of having such tests. Some allergies disappear as you grow up: others may be with you for a lifetime.

How are allergies treated? There is some debate about this. Some physicians feel strongly that patients should have desensitization shots. This series of injections, which may go on for years, unusually on a weekly basis, helps build up protection against an allergen and makes allergy symptoms less severe. This traditional approach is becoming less practiced as these shots not only require a regular, long-standing time commitment, but they may also be very expensive. Often, avoiding a particular allergen whenever possible may be quite effective in the long run and much less costly than desensitization shots.

Many physicians advocate treating allergy symptoms with drugs such as antihistamines. This treatment may be especially helpful for the patient with occasional allergies. Also, there are now more new drugs and nasal sprays that do not have the undesired side effects of drowsiness and can be taken just once daily. Ask your doctor about these.

You can help yourself in specific ways, too. Probably the most important part of managing an allergy is avoiding your specific allergens as much as possible. This may mean working with your family to keep your homes as dust-free as possible, parting with (or keeping your distance from) the family pet, avoiding offending foods, and, especially, staying away from friends who smoke or smoky rooms, which often can trigger allergies.

ANEMIA

I've been sort of tired lately and was wondering if I might be anemic. Can anemia be caused by heavy menstrual periods? How can I find out if I'm anemic and what can I do about it.

Brittany F.

I've been hearing a lot about sickle cell anemia the past couple months. What is it? Can anyone get it? What are the symptoms?

Tanisha W.

Thanks to certain television commercials, the word *anemia* is often used to describe everything from depression to the legendary "tired blood" malady. We obviously do not support such television diagnoses. Anemia is a very specific problem that must be diagnosed by a physician (via blood test) rather than by symptoms alone, since some victims have no unusual symptoms. There are many types of anemia, and while it is beyond the scope of this book to cover every type, we will discuss two forms that are commonly seen in teens and young adults: iron-deficiency anemia and sickle cell anemia.

Iron Deficiency Anemia

This type of anemia is often mislabeled as "tired blood." When you have this condition,

your blood is not tired, but is lacking sufficient iron supplies to manufacture a constant supply of red blood cells. When the body lacks sufficient iron, the number of red blood cells may decrease, causing so-called iron-deficiency anemia.

What causes it? Many factors can cause the body to lack iron. Among these may be a heavy menstrual flow. While actual blood lost during menstruation does not have to be replaced, lost iron may need to be.

One of the best sources of iron is a good, well-balanced diet. However, many young adults favor junk foods, which do little, if anything, to help replenish the body's nutrients and iron supplies.

It is quite common, then, to see an active teen with regular menstrual cycles (and often a heavy menstrual flow) who favors a predominantly junk food diet develop iron-deficiency anemia.

How do you know if you have it? You may feel fatigued. But it is also possible that you will have no symptoms at all. A simple blood test is the only reliable way to tell whether you have this form of anemia.

What can you do about it? For some, if it is only a mild anemia, diet may correct the anemia. Others may require additional iron supplements. You and your physician together need to work out the best treatment method for you.

Sickle Cell Anemia

Sickle cell anemia is an inherited disease, most often seen in African Americans, in which there is a genetic defect in the structure of the red blood cells and, as a result, a decrease of healthy red blood cells in the body. An estimated 80,000 African Americans suffer from this disease.

Due to this structural defect, the red blood cells are shaped like sickles or quarter moons, instead of being round, and cannot carry on the functions of normal cells—specifically, that of oxygen/carbon dioxide exchange in the lung tissues. Because theses red blood cells have an unusual shape, they cannot pass through the rounded blood vessels easily and may become lodged in them, causing congestion in the part of the body where it occurs. This congestion can become very uncomfortable, with leg, abdominal, or chest pain, impaired circulation, and possibly skin ulcers.

This serious disorder may become even more critical in instances where the oxygen level of the blood is affected—for example, during anesthesia or when an infection occurs in the body. For this reason, it is vital to know whether you have sickle cell anemia or may be a carrier. It is estimated that one in every twelve African Americans may be a carrier of the sickle cell trait.

If you are African American, we strongly urge you to be tested for this trait. In many cities, there are testing centers for sickle cell anemia and even vans that enable medical personnel to do free testing in certain neighborhoods. Today, many states require that all newborn infants be tested for sickle cell disease. The test for sickle cell anemia is a simple but important blood test.

You may not have the disease yourself, but you may be a carrier. If you conceive a child with a person who is also a carrier, it is possible that the child will have sickle cell anemia. It is important to know the possibilities—and the risks—in advance. It is also important to know whether you have the disease or are a carrier, since it does require the ongoing care of a physician.

There have been some promising breakthroughs in the treatment of this disease. Although bone marrow transplants have given some severely ill children healthy new lives, relatively few get this treatment because it can be dangerous and requires a sibling who is a good tissue match as a bone marrow donor. Only about 7 percent of sickle cell patients qualify for this procedure. However, the most promising research is in the area of gene therapy. Here physicians remove some of the patient's bone marrow (via a needle and usually from the hip). This bone marrow is then treated with DNA/RNA fragments, dissolved in fat globules to enable them to get into the cells, which then correct the genetic defect. The marrow is then infused back into the patient. As of this writing, this new therapy is still being tested, but shows great promise for the future.

ASTHMA

I first got asthma at the age of 2. I'm now 15. I've heard things about its causes, but nobody has really talked to me about it. Is asthma an allergy or tied to the emotions or inherited?

Sue A.

Asthma may mean an occasional wheeze or, in its most severe form, it can kill. In fact, over the past ten years, there has been a worldwide increase in deaths from asthma. This is causing medical science to take a closer look at the causes and complications of asthma and to begin to treat this disorder in entirely new ways.

Anyone with asthma should have a regular physician and work with him or her in a team effort to monitor and control the asthma—not just to manage crises. In the past few years, there has been a significant change in asthma treatment. The focus used to be on bronchial dilation, opening up the airways. Today, it is on reducing the underlying inflammation of the airways with new drugs, preventing inflammation with new drugs, and closely monitoring air flow. Inflammation and swelling are predominant features of asthma: reducing these in addition to treating bronchial constriction can lead to better management of the disorder.

Close monitoring of air flow is vital. More physicians are monitoring asthma patients—not just during or after an acute attack, but also regularly to see whether medication is helping. Air flow is measured in the physician's office (and can also be monitored at home) with the use of a *peak flow meter*. These readings—which, ideally, are kept in *peak flow diary cards* by the patient on a daily basis at home—are important in two ways: first, they can tell your doctor if your medication is working: second, they can serve as an early-warning system to help you get treatment early on and, quite possible, avoid a major health crisis. (Studies of young people who died during a severe asthma attack have found that these young people and their families often didn't pick up early-warning symptoms or realize the severity of the problem until it had become a life-threatening crisis.)

New guidelines for self-monitoring from the National Institutes of Health were stated in its

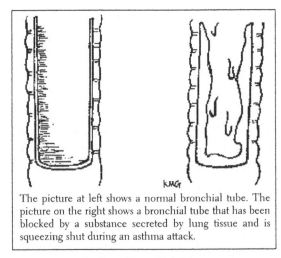

The picture at left shows a normal bronchial tube. The picture on the right shows a bronchial tube that has been blocked by a substance secreted by lung tissue and is squeezing shut during an asthma attack.

Asthma/Bronchial Tubes

National Asthma Education and Prevention Program in 2007. This system involves using peak flow meters at home and recording the readings on a daily basis, using a traffic-light concept of rating how you're doing and what action, if any, may be required. For example, if your readings are 80 to 100 percent of expected flow, you are under a "green light." This means that things are going well and that no special actions, beyond your usual self-care and regular medications, need to be taken. If, on the other hand, you have a reading between 50 percent and 80 percent of predicted flow, you're in the "yellow light" category and should increase medications as previously directed by your physician. Your "red light" alert is triggered by any reading below 50 percent. That means you or your parents should call your doctor *immediately*.

While asthma is usually considered a severe form of allergy, recent research reveals that viral infections may play a major role in triggering asthma attacks in young children. According to researchers, a genetic predisposition to a defect involving the airways in the lungs or the bronchial tubes may underlie the reaction to the virus. However, when asthma develops after early childhood and before middle age, it may indeed be caused by an allergy. As an allergy, asthma can run in families.

What happens during an asthma attack? The lung tissue begins to secrete a substance that causes the air passages of the lungs to become blocked. The tiny bronchial tubes squeeze shut, making the victim fight desperately to breathe. The victim may experience a sensation of tightness in the chest, shortness of breath, wheezing, rapid breathing, or all of these symptoms at once: it can be very frightening.

The attack may be brought on by a specific allergen, such as being in a room with people smoking, or by the flu or an upper respiratory infection, or even by a stressful situation. Stress may involve a specific situation in the young person's life or may be the result of ongoing family problems. Because of this, some physicians may treat asthma patients with a combination of drugs, psychotherapy, and family counseling. In severe cases, the asthma patient may be removed from the home for a time. Asthma can be an extremely serious lifelong problem for some, while others find that symptoms ease or disappear as they get older.

If after removing specific allergens such as a pet, smoke, or dust or mold in the house, you still have asthma attacks, then specific drugs may help prevent or alleviate your symptoms. Today, we know that a combination of drugs may work better for many patients. Physicians often combine drugs such as inhalers, which prevent asthma attacks, with specific drugs that work during an asthma attack.

Today much new treatment is aimed at using inhalers rather than oral medicine, since these drugs work directly *in* the lungs, rather than on the lungs through the bloodstream and thus via the whole body, where the drug is not needed. Many drugs such as albuterol (Ventolin, Proventil) are *bronchodilators*: that is, they are inhaled by the patient and open up the air passages of the lung directly in an acute attack. Other inhaled drugs are *anti-inflammatory*. For example, Azmacort, an inhaled steroid, is inhaled through a dispenser called a *metered-dose inhaler*. These drugs work to prevent asthma attacks in most cases. Also, attachments known a *spacers* hook onto the inhaler and provide better penetration into the lungs.

No matter how mild or severe your asthma may be, teamwork is essential. It's important to understand your disease and how to make self-monitoring a regular part of your life. Your physician, your family, and your environment are all important in the unified effort to make treatment effective. But your efforts, most of all, are crucial in controlling this disorder.

BED WETTING (NOCTURNAL ENURESIS)

I'm almost 16 and wet the bed sometimes. I'm so ashamed I could die! I've thought about asking my doctor about this, but I'm too embarrassed.

J.B.

It's easy to feel embarrassed or like a baby if you have a problem with bed wetting (medically termed nocturnal enuresis). It may be some consolation, however, that you are far from alone. This condition is not uncommon in teens and young adults. In fact, a recent survey found that 3 percent of all 12-year-olds have this condition. Another note of optimism: nocturnal enuresis is *not* a sign of emotional immaturity and it *can be treated*.

What causes this condition? Some research has found that nocturnal enuresis is related to a specific stage of sleep. The fourth stage (deep sleep) may be so deep for some people that muscle control of the bladder may be lost, causing urination during sleep. Other studies are conflicting and do not relate bed wetting to sleep stage.

What can you do if you have this problem? First, don't let embarrassment keep you from asking your doctor for help. Remember: this is not uncommon and it can be treated.

There are two medical therapies now used. One of the most common medical approaches to nocturnal enuresis is a drug that, when taken before bedtime, causes the sleep level to be more active, preventing the sleeper from going into such a deep fourth stage. It has been clinically proven that these drugs, by elevating the sleep level, decrease the incidence of bed wetting.

Another more recent medical treatment for bed wetting is a nasal spray called *desmopressin acetate* (DDAVP or Stimate), which is an antidiuretic hormone effective in treating adolescents. One spray in each nostril at bedtime has reduced bed wetting in as many as 75 percent of adolescents with this affliction. At the time of this writing, there has been some controversy over DDAVP and you should con-

sult with your physician regarding medication for this medical concern.

These are some commonsense ways you can help yourself, too. Don't drink fluids, or at least cut down on fluid intake, in the evening. And don't forget to urinate just before you go to bed. Also, if someone in your home goes to bed later than you do, you might ask them to wake you just before they go to bed so that you can urinate at that time, too.

DIABETES

I have diabetes and I hate it. It's too hard to do things with my friends. I'll have eaten dinner and then some friends come by and say, "Let's go have pizza." I feel embarrassed not being able to have any. I have to wait until later in the evening for a snack, but I feel silly telling them that. What can I do?

Casey K.

Even though Casey, and many other teens who have been diagnosed with diabetes, may be feeling embarrassed, painfully different from peers and very much alone, they have lots of company. More and more teens are being diagnosed with diabetes—increasingly with Type 2 diabetes—causing great concern among health professionals nationwide.

What are the real facts about diabetes—and the realities of living as a teenager with diabetes? *Diabetes mellitus* is a chronic metabolic disorder that occurs when special cells in the pancreas are inactivated or severely impaired and are thus unable to manufacture *insulin*, a hormone necessary to convert food into glucose, the body's major energy source.

There are two major types of diabetes. Type 1, or insulin-dependent diabetes, can occur at any age, but most of those with this form of diabetes are first diagnosed in childhood or adolescence. Type 1 diabetes is considered an autoimmune disorder where the pancreas ceases to produce insulin. With little or no natural insulin production, those with Type 1 must take insulin shots.

Those with Type 2 diabetes, on the other hand, tend to be children, adolescents and adults who are overweight and inactive and whose insulin production is impaired. Because those with Type 2 diabetes may still produce some natural insulin, they can often control the disorder simply with oral medications, diet and exercise.

The symptoms of diabetes include sudden excessive hunger and thirst, unexplained weight loss, frequent urination, fatigue, irritability, confusion, genital itching, skin infections, and/or sudden vision changes.

WARNING:
DIABULIMIA IS AN EXTREME HEALTH HAZARD!!

What IS diabulimia? It isn't an official disorder you'll find in a medical text, but it is a health hazard that is increasing among diabetic teens and young adults. This is diabetes, most commonly the Type 1 variety, that occurs *along with* an eating disorder.

Quite often, those with Type 1 diabetes are diagnosed just about the time puberty—and the desire to be thin—hits. A common symptom of Type 1 diabetes is weight loss. Once a diagnosis is made and insulin started, the teen regains the weight lost and may experience some temporary puffiness and water retention. Some girls and young women are so concerned about this that they start taking much less insulin than they need in order to keep their weight down. Physicians have begun to regard taking too little insulin on purpose as a form of purging behavior.

Why is it so dangerous? Playing with insulin dosage can have devastating health consequences. Too little insulin resulting in high blood sugar can, over a shorter time than you might imagine, damage vital organs and blood vessels all over the body, leading to heart and nerve damage, blindness and kidney failure. Diabetic ketoacidosis or DKA is life-threatening and can develop in as little as 24 hours after missing an insulin injection. In a Scotland survey, 14 women with Type 1 diabetes and eating disorders were studied over a 12 year period and the findings were alarming: at the end of the study, five of the 14 women (some as young as the mid-twenties) had died. Of those who survived, two were blind and three had experienced kidney failure and were on dialysis.

Our Advice: Do NOT risk your health and life by under-dosing on insulin! You can regulate your weight with healthy diet and exercise.

If you have such symptoms, your doctor will test your blood and urine to discover whether there is excess sugar in your urine and bloodstream and to determine how well your body absorbs and utilizes sugar. By the way, have you ever wondered why so many school, camp, and sports physicals require a urine test? Now you know: it's to detect diabetes. Many cases go undiagnosed for quite some time. But the earlier you're diagnosed, the sooner you can begin to safeguard your health.

What causes diabetes in a young person? Many researchers now believe that Type 1 diabetes may occur in those with a genetic predisposition as the result of a viral infection. A number of researchers, too, are beginning to regard Type 1 diabetes as a possible autoimmune system disorder: that is, for reasons not yet fully understood, the body's own immune system produces antibodies that attack the insulin-producing cells of the pancreas as foreign invaders. Much more research needs to be done, however, before the exact causes of diabetes are known.

Again, those who develop Type 2 diabetes are most often significantly overweight and inactive. Type 2 diabetes used to be an affliction of middle-age and was rarely seen in adolescents. However, the number of children and teens who are overweight or obese has increased to nearly 20% of the young population—or 1 in 5 children and teens. Many of these young people are inactive as well, putting them at an even greater risk for diabetes. Being diagnosed with diabetes does not mean that you can't live a full and active life—doing what you love to do, having a satisfying career and, someday, marrying and having children.

But your life does change in some ways.

There is the challenge of keeping the amount of glucose in the body—measured in the blood—as close to a normal level as possible. Insulin injections, replacing the body's normal insulin production, or daily medication to increase natural insulin production are part of this. But since oral medications or insulin injections can never quite replace the body's fine-tuned accuracy in calculating how much insulin is needed, people with diabetes must monitor the level of glucose in the blood several times a day. This can be done very easily, at home or at school, with a special portable blood-testing device called a *glucometer*. A drop of blood from the finger applied to a special monitoring strip can tell you whether the glucose level is too high (more insulin may be needed) or too low (you need to eat more food to increase the amount of glucose in the blood). This home blood-monitoring device can help you to control your diabetes better and possibly avoid some of its medical complications.

If taking blood from your finger proves too painful or difficult on a several times daily schedule, some of the newer glucometers require less blood, allowing you to take samples from less sensitive areas, like the forearm.

There are also other considerations. You need to eat well-balanced meals on schedule. You must learn how to adjust the amount of insulin you'll need depending on how much exercise you'll be getting on a certain day or what foods you may be eating. Also, a cold or attack of the flu may increase your insulin needs. While all this may sound complicated at the beginning, it doesn't have to be. With time and guidance from your physician and/or nurse practioner, you may find that these special needs quickly fit into your normal daily routine.

You will find, too, that controlling your diabetes and having a decent social life are possible and manageable. For example, if your friends want to go for pizza and you've already eaten, go along and have a diet drink. Many people who are watching their weight would do the same thing. Your friends may be so busy enjoying the pizza and your company that they won't notice that you're not eating. Taking good care of your diabetes does not mean that you can't have fun with your friends.

Think about it this way: caring for yourself—with insulin shots for Type 1 or oral medication for Type 2 diabetes, blood testing, and meal planning—doesn't have to take more than 20 minutes a day. The rest of the time is yours to do just about anything you want. You can enjoy sports, eating out with your friends, and going to parties. Some of the things you *can't* do and stay healthy—such as drinking a lot of alcohol or eating a lot of junk food—aren't healthy for *anyone*.

It's important, in taking responsibility for your health, to be aware of the symptoms of an *insulin reaction* (too little sugar in the body), which could lead to a *hypoglycemic seizure*, as well as the symptoms of too high a sugar level (which, if ignored for days, could lead to serious consequences such as *diabetic coma*). While diabetic coma is quite an unlikely event in someone with a well-controlled diet and insulin intake, an insulin reaction or insulin shock leading to loss of consciousness or a seizure can happen on occasion. So it's important to be prepared with a snack—for example, carry a small box of raisins around with you—that will boost your blood sugar level rapidly.

In the past, many people thought that this meant carrying extra sugar cubes or candy around all the time, but many experts insist that this is not the best measure. A sugar cube will quickly raise the blood glucose, but the glucose can fall again quickly unless you also eat some form of protein. Milk is good for these reactions, as are raisins, other fruits, and cheese.

It's important, also, to wear an ID bracelet giving your condition, name, doctor, and instructions for emergency treatment. This could safeguard your health or maybe even save your life if you were found unconscious, as in insulin shock or diabetic coma, or if you were injured in an accident, since there are certain drugs diabetics should not take.

This may seem like a long list of requirements. Some diabetic teens feel helpless and overwhelmed at first. Some try to ignore the reality of their special medical needs. Many teens rebel. It's tough to be different and have to remember so many things. It may be difficult, too, to assert your independence when you are dependent on a drug for your life and when your parents may be concerned and even overly protective. However, making the decision yourself to know and regulate your disease can be a real life-enhancer.

What is in the future for diabetic teens? Many wonder if they can have normal lives and fear suffering from serious complications.

The possible complications are not to be minimized. Diabetes is the third leading cause of death in the United States, after heart disease and cancer. It can lead to kidney disease, nerve damage, heart disease, gangrene and stroke. It is also the leading cause of blindness in adults. Damage to the blood vessels in the retina is common among the majority of those who have had diabetes for 20 years or longer.

But it's important to remember that excellent control of diabetes is possible with the more accurate monitoring of home blood tests. And this better control will diminish or delay the more serious consequences of this disease.

A lot of ongoing medical research may also help you in the future. For example, insulin pumps, which deliver measured doses of insulin throughout the day without the need for insulin injections, are being improved. These pumps were once worn only on the outside of the body, but newer programmable pumps implanted under the skin of the abdomen, delivers correct amounts of insulin on a regular schedule.

Today chances of living a full, active and happy life are much greater than the prospects faced by young people with diabetes a generation ago. Along with the responsibilities your special medical needs require can also come some positive changes. Taking responsibility for yourself can give you a new feeling of independence. You may find, too, that little things like taking your own supply of sugarless diet drinks to a party will not set you apart in a major way. Some of your weight-conscious friends may be doing the same thing. You may find, too, that by keeping your diabetes under good control, you'll really start to feel better—and able to do more things you enjoy. Being in control will give you the freedom and the opportunity to live an active, normal life.

In fact, by keeping your weight down, your body trim and well-exercised and your diet balanced and nutritious, you may even be in better shape and live longer than people without diabetes who eat junk foods, get overweight, don't exercise, and otherwise abuse their bodies.

EPILEPSY

I'm 14 years old and have epilepsy. I'm afraid to ask my doctor some of theses questions, so I'm asking you. What is epilepsy? (I know what it is, kind of, but want to know more.) Is it hereditary? Will I have to take pills all my life?

Wants to Know

I'm 15 and my boyfriend is 16. I found out that he has something called "temporal lobe epilepsy" and gets stomach pains because of this. I don't understand and he doesn't want to tell me about it. Could you please tell me what it is? (In English, if you know what I mean!)

Anne A.

Epilepsy, a general term used to describe a variety of seizure disorders, is an often misunderstood disorder of the central nervous system that, due to uncontrolled electrical discharges in the brain, will cause seizures. That's it. Epilepsy is *not* a mental illness. It is *not* an invariable sign of developmental disorders (although some people with developmental disorders do experience seizures). It is not a condition that will prevent you from living a full and happy life.

There are a number of possible causes of this disorder. It can be caused by head injuries from accidents, birth injuries, or brain tumors. Other causes of epilepsy are still being explored.

There are also a number of different types

of seizures. The most common fall into three general categories:

- *Grand mal seizures* cause the victim to experience a blackout and convulsions of the entire body. This can be frightening, not only to the patient having the seizure, but also to those around the patient who do not know what to do or how to help.
- *Petit mal seizures* may be mistaken for a period of staring or daydreaming. The patient, usually age 6 to 14, will stare, blink the eyes rapidly, or have minor twitching movements before resuming normal activities. Prior to diagnosis, some young people raise the ire of teachers for "daydreaming" in class.
- *Psychomotor* or *temporal lobe seizures* may involve staring, abdominal pains and headaches, chewing and lip-smacking movements, picking at clothing, pacing, buzzing and ringing sounds in the ears, dizziness, and, in some cases, sudden feelings of fear or anger followed by a desire to sleep and, later, amnesia about the whole episode.

In many cases, seizures can be controlled. While there is no cure for epilepsy, it is estimated that 50 percent of those with some form of this disorder achieve complete control of seizures with anticonvulsants, and lead essentially normal lives. Another 30 percent gain partial control of seizures through medication. In fact, some people with epilepsy have not had a seizure for ten years or more, and according to a study at Washington University in St. Louis, some (though not all) of these patients may even be able to stop taking medication after a certain number of seizure-free years.

People with temporal lobe epilepsy may also have one or more psychiatric symptoms. The most common is depression, followed by anxiety, attention-deficit disorder and personality disorders. Some with temporal lobe epilepsy will also exhibit symptoms like being extraordinarily religious or writing compulsively (this cluster of symptoms is sometimes called "interictal behavior syndrome"). If you have temporal lobe epilepsy and have been having problems with moods, talk with your doctor about additional medication. With a careful mix of medication, those with temporal lobe epilepsy can live normal, happy lives.

Many teens with epilepsy are upset about the possibility of a lifetime of medication, especially if they continue to have seizures.

The need for continual medication, the fear of having a seizure, and a feeling of being different plague many people with epilepsy, but this can be especially painful in adolescence.

You may rebel at having to take medications. You may feel smothered and angry when your parents remind you about your medications or show unusual concern. You may feel ashamed about having epilepsy and may be afraid to tell anyone. You may be terrified of having a seizure at school and may be mortified if you do. Some kids, it's true, can be pretty cruel and callous about other people's pain. Often, however, such a reaction may be due to fright, ignorance, and embarrassment.

You may feel embarrassed about feeling different in rather obvious ways. It can be particularly tough when everyone else is getting a driver's license and you're stuck trying to make excuses about why you don't have one yet. While those with epilepsy may get driver's licenses in most states, you most submit written proof from your physician that you have been free of seizures for a certain period of time (two or three years in many states). If you have to wait for this time to pass, it can be difficult.

A spokesperson for the Los Angeles County Epilepsy Society observes that more and more young people are getting epilepsy as the result of head injuries from auto, motorcycle, or skateboard accidents. So it can happen to anyone. That's why it's important to understand what epilepsy is—and it not.

INFECTIOUS MONONUCLEOSIS

I'm 20 and a college student. I have just been diagnosed as having mono. My doctor was most emphatic about my getting a lot of rest. He said something about complications if I don't take proper care of myself. What complications can happen? Is there something I can do for myself besides just resting?

Doug W.

Infectious mononucleosis is a very common problem among young adults, especially college students. A lot of research has been done on the disease that most young people call "mono." It has been found to be caused by a virus. How this virus is spread, however, is still subject to debate.

In the past, mononucleosis was often called "the kissing disease," but that has proved to be something of a misnomer. You can have close contact with a victim of mono and not get it. Some evidence suggests that people who are fatigued and exhausted may be predisposed to the disorder because their immune system is weakened, which makes them more suscepti-

ble to certain infections. Infectious mononucleosis is caused by the *Epstein-Barr virus*. The exact method of transmission is unknown.

What are the symptoms of mono? They vary a great deal, but the most common tend to be extreme fatigue and the need for a lot of sleep. Of course, if you're exhausted to begin with, it may be difficult to tell whether your problem is simply fatigue or whether it is mono. However, when you're tired, you can usually pull yourself together and function pretty well when you want or need to do so. If you have mono, on the other hand, you may not be able to function even if you want very much to be awake and alert.

Other symptoms of infectious mononucleosis include swelling of the lymph glands (especially those in the neck), headaches, and a very severe sore throat. There may also be a skin rash and, in some cases, enlargement of the liver and/or spleen. Sometime you may have a fever, and with a severe sore throat this may be confused with a strep throat. It is important to have this condition diagnosed by a physician, which he or she will do via a physical exam and a blood test.

How is mono treated? With lots of rest and a good diet. These simple instructions are important. If a patient doesn't get proper rest, avoid contact sports (if so directed by the physician), and eat well, enlargement and possible rupture of the spleen could result.

How serious is that? While rupture of the spleen would mean emergency surgery, one can live a normal life without this organ. But *who needs* complications like that?

Many teens with mononucleosis risk such complications by resuming normal activities too soon. It's sad but true that mono seems to strike at times when you don't really have time to be sick—such as around exam time or graduation. Yet sufficient rest is vital to complete recovery.

How long could mono keep you sidelined? This can vary a great deal. Some are only out of step with their normal activities for a week. Others may take a month to recover. It's a highly individual matter. Your body will usually let you know when it's ready to function at full capacity again.

OSGOOD-SCHLATTER DISEASE

I have been having a lot of swelling and pain in my knee and lower leg. I'm active (co-captain of our varsity basketball team) and hate having this pain. What could it be and what can I do to get rid of it?

Rusty C.

Osgood-Schlatter disease, a disorder of the mineralization of the leg bones, it quite common, especially in active young people between ages 10 and 15.

This condition, which can cause swelling and tenderness around the knees and pain in the lower leg, may be caused by stress on the tendon that attaches the *patella* (knee bone) to the *tibia* (front leg bone). The stress is due to the changes of puberty: increased muscle mass in the legs and active use of the upper leg muscle, the *quadriceps*. The stress of the patellar tendon on the upper prominence of the tibia, and irregular calcium deposits in the upper tibia cause the painful swelling and pain

in this part of the bone. This is a common condition of early puberty when growth is very rapid. It is also a *temporary condition* that is usually self-healing.

To facilitate healing, a physician will usually recommend that you stay away from vigorous sports and exercises involving bending for a certain amount of time—usually a few weeks or sometimes several months of inactivity. It depends on you. If you find that after a few weeks, you can play sports without pain and without increasing the swelling, then it may be OK for you to resume playing. However, if playing a sport causes the pain and swelling to increase, then you will need to take additional time off. This doesn't mean that you can't still be active. Just limit your activities to those—such as swimming—that don't put stress on the knees.

Those with unusually severe cases of Osgood-Schlatter disease may require casts to help healing, but usually a relatively brief period of rest and taking an anti-inflammatory medicine, such as Ibuprofen (Advil) is enough. While this period of reduced activity may seem to go on forever, it may be some consolation that, once healed, you'll be as good as ever—is the following testimonial from a teen named Beth shows:

I'm 16 and two years ago I had Osgood-Schlatter disease bad enough to have a cast on my knee for two months. But now I'm going strong. I'm a cheerleader, a majorette, and I'm on the girls' basketball team. I just wanted to tell other teens to follow their doctors' instructions and take care. You'll be OK, too!

Beth

SCOLIOSIS

I'm supposed to get a brace at the end of
July for my back because I have a curvature
of the spine—scoliosis—and I'm scared. I
know I'll feel like such a jerk running around
with a thing like that on my body!

Scared

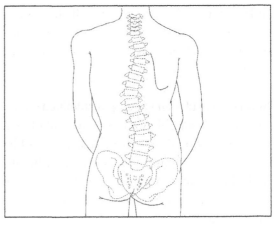

Scoliosis

Scoliosis is a correctable deformity in which
the spine curves to one side instead of growing
straight, is especially common in girls (who
are eight times more likely to have it) in the
growing years between ages 10 and 16. The
usual ages of onset are 9 to 10 for girls and 11
to 12 for buys. There is some evidence that this
condition may be inherited, although certain
diseases such as rheumatoid arthritis and cere-
bral palsy as well as spinal injuries may also be
factors. Most cases of scoliosis, however, have
no easily determined cause. But we do know
that this condition afflicts about 10 percent of
young adolescents to some degree.

Early symptoms include shoulders that are
not level, uneven hips, and prominent shoul-
der blades. An "S" curve in your spine may
also be observed if you have a friend or family
member look at your back as you bend over.
A number of school districts across the nation
have special screening programs to detect scoliosis in its early stages.

When there is less than a 20-degree curvature of the spine, no treatment is necessary.
However, the physician must watch the curvature over a period of time to make sure that
it is not increasing. The possibility of increasing curvature can depend largely on your age
at diagnosis and how much growing you have
left to do. For those diagnosed with scoliosis
before age 12, there is about a 75 percent risk
of curve progression, compared with 30 percent for those between ages 12 and 15 and only
10 percent for those over age 15.

If the curve progresses or is more pro-
nounced to begin with and is greater than
20 degrees, you may need to wear a *Milwau-
kee brace* for a period of time and do special
exercises. The brace, while it may look cum-
bersome, doesn't have to interfere with your
normal activities and may help a great deal to
move your spine back into a normal position.

In severe cases of scoliosis, if the curve of the
spine is greater than 40 degrees, surgery and casting are required. Here, an adjustable *Harrington
rod* is surgically implanted to help straighten the
spine. However, this procedure is quite rare.

Treatment for scoliosis—whatever the
method—will keep the curvature from pro-
gressing and causing serious deformities in
later life. So if you notice any indications of
scoliosis, don't be afraid to tell your parents
and your doctor. Treatment now will be of life-

long benefit, and the earlier you seek help, the less help you're likely to need.

URINARY TRACT INFECTIONS

I have pain and burning when I go to the bathroom and a friend of mine told me that this is a urinary infection. How do you get it? I heard it may have something to do with sex, but I don't have sex! How do you get rid of it?

Ally D.

Urinary tract infections are common in young adults, most often in young women. Quite frequently, these may be young women who are having their first sexual experiences. But sex is not the only factor in urinary tract infections. Bubble baths may cause irritation of the urethra and, as a result, a urinary infection. Careless wiping after a bowel movement can be another cause. The rectum is close to the urethra (urinary opening) in the woman and it's easy for bacteria from the rectum to invade the urinary tract. This is especially likely if you have a habit of wiping toward the vagina (forward) after a bowel movement. Wiping *away* form the vagina and urethra (backward) will minimize this risk.

How can sexual activity increase your likelihood of developing a urinary tract infection? During intercourse, the man's penis—while thrusting—may touch areas near both the woman's rectum and urethra and may this spread bacteria from the rectum to urethra. For some sexually active women, this may mean almost continuous urinary infections.

How can you avoid such problems?

- *Use good hygiene.* Bathe or shower regularly, taking care to wash the genitals and rectal areas thoroughly.
- *Urinate as soon as possible after sex.* This can help to wash out any bacteria that may be present in the urinary tract.
- *Drink water after sex.* Some urologists recommend drinking water after sexual intercourse. This will be flushed rapidly through the kidneys. This further urination will help to wash any remaining bacteria out of the urinary tract before the bacteria have a chance to multiply.

How do you know if you might have a urinary tract infection? In some cases, it may be difficult to distinguish a urinary tract infection from a vaginal infection. However, with a vaginal infection, you will usually have a vaginal discharge as well as painful or burning urination.

Symptoms of a urinary tract infection include pain and burning on urination and greater frequency of urinating (not as a result of drinking lots of fluid), blood in the urine (when you are not having your menstrual period), and in some cases a concurrent kidney infection with pain in the lower back.

If you have such symptoms, don't just wait and hope that they will disappear. See a physician. A urinalysis will reveal whether you have such an infection. If you do, your physician will usually treat the condition with antibiotics.

LIVING WITH SPECIAL MEDICAL NEEDS

Anyone can have a special medical problem. But it can be especially hard to cope with if you're a teen and if your problem is *chronic* and not likely to change. Besides whatever discomfort your physical condition may bring, there will be trying times emotionally.

There will be times when you'd like to throw your medicine out and pretend that you don't need it. There will be times when your parents seem to nag or overprotect you, or take over your illness instead of giving you the space and the responsibility to care for yourself. There will be times when you feel guilty about the time, expense, and emotional strain that your special needs may be putting on your family and times when you try to reassure your parents.

And there may be times when you find yourself almost enjoying the attention and special privileges or considerations you may get because of your condition, times when you may use your illness as an excuse to get out of doing things for yourself that you know you can do. There will be other times when you may feel enraged at being different. You may feel like screaming "I hate this! Why me?" And there may be times when you fear the future and what it may bring.

The fact is, though, that not one of us knows what the future will bring. For example, most teens who die this year will do so in accidents. Discovering that you have a chronic disease such as diabetes or epilepsy does not mean that your life is over. Part of living fully with (or despite) a special medical need means accepting your feelings of rage, rebellion and depression as entirely normal.

If you've ever wondered "Why me?" you're far from alone. It can help a lot if you talk these feelings over with someone who understands—a special friend, a family member, your doctor, a counselor, or a medical center social worker. Once you begin to accept your feelings,

it is usually easier to get past the negative ones, to accept your special needs, and to take responsibility for your own care as much as possible. Control of your condition—even in little ways—can give you new feelings of power in your life. When you have a chronic medical condition, it's easy to start feeling that things are constantly being done to you rather than doing things for yourself. It may help you achieve a real sense of independence if you can assert your right to be involved in your own treatment and to manage your own life as much as possible.

Keeping your condition—whether it's asthma, diabetes, epilepsy, or something else—as well controlled as possible will free you to do other things. You will be able to see past your special needs to your special potential—and the full range of exciting possibilities in your life!

YOUR SPECIAL MEDICAL NEEDS

✔ Doing what you need to do to take care of your special medical need can free you to enjoy the rest of your life.

✔ If you assert your right to be involved in and to control your condition, even in little ways, you will have a new feeling of power in your life. For up-to-date information on your special medical need, check the appropriate section of this chapter!

✔ For up-to-date information sources for special medical needs, see the Appendix.

ELEVEN
You And Your Sexuality

I'm confused. People talk about sex. And then they talk about sexuality. My friend says that everyone has sexuality even if they don't have sex. I always thought that the two words meant pretty much the same. Is sexuality something everyone has? Even old people and kids?

Wondering

Many people confuse sex with sexuality and many, too, think that sex automatically means intimacy as well.

It's more important than ever to know exactly what these differences are in order to make wise, responsible sexual choices.

Sexuality, which includes sexual *feelings* and how you feel about yourself as well as others (as well as sexual activities), is a major part of who you are all your life—from infancy to old age. All too often, however, people see it only in a limited sense. Some see sexuality as a synonym for sexual intercourse. But there is so much more to it than that. Sexual actions are only a *part* of your sexuality. You can be a very

normal, happy sexual person without having sex—right now or even for years!

Some people define sexuality in terms of sex roles. They are very concerned about being masculine or feminine to society's traditional standards and may be afraid of any feelings or actions that might seem to contradict society's images of how a man or a woman should be. A young man may hide tender feelings to protect a macho image. A young woman may feel guilty about having strong sexual desires or may take great pains to hide her intelligence. Yes, despite all the social changes in the past two decades, we still get letters describing these feelings and choices. And when men and women get stuck in these old ways of thinking and acting, they may be sacrificing personal honesty to maintain old stereotypes.

Caught up in roles where "sexuality" may be seen in terms of "sexiness," people may relate to one another as sex objects, forgoing the friendship that gives love and sex new meaning and bypassing the tenderness that makes an intimate friendship so special. Indeed, someone who defines himself or herself in terms of traditional sex roles may have trouble maintaining close relationships with the same or opposite sex, afraid to show tenderness in a same-sex friendship or honest friendship in a dating or sexual relationship.

SEXUALITY AS PART OF YOUR LIFE

Some people see sexuality as a separate entity in their lives. It isn't. Your sexuality goes far beyond labels and stereotypes, far beyond sexual relationships, far beyond whatever sexual actions and options you might choose. The fact is, despite the choices you make regarding sexual activities—even if you choose *never* to have sex with another person—you are an innately sexual being, just like everyone else.

There is nothing strange or mysterious about your sexuality. It just *is*. Like you. How you choose to *express* yourself sexually, on the other hand, does involve value judgments. Who you are, how you feel, and what you think can't be judged. But you are responsible for your choices and activities.

Sexuality is shared equally by males and females. No one sex is more sexual than the other. We're all simply people. And people feel tenderness and passion and love. People feel sexual desires. People have all kinds of sexual fantasies. People of all ages—even infants— feel sexual sensation.

Accepting your sensations, your fantasies, your desires, and your feelings—from tenderness to passion—as normal and natural can help you feel more at ease with others and with yourself. Feeling such comfort with your sexuality can help you make more responsible

choices regarding any sexual activities. For example:

- *You can have and enjoy a sexual fantasy without ever needing to act on it and make it reality.* We fantasize about all kinds of things—why not sex? Feelings and fantasies can't be judged. They just happen. However, you *are* responsible for the choices you make and what you *do*. You may have fantasies about things that you wouldn't dream of doing. That's OK. You may find yourself having warm feelings toward someone of the same sex or someone of the opposite sex. These feelings don't necessarily define you one way or the other. Most of us are capable of responding emotionally to people of both sexes with warm feelings, deep friendship and love, and, at times, somewhat erotic feelings. This can happen with people whose primary sexual orientation is heterosexual as well as with people who are primarily homosexual. Most people, whatever their sexual orientation, age, or marital status have a rich and varied fantasy life.

- *Fantasies can help you act more responsibly by putting sexuality in perspective and balance with the rest of your life.* In a study at Trinity University, for example, people were told either to think about sex or to attempt to keep all thoughts of the subject out of their minds. The mere mention of sex was arousing to all people in the study, but the excitement level gradually diminished among those who were encouraged to think and fantasize about sex. Those who tried *not* to think about sex felt themselves fighting constant, unexpected thoughts about sex and a continuous level of sexual excitement.

- *Real love and intimacy do not need sex in order to grow and thrive in a relationship.* Sexual sharing may be simply a part of some of these relationships when the time is right. If you know the difference between love and sex, you're not likely to get the two confused and, in search of love, to enter prematurely into sexual relationships.

- *If you feel good about your sexuality, you won't be in a rush to have sex.* You can enjoy all your feelings and sensations. And, when you do have sex eventually, your positive feelings about your choice will lead you to make wise decisions about birth control. (People who don't use birth control because they think that such "planning ahead' is wrong don't feel good about having sex or about the sexuality. So they need to pretend that sex is, invariably, a passionate accident.)

YOUR SEXUAL ORIENTATION

I'm 15 and gay. (It feels funny and yet very normal to write that! It's the first time I've written that on paper yet it's like saying what's been in my heart as long as I can remember.) I knew I was different in some way when I was just five or six, but really started knowing by sixth grade. Just last week, I came out to my parents. They were pretty cool about it overall, but keep saying "Are you SURE? You're so young! How do you know for sure?" I tell them that I'm as sure as anyone else my age who is into dating girls. They have some gay friends who didn't come out until they were in their thirties—one of the guys was actually married

and has a son! So I think that's why they're surprised I know so early, but I keep telling them that times are different now and that maybe their friends always sort of knew, but couldn't accept that they were gay because it was so looked down on when they were young. What do you think?

Jason O.

Sexual orientation is a major aspect of our sexuality. Even though, ideally, sexual orientation should be just another part of who we are, some gay people—young and older—still feel the sting of society's disapproval. This is more prevalent in some communities, some schools, and some social circles than others. What it can mean is that some heterosexual teens worry about the fact that they may have warm emotional feelings—and maybe some erotic feelings—about certain people of the same sex: perhaps a much-admired teacher or an especially treasured friend. And some young people who know in their hearts that they are gay may worry about being socially isolated and ostracized by school friends and rejected by their families if they let people know who they are and how they feel.

In both instances, these young people's worries stem from the reality of social prejudice against people whose sexual orientation is gay or lesbian. In both instances, too, these young people are experiencing feelings that are entirely normal for them.

Crushes on teachers or others of the same sex are normal. We admire and love many people, especially in adolescence. Everyone has idols and secret crushes. Admiring someone else may help you discover more about what you would like to grow to become. It can be a positive step in your growth toward maturity.

Close friendships with those of the same sex are vitally important, too. Closeness with a best friend can be great mutual comfort at a time in your life when you face so many changes. In friendships, people express affection in many different ways. Some express their feelings with thoughtful acts or gentle teasing. Some can say how they feel. For others, a touch or hug or kiss says, "You're special. I care." And our sexual orientation—whether heterosexual or homosexual—is a normal part of the people we happen to be.

It may help to know that, although most of us have a definite sexual orientation that is either heterosexual or homosexual, very few people are 100 percent heterosexual or 100 percent homosexual. The Kinsey Institute has devised a scale to rate sexual orientation. An extreme heterosexual, someone who has never responded emotionally or physically to someone of the same sex, would be a "zero," while a "six" would be the other extreme—someone who is and always has been exclusively homosexual. A 1970 Kinsey survey revealed that at least 60 percent of American men and 30 percent of American women have had at least one overt, intentional homosexual experience by age 15. Other studies have placed these figures even higher.

So a high percentage of the American population would be neither a zero nor a six, but somewhere in between. They would include people who are almost exclusively heterosexual, but who have had a minor homosexual experience; people who have had experiences with both sexes, but who prefer the opposite sex; people who have no special preferences;

and people who prefer those of the same sex, but who are not exclusively homosexual.

What about the men and women whose sexual orientation is primarily homosexual? There are a lot of them. In fact, 7.2 million Americans under the age of 20 are gay, lesbian, or bisexual, according to the Statistical Abstract of the U.S. Bureau of the Census.

How we develop our sexual orientation is still being studied, and so far the findings have been fascinating, if not definitive. We do know that you find your gender identity—seeing yourself as male or female—by age 2. Most of us see ourselves by our anatomically correct gender. (Those who see themselves as the opposite sex are called transgender; we will be discussing gender identification and all its variations in the next section. We would just like to say here that transgender people are *not* transvestites, who are either heterosexual or homosexual and identify themselves congruently with their male or female genitals, but who enjoy dressing in the clothing of the opposite sex.)

Those who have a homosexual orientation see themselves as the gender congruent with their genitals, but simply grow up finding that they are physically attracted to those of the same sex.

We know that some people may not come to terms with their true sexual orientation for years. In fact, especially in the past, when being gay wasn't something one could talk about or reveal openly, especially at a young age, some gay people married and had children before coming to terms with the fact that they were primarily homosexual. This may have had much less to do with "turning gay" or choosing to be gay and much more to do with the fact that, in years past and even today, there is so much social disapproval of homosexuality that it may take years for a gay man or lesbian woman to come to terms with his or her sexual orientation and to find the courage to come out of the closet. It's quite possible that this scenario may change for today's teens—some of whom are growing up in a much more supportive social environment than those who came before them. But, as many gay and lesbian teens know, it still isn't easy.

The prevailing wisdom used to be that a person couldn't be totally sure of his or her sexual orientation until young adulthood. Now we know that most teens are quite aware of their own sexual orientation at a very young age.

Dr. Gary Remafedi of the Adolescent Health Program at the University of Minnesota headed a team of researchers that surveyed 34,706 teens in grades seven through twelve in that state. His findings: most teens know their sexual orientation by age 17 or 18. At age 12, only 26 percent of young people were unsure of their sexual orientation. By age 17, those who were still unsure had dropped to 5 percent.

Some religious counselors feel that sexual orientation may be learned behavior and, as such, can be changed. Some mental health therapists believe that sexual orientation *may* be changed in instances where the individual is highly motivated and wants very much to change. But mainstream experts are skeptical. There isn't much conclusive evidence that such therapy changes a person's actual sexual orientation, but simply his or her sexual behavior. That is, you may learn to behave in a dif-

ferent way, but will your real feelings change? Other unanswered question: how long can you behave in a way that may be contrary to your true sexual orientation? And what will the psychological cost be?

May other therapists emphasize the importance of authenticity and self-acceptance. A lot of therapy these days is supportive: helping gay people deal with social pressures and disapproval, to understand and to accept their feelings. Some wonder to begin with, "*Why am I gay?*"

There are many theories. Some controversial studies are focusing on hormonal influences in the womb that may predispose a person to become homosexual. Some experts believe that whether one actually becomes homosexual may depend on these prenatal hormonal influences combined with certain environmental factors. A recent study at a medical center in Boston found that there seems to be a tendency for male homosexuality to run in families. The researchers studied 51 homosexuals and 50 heterosexual men as well as their siblings. About 4 percent of the brothers of heterosexual men were gay. Among the brothers of homosexual men, some 22 percent were also homosexual. The researchers have said that, in this particular study, it was not possible to show whether heredity or upbringing was more important in determining sexual preference. Curiously, these differences were not apparent in the sisters studied. The sisters of homosexual men were not any more likely than sisters of heterosexual men to be homosexual.

In another study, this one at Northwestern University, researchers studied the sexual orientation of twins. They found that, among identical twins—those who share the same DNA—if one twin was gay, the other had a 50% chance of being gay. Among fraternal twins—who share the womb and are born at the same time but no more closely related DNA-wise than any other siblings—there was only a 20% chance of a twin sharing his or her gay twin's sexual orientation.

Research into whether a "gay gene" is present in the DNA, perhaps on the X chromosome contributed by the mother (since some studies have shown that when homosexuality appears to be genetically linked, it has appeared to be on the mother's side) is ongoing and it may be years before we have any solid conclusions. There is also research into the "brother" factor—and the fact that men who have older brothers are somewhat more likely to be gay. A study at the University of Toronto found that for every older brother a man has, his chances of being gay increase. Researchers theorize that there may be changes in the mother's uterine environment with each male child and that the mother's immune system may start reacting differently to male specific proteins and this, in turn, might trigger some changes in the brain of the developing fetus. But none of these theories are conclusive at this time.

There's a lot more we need to learn about what makes us who we are—whether we're primarily heterosexual or homosexual. What's important to remember in the meantime is:

- Many gay people are at least vaguely aware that they are somehow different in very early childhood.
- While a lot of people worry about gays molesting or "recruiting" young people, the fact is that the vast majority of child molesters are heterosexual.
- There's no reason to fear someone who is gay or lesbian. Generally, they don't want to be rejected socially or physically any more than you do, so they're likely to be attracted to people who share their sexual orientation. If someone does show an interest that makes you feel uncomfortable, all you need to say is "No, thanks."
- Homosexuality is not a disease nor a mental illness. In the past few decades, important professional organizations—such as the American Psychological Association—have accepted this fact as policy. There is nothing inherently wrong with someone who is gay or lesbian. Sexual orientation is just another part of who we are as human beings, like having blue eyes or red hair or a family-shared talent for music.
- Reading and learning about gays and lesbians is not going to turn your sexual orientation in that direction unless it was there already. Some people fear that if teens read or hear about homosexuality—for example, in a school sex education class—they will want to become homosexual. Not likely! Given the physical and verbal abuse that gay and lesbian teens still face on some school campuses and the anger and rejection they often face at home when they try and discuss their sexual feelings with their parents, it's unlikely that many teens would be eager to make that choice—if, in fact, being gay were truly a choice.

Think about it. Who could influence a person strongly enough to make such a difficult choice? Studies show that even parents—who, perhaps, influence us more than we ever know—don't have a definitive influence on their children's sexual preferences—with most homosexuals coming from homes headed by heterosexual parents and gay parents no more likely to raise children who grow up to be gay.

If you feel you may be gay or lesbian, accepting this reality can be a painful and confusing process. It may begin when you're very young and realize that you're different in many ways that you can't explain. Or you may only gradually become aware of your feelings, longings, fantasies, and consistent attraction to those of your own sex. You may have times of feeling terribly alone, like you're the only person who feels so different and like if you breathe a word to anyone your whole world as you know it—family relationships, friendships—could fall apart. You may have times of denying your feelings to yourself and to others as a way of being accepted. You may date and even have sex with people of the opposite sex (studies of adult gay men and lesbian women show that most have had heterosexual experiences). You may work very hard to act like everyone else, keeping an important part of who you are hidden even from those close to you for a long time. Then, as your sexual identity seems to be an intrinsic part of you, you may begin to share this part of yourself with others—with widely varying results ranging from loving acceptance to angry rejection. The process of accepting yourself, with such mixed reactions even among those you love most, is not easy. You may need to talk with a counselor or someone else you feel could help you through this time.

As you begin to accept your sexual orientation as part of the complex and fascinating person you are, you may feel less overwhelmed by your feelings. Your sexual orientation is only a *part* of your total identity—not the whole thing. You are still the unique individual you have always been, with your own special array of skills, talents, and strengths. Once you realize this—and once your family and friends realize, too that you're still the same person they've always known and loved—you will begin to move past your pain to new peace. Growing in self-acceptance and in your capacity to relate to others in a non-exploitive way, to give and receive love, is vital—whatever your sexual orientation.

YOUR GENDER IDENTIFICATION

I'm 16 and confused about all this stuff I'm seeing on television and the Internet about people who are trans—like a woman trapped in a man's body. Are these people just crazy? Or is there something to it? I saw a little of a show about a guy who is, like 70 or something, and decides to be a woman and expects his family to just accept it. I mean he looks like a man in a dress. Just gross. Of course, Caitlyn Jenner looks pretty good. But still, why would someone who won an Olympic Gold Medal, has a lot of kids and money and is famous and kind of old DO something like that?? I guess what I want to know is, what is it with these old guys wanting to be women? Is this something that just strikes like lightning sometime in your life? Could it happen to anyone, anytime?

Bailey F.

With the increased discussion of gender in the media in the wake of Caitlyn Jenner—who won the 1976 Olympic Decathlon, one of the most macho events imaginable, as a man named Bruce Jenner—coming out as a transgender woman in 2014, there are a lot of teens—and even older people—scratching their heads and wondering what this is all about.

It's all about gender identification: how you see yourself internally, regardless of what genitals you have. For most people—called *cisgender*—the genitals and internal sense of self match. You're male; you're female. You don't even have to think twice about it.

But that isn't the case for everyone. In recent years, researchers have been confirming what transgender people have been insisting for many years: it's entirely possible for someone to have the genitals of one sex but a vastly different internal sense of being the opposite sex...or somewhere in between.

There is growing acceptance of the reality that, just as there is a certain fluidity in sexual orientation—with a great number of people falling on neither extreme of heterosexual or homosexual, but rather somewhere in between—there is also fluidity in gender orientation, with many people ranging from displaying the traits of a gender that does not agree with their physical sex, to feeling strongly that they truly *are* of a gender that is in conflict with the physical evidence of being male or female.

After all, we all have friends and family members who haven't fit the macho male or girly-girl modes: the girl who is a tomboy and prefers climbing trees to playing with dolls; the quiet, sensitive boy who abhors rough-and-tumble play and sports in general, and longs

for a doll house for Christmas. There are even kids who seek to dress as the opposite sex when they're younger, then lose interest in all that when they become teens and more comfortable with themselves as their bodies grow and change. These kids, who show signs early on that they may be transgender but who turn out not to be, represent about 75% of children who show some unease with assigned sex roles. Some of these children, as they grow into adolescence and beyond, may come out as gay or lesbian. Others turn out to be heterosexual and simply have masculine or feminine traits that mix in an endless variety of ways to produce the individuals they grow up to be.

But for the remaining 25% of young people, who often from an early age are certain that a major mistake has been made, that the way the world sees them is *not* the way they truly are, *do* turn out to be transgender.

Being transgender in a world that truly doesn't understand can be an emotionally devastating experience. It isn't just a question of the frustration involved in knowing you're one way, despite all physical evidence to the contrary; there's also the terror of being bullied relentlessly, marginalized, ridiculed and, in some cases, brutalized and even killed. So, many transgender people show signs of distress, heightened anxiety and depression as reactions to the difficulties of being different. Being transgender is *not* a mental illness. Researchers are beginning to find physical reasons for physical and psychological senses of gender not matching.

When a fetus is in the womb, its sex/gender is not immediately apparent. It isn't until about six weeks into the pregnancy that a release of hormones causes the external and internal reproductive systems of the fetus to develop. Soon thereafter, this allows excited parents to get a preview, via ultrasound, of whether their baby will be a boy or a girl. But despite this sneak peek, it's not until later in the pregnancy that the sexual differentiation of the brain occurs, triggered by another release of hormones. This is what researchers believe determines the gender identification and gender-based behavior of the child-to-be.

In most instances, the genitals and gender identification of an individual are a match. But sometimes, male or female anatomy (or some variation) are paired in one small body with a brain that is conditioned to be the opposite gender, or some variation along the continuum.

In fact, in some recent studies utilizing scanning technology, researchers have been able to see into brain structures of people who are cisgender (genitals and gender identification are in sync with each other) and those who are transgender (but who have not yet taken hormones to begin a sex change). The findings have been interesting: in a number of cases, the brains of transgender individuals differ in structure from those of cisgender people—sometimes resembling those of females more than males, sometimes the opposite, but always on a continuum. There is much we don't yet understand, and a lot more research needs to be done, but there appears to be a growing amount of evidence to support the fact that being transgender is a physical trait, like blue eyes or brown hair.

One of the most fascinating accounts of possible physical/hormonal influences determining who is male and who is female is the story of the Maines twins, born as identical twin boys. However, as soon as she could speak,

one of the twins began to insist that she was a girl, not a boy. And the other twin, forever male, grew up insisting, "You were always my sister, never my brother." Their parents were initially confused, upset, completely puzzled, but always loving and supportive. After some expert medical consultations, the family decided that the twin who identified as a girl would get medication when she was about to show signs of puberty—at about the age of 12—to postpone male development and prepare the way, when she was older, to have a surgical sex change, if that was what she chose to do. That was her choice. She started taking female hormones after her sixteenth birthday and, when she was 18, just before starting college, she made the final transition to bring her physical body in line with her gender identification. This fascinating story is described in the book *Becoming Nicole: The Transformation of an American Family* by the Pulitzer Prize winning medical journalist Amy Ellis Nutt.

The notion of giving pre-teens hormones to stave off puberty and buy time while they make a decision about whether or not they want sex reassignment surgery (usually not done before the age of 18) is controversial. Those against this are concerned about introducing puberty-suppressing drugs to young people who may not turn out to be truly transgender. Those who are in favor argue that the effects of the drugs are reversible and that it is much easier to transform the physical appearance of someone transitioning to the opposite sex if the changes of puberty haven't taken place. Both sides have valid points, and it's obvious that there is much more we need to learn—as medical professionals and as a society.

The fact remains, however, that it isn't easy being on the transgender continuum. And it *is* just as varied as sexual orientation. Some physical males clearly see themselves as female; some physical females clearly see themselves as men. These are *transgender*.

Then, there are those who don't see themselves as any particular gender, as being somewhere in between male or female or completely free of gender altogether. This group of people is known, as a matter of personal preference, by a number of descriptions, including *genderqueer, agender, gender-free*. Some see themselves as being a distinctly third gender, and a number are resistant to any labels being attached to their gender identification.

There are, as you can see, a number of variations of individuals in the trans community. Some opt for sex change surgery—whether full or in part. Some dress and act in accordance with their gender identification but retain the genitals they were born with. Some know and express their differences at an early age; others are much older when they come to terms with the difference between their apparent sex and the way they feel inside.

The award-winning writer and college professor Jennifer Finney Boylan had always had a notion, from vague to nagging, that there was a discordance between who she was and the person she appeared to be. But she lived a quite traditional life, advancing in her writing and teaching careers, getting married to the love of her life and being a devoted father to two sons before coming to terms, with great anguish, with the person she really was. Now, years later, she has fully transitioned from a man to a woman, is still married to the same woman, and has an excellent relationship with both sons. Her journey to this point was far from pain-free, but it is probably the best public example of an excellent outcome of the transgender experience.

It's a much harder road for others—especially, as Jennifer Finney Boylan pointed out herself in a recent New York Times article—those who are people of color and/or who live in poverty and are at greater risk of violence. Transgender people in general have a significantly higher risk of suicide and suicide attempts. While studies have found that 4.6% of the overall U.S. population has reported a suicide attempt and 10–20% of gays, lesbians and bisexuals report a suicide attempt, 41% of those transgender or gender non-conforming people have attempted suicide. This higher rate of suicidal thoughts and behavior is not due to a higher rate of mental illness but is rather due to the ostracism, bullying, rejection and physical threats gender non-conforming people face in this society. The risk of suicide is particularly high in those who feel rejected by their parents and extended families.

One mother, whose daughter has become her son, says that, "The decision to love and support him is a decision that could make the difference between life and death."

Support can make such a difference. A recent Canadian study examining the impact of Gay-Straight Alliance groups in high schools nationwide came up with a surprising finding: the presence of and participation in such groups brings down the rate of suicide attempts among gay, lesbian, bisexual *and* straight teens! It was thought that the more open and tolerant environment that the presence of such groups creates in schools enables all students to feel less labeled and more free to be themselves.

There is evidence, too, that acceptance of the fluidity of sexual orientation and gender identity—the two aspects of our sexuality about which none of us has a choice—is much more common in the younger generations. While not every young person is as free-thinking as Miley Cyrus, who refuses to label herself on the gender identity scale or to commit to a specific sexual orientation (saying that she is up for anything with someone over the age of 18 and that doesn't involve an animal), fewer young people today see themselves as sexual orientation or gender-trait extremes. A recent report from YouGov found that 93% of adults over 65 identified themselves on the sexual orientation scale as either a zero (completely heterosexual) or a six (completely homosexual) while 7% described themselves with varying degrees of bisexuality (between one and five on the scale). In contrast, among those between the ages of 18 and 29, 66 percent described themselves as a zero or six while 29% considered themselves somewhere in between the two extremes.

Since both sexual orientation and gender identification are intrinsic parts of the people we are, it makes sense to take steps to accept, support and even celebrate our differences.

SEX EDUCATION AND YOUR SEXUAL CHOICES

I can't talk to my parents about sex. Their only sex education is "Don't you dare!" Now they're upset about a new sex education class offered next year at my school and I'm afraid they won't sign a permission slip for me to be in the class, which would be so embarrassing, plus I want to know the facts about sex. I don't have any plans to do anything because I do want to be a virgin when I get married. I really believe in that. But I feel really stupid around my friends and confused. I think a sex education class would help. How can I convince my parents to let me take it?

Sarah H.

Our sex education comes from a wide variety of sources—some helpful and some not so helpful. We get impressions about sex by what we see on TV and in the movies. We pick up certain ideas and attitudes from what our parents *don't* say as well as from what they *do* tell us. We learn many things—some correct, many not—from our friends. And, despite the controversy surrounding school-based sex education programs, we can also learn a great deal from these.

Ideally, a sex education program at school or, less formally, at home from parents, needs to include discussions of all aspects of sexuality, *including* the option of abstinence. There are many good reasons for abstinence from sexual intercourse during the teen years: we'll be discussing these later in this chapter. However, to limit all discussion to this highly suggested option neglects the needs of teens whose values and choices differ. A good sex education course needs to discuss the following:

- *Sexual choices*—including abstinence.
- *Respect for yourself and others*, whatever your sexual choices. Teens of both sexes

need to be educated about the necessity of respecting another's feelings and values. Both boys and girls need to respect another's right to say no without ridicule. Both sexes need to discuss and to learn what responsible sexuality is all about—and what intimacy means, with or without sex as a component of an intimate relationship.

- *Facts about the body and about sexuality.* This includes understanding how males and females differ biologically and socially. Understanding biological differences—such as the fact that males may become sexually excited faster and more urgently during a kissing or making-out session and, on the other hand, that their health and sanity are not in danger if their sexual urges are not fulfilled on the spot—can help young people of both sexes avoid trouble. Understanding the social pressures of being male or female in junior high or high school—the pressures on guys to be macho and "perform," and on girls to have a boyfriend—may lead to more mutual compassion and good communication.

- *Practical facts about sexuality*—including information about birth control and sexually transmitted diseases. In many ways, education about birth control underscores one's risk of getting pregnant if one has sex—and may lead to sexual responsibility, not wild abandon. Education about sexually transmitted diseases is also vital—and may deter some teens from having sex at this point in their lives while helping others protect themselves against various health risks.

It is also vital to know about how one thing can lead to another if you don't realize what's happening. The fact is, some teens engage in activities such as deep kissing, petting, and oral sex without realizing that these are part of sexual foreplay and can lead to unplanned intercourse unless you know specifically know far you're prepared to go and stick to your decision. So knowing explicit details about sex, rather than inciting impulsive action, may actually help you make more responsible choices.

WHAT IS SEX ANYWAY—WHEN YOU'RE MAKING CHOICES?

> I have a friend (we're both 15) who claims she's a virgin because she's only had oral sex with her boyfriend. I say I'm more of a virgin because I haven't done anything like that. We both took abstinence pledges, but I think I'm sticking to mine better. She said that the oral sex doesn't count as sex at all because she has only done it to her boyfriend (he doesn't do it to her) and she has never "come." She said for something to be sex, you have to "come." This all sounds bogus to me!
>
> Emily A., 15

Emily and her friend raise some interesting points about what people consider abstinence and what people consider having sex.

By a number of definitions, not having had vaginal sexual intercourse (if you're heterosexual) makes you a virgin and abstinent. If you're gay or lesbian, a definition of virginity just might extend to specific homosexual practices and exclude heterosexual sex! One recent study conducted by researchers at the Prevention Research Center in California. and the Pacific Institute for Research and Evaluation in Maryland found that 83.5% of teens polled believed that an adolescent was still a virgin if he or she performed any genital touching, and over 70% believed that you could participate in oral sex without losing your virginity. Some 16.1% believed that you would still be a virgin despite engaging in anal sex. The study also found that those who reported having prior sexual experience (like touching or oral sex) were three to eight times more likely than less sexually-experienced teens to agree that peers engaging in those behaviors were virgins. In terms of what entailed abstinence, 89% of teens in the study agreed that those having vaginal intercourse were *not* abstinent. (We'd be fascinated to know what the other 11% considered to be sex—and abstinence!)

The fact is, one can do a lot of talking about what it means to be a virgin or to be abstinent, but the important thing to remember is that every sexual activity you engage in is a choice—and not without risks.

You can get sexually transmitted infections—even HIV—from oral sex or anal sex or from genital contact that doesn't involve penetration. And even though getting pregnant as a result of sperm being deposited just outside the vagina isn't the easiest way to conceive, it can happen. It's also true, as we said before, that engaging in one sexual activity may lead to another, whether you planned on it or not.

Another important thing to consider: your own values and how important being abstinent is to you at this time in your life.

All the thoughts and feelings that go into making such important choices in your life can be difficult to discuss with people. Your friends may or may not share your values and feelings about what is right for you. And, as much as you love your parents and know they love you, sexual choices can be a tough subject to bring up with them. And they may have difficulty talking with you about sex, too.

It's important to realize that many parents have difficulty talking about sex because *they* weren't raised to be open about the subject. (Their parents couldn't and didn't talk to them either!) When parents do talk, they may stress abstinence because of their love and concern for you. Most parents are well aware of the bad things that can happen as a result of sex too soon or with the wrong partner: not only the risks of AIDS and other sexually transmitted diseases and pregnancy, but also of the emotional pain that can come when and if the relationship ends. As much as they may want you to become independent, your parents still have a strong inclination to want to protect you from danger and from hurt. So their negative feelings about teen sex may not be coming from lack of caring or from prudery, but from their love for you.

These parents need to understand that correct information—from them and/or from school programs—will help you make more responsible, life-affirming choices. Studies have shown that teens who scored highest on tests of sex knowledge were much less likely to be having sex than their lower-scoring peers. Other studies have found that teenagers who have had complete sex education courses in school that cover all options and areas of information are more likely to use birth control if they do decide to have sex.

■ *How to make your own choices and decisions.* Some choices are too important to be left to chance—including choices about sexuality. And these choices aren't always easy. For example, making a decision about whether or not to have sex with someone you truly love, someone who cares about you, respects you, and loves you, too, is quite different from making the decision not to have sex with a casual date who is coming on strong. Your choice, in both cases, may be *not* to have sex, but saying no to someone who really matters to you is very hard. And saying yes to sexual involvement can be difficult, too, and is not necessarily just a matter of going with the flow and letting your hormones take the lead.

Some people have difficulty accepting the fact that teens have—or should have—choices about their sexuality and feel that parent-mandated rules should be the law. While parental values and wishes *do* need to be respected and considered (because, more often than not, your parents, above all others, have your best interests at heart), your parents can't be with you 24 hours a day or on every date. You will be faced—and probably already have been faced—with making choices on your own. That's why it's so important that you know how to think and decide for yourself what's best for you. Many times, this may coincide with what your parents want for you. Sometimes it may not. Either way, you need to feel confident and empowered by your own decision-making ability. You need to be able to stand up for what

you want and not let someone else—including a partner—talk you into anything that doesn't feel right for you.

Whatever your choices—right now and in the future—making them with as much information at hand at possible will help ensure that you will make wiser, more responsible decisions.

MAKING SEXUAL CHOICES

I'm 13 and confused. Well, I want to know if you could have any idea when you are ready to have sex? I want to but I'm scared, and all the risks that are involved are holding me back. Can you help me out?

Confused Greatly

You have sexual choices all the time. You don't have to be sexually active to do this. Deciding that you would rather be a virgin until marriage or, at least, for a while longer is a sexual choice—and can be a very positive one!

Deciding how to deal with your sexual feelings is a choice, too. Some people enjoy fantasies. Some masturbate. Some choose to have sex with other people. And some choose all three or varying combinations.

Sexual decision making is an important part of deciding who you are and what your values are. It's vital that your actions match your values. Otherwise, you will feel bad about yourself and guilty about your choice. All sexual choices—from choosing to have sex with someone or choosing, at least for now, to abstain from sexual activity—can and should be joyous ones, made after careful reflection and with a strong sense of what's right for you.

MASTURBATION

Is masturbation normal? Can it harm you? Can you do it too much (and maybe use up all your sperm so that you can't have children when you're grown up and married)?

Just Asking

Masturbation is a natural expression of sexuality for males and females, young and old. It means sexual stimulation of oneself—in some instances, to the point of orgasm. It is estimated that about 97 percent of males and 90 percent of females have masturbated by the age of 21. Contrary to old wives' tales, masturbation will not cause hair to grow on your palms; make you sterile, blind or insane; give you acne; or take your virginity. It can offer release from sexual tensions, particularly if you are not sexually active in other ways. Of course, many married people and others with satisfying sex lives may masturbate as well.

Masturbation is also the safest form of sexual activity is you're concerned about avoiding the risk of AIDS. (Between two people, the safest sex is in a long-term, mutually monogamous relationship in which both partners were virgins coming into the relationship and who have no other risk factors—for example, IV drug use or a history of blood transfusions before 1985.) Other benefits of masturbation include releasing sexual tensions, growing to learn what you enjoy, and experiencing orgasm.

Orgasm, a normal sexual experience, means reaching a height of sexual excitement. For the male, this means ejaculation. Women, of course, don't ejaculate, but have feelings of intense excitement and, sometimes, a throbbing feeling in the genitals followed by the same sense of relaxation and peace that a man may feel after ejaculation. Orgasm may occur when you're fantasizing about sex or masturbation or when you're having some sort of sexual contact—from petting to intercourse—with someone else.

Can masturbation ever be harmful? Only in a few instances. First, if you are extremely religious and/or your values and beliefs are making you feel extremely guilty about masturbation, this may be a problem for you. The self-hatred that may be a by-product of extreme guilt may drive you to masturbate even more. And so you're caught in a cycle of misery.

How can you deal with this? You may want to talk about your feelings with your physician, clergyperson, or someone else you can trust to listen and who may reassure you that you are, indeed, quite normal. Whether or not you do masturbate is very much a matter of personal choice. If you do, it doesn't make you bad. If you choose not to, due to your personal beliefs, it doesn't make you strange. It's up to you.

Many teens wonder if it's possible to masturbate too often. How often is too often? That's a good question—and one that's difficult to answer. In general, however, masturbation—though healthy and normal—is not meant to take the place of other things in your life. If you find yourself using masturbation as a crutch to avoid problems, facing feelings, challenges, or social encounters with others, you may want to re-evaluate its place in your life and make some changes.

A number of young people feel very guilty about group masturbation, which is quite common especially in early adolescence, especially in boys. This may mean masturbating in the presence of a friend or friends or touching each other in erotic ways. Among boys, some of these group masturbation sessions are almost competitive games to see who can ejaculate fastest and farthest. This can all seem like a good idea at that time, but some teens are plagued with guilt afterward, wondering why they did it and if this means that they're gay.

Especially in the early teens, such group masturbation is quite common and is not considered abnormal. As your own body is developing, you may have an intense curiosity about others, wanting to see if they have the same feelings you do. Finding out that others may look, feel, and respond much like you do may help to reinforce your own positive feelings about yourself and your ability to function sexually. Testing this ability around friends of the same sex may be somewhat less threatening if you happen to be quite young and still a bit uncomfortable with the opposite sex. But remember: it's important not to label yourself. Participating or not participating in group masturbation is very much a matter of personal choice. Some do it more than others, and some never try it at all—and that's OK, too.

RELATING TO OTHERS

My boyfriend is trying to talk me into having sex with him, but I'm scared of being used.

It isn't that I don't love him, but I don't feel ready to have sex. But I don't want to lose him. What should I do?

Maureen M.

Making decisions about whether to become sexually involved with another person and building non-exploitive relationships with the opposite sex can be extremely difficult when there's so much peer pressure to be sexually active, to "score" and to be popular, and, especially for girls, to have a special boyfriend. In such a pressure-filled atmosphere, it can be difficult to make a few choices about your sexuality, about what you will—or won't—do at this time. Yet free choices are what non-exploitive relationships are all about.

Many young people are choosing to postpone sexual activity these days. A recent government study found the numbers of teens overall who have had sex has dropped noticeably since the early 1990s. A recent government study announced by the National Center for Health Statistics revealed that in 2005 (the last year for which statistics were available) 47 percent of high school students reported that they had had sexual intercourse, compared with 54 percent of high school students who were sexually active in 1991.

So, right now, it's likely that the majority of people you know have not had sex. In some way, though, that's less important than what feels right for you at this moment. In fact, you may discover that there are some very good reasons for you to say no to sexual activity right now.

12 Reasons to Say No Right Now
1. *You don't feel ready.* This is one of the most important reasons *not* to have sex. Feeling ready—instead of pressured—can make

sex a whole different experience, when you freely choose to engage in it.

2. *Premarital sex is against your beliefs and values.* Your values matter—a lot! And if you violate them, the guilt and anxiety you would feel would override any enjoyment. Why put yourself through such an emotionally taxing experience?

3. *You're in love for the first time.* Be cautious. Go slow. You're emotionally vulnerable to pain when your feelings are so strong and new and when you have so little experience with love and loss. Work on building a strong, stable relationship as well as on your own self-esteem before even *thinking* about having sex.

4. *Your partner is pressuring you.* Beware of the person who ignores your feelings and tries to threaten or bully or cajole you into sex before you feel ready. If he or she really cares, your partner will respect your values, even if they don't agree with his or hers.

5. *You don't know anything about and/or are too embarrassed to use birth control.* This is a splendid reason to wait. Until you can learn which methods of birth control work and which ones don't, you don't know enough to have responsible sex. Furthermore, until you can admit that you are —or will be—sexually active and use a reliable method of birth control, you're not mature enough to cope with the many responsibilities of a sexual relationship.

6. *Pregnancy would be a personal disaster for you.* No birth control method except abstinence is 100 percent effective. If a pregnancy would be a real disaster right now—for reasons of health, education,

family, relationship or other personal matters—abstinence is the best way to avoid this.

7. *You want your first time to be extra-special.* You will probably always remember—for better or worse—the first time you have sex. Do yourself a favor and wait for the right time, the right person, and the best possible circumstances. Do you really want your first time to be in the back seat of a musty old car? Or a rushed encounter before your parents get home from work? Don't create never-to-be-forgotten memories you'd really rather forget!

8. *Your relationship is in jeopardy.* Relationship problems are not solved by having sex—even if your major problem is the fact that you and your partner differ over sexual choices.

9. *You don't know each other well.* The best sexual sharing comes with someone you know and trust. Sex, under the right circumstances and with the right person, can be very special. Why do it with someone who *isn't* special to you?

10. *You're concerned about sexually transmitted diseases.* You're right—and you're smart—to be concerned. Besides the risk of HIV, a number of other sexually transmitted infections can threaten your health and your future fertility in addition to your dignity. If you're sexually active, you are at risk for sexually transmitted diseases. The more sex partners you have, particularly people you don't know well, the greater your risk. It's smart to consider these risks beforehand—and these can be an excellent reason not to have sex right now.

THE TEENAGE BODY BOOK

11. *You don't know much about sex.* Read. Take a sex education course. Talk with your parents or other informed adults. Bring a list of questions to your doctor. Become a theoretical expert first. Knowing the real facts about sex can help safeguard your health and your future.

12. *You're tempted to have sex for nonsexual reasons.* Maybe you're not especially popular and think that being sexually active will change all that. Despite what you may think, having sex cannot make you genuinely popular, ensure a lasting, loving relationship, boost your self-esteem, or decrease loneliness. If you have sex to get what you can really only give yourself, you will be disappointed.

Taking the time to learn how to build and nurture friendships can help you grow into a giving and mature person who can fully share with another when the time, person, and circumstances are right.

How to Know When You're Ready for Sex

The decision when and with whom to have sex is, ultimately, entirely yours. How do you make a responsible decision regarding sexual involvement? You might start by asking yourself a number of questions.

■ *Am I trying to prove something to others? To myself? How do I really feel about having sex right now? How does my partner feel?* It's important to know why you're thinking of having sex and how you feel about it—and how your partner feels. If you're in a loving, committed relationship and the choice seems right to both of you, it may well be the right decision.

But it's also important to know what sex cannot do for you—in case you may be thinking of sex for nonsexual reasons. Sex cannot fill gaping holes in your self-esteem or make you instantly wise, mature, and adult. Sex also cannot necessarily bind you to another person forever or make love, commitment, and intimacy grow where these qualities never existed before.

■ *What feelings do I have for the other person?* If you see your potential sex partner as a challenge, a conquest, or someone who's simply there and available—stop and think before acting. For the best possible sexual experience, wait for someone you like very much or love, someone you know well and with whom you can be comfortably yourself.

■ *Do we communicate well?*

Can you talk openly and honestly?

Can you share what you're really feeling?

Can you talk about what sex means to you individually and as a couple?

Can you make a responsible decision together, sharing the responsibilities for being involved and for whatever consequences may occur? Can you talk to one another about birth control, for example?

Can you tell each other if something hurts, is uncomfortable, or is distasteful to you?

Can you talk about your expectations—and your fears?

■ *Do I have accurate information about sex?* Sexual/anatomical ignorance can cause a lot of unplanned pregnancies *and* a lot of grief and disappointment when the people involved don't have enough information about their own bodies—and each other's bodies—to fully give and receive sexual pleasure.

■ *Are we willing to take full responsibility for our actions?* Responsibility means reviewing all possibilities—and options—in advance. Pregnancy and sexually transmitted diseases are two very real risks of sexual involvement.

What will you do in the event of an unplanned pregnancy? Could you be supportive of one another? What options would you have?

If one of you noticed symptoms of a sexually transmitted disease, could you take the responsibility of telling your partner and suggesting that you both get tested?

Do you know how to prevent an unplanned pregnancy? Have you learned what the most reliable methods of birth control are and how they can be obtained and used?

More to the point: *will* you take the responsibility of using a reliable method of birth control? Are you mature enough to plan ahead to prevent a pregnancy?

"Birth control is like planning for sex, and I feel that such planning is wrong. Sex should be romantic and just happen..." is a comment we have heard a lot—often from teenage mothers. Some of these teens are victims of the old double standard, which see the man as the seducer and the woman as the seduced. This old myth seems to say that, unless a woman is quite literally swept off her feet, she's no lady.

A variation on this theme is the romance myth that says that sex is romantic only when it is totally unexpected. Some victims of the "He swept me off my feet!" school of thought feel that they have to get drunk or stoned to make sex OK.

Others feel that just getting carried away with passion justifies the act. This attitude is reinforced by many popular TV shows—especially the daytime and nighttime soaps—where characters lead active sex lives, but only rarely seem to concern themselves with birth control

The fact is, planned sex can be extremely romantic. In some cases, it may be much more so than the so-called spontaneous variety of sex. Taking birth control precautions to avoid an unwanted pregnancy and to help alleviate the fear of such pregnancy can free you both to enjoy such sex.

Birth control should be a mutual decision and discussed well *before* having sex, not during or after. Seeking a reliable method of birth control means admitting to yourself and, possibly, to others that you are—or soon will be—sexually active.

Can you do this?

If you're not ready to face this responsibility, you're not ready to have sex.

■ *Are we loving, caring friends?* There's a lot to be said for waiting until you can have sex with a very special friend:

A friend will not make fun of you or criticize you if you're clumsy, uncertain, or scared.

A friend will enjoy sharing all kinds of experiences—some sexual and some not—with you.

A friend is not likely to say "You got pregnant? That's *your* problem!"

A friend will not brag and tell all.

A friend will ask,"How do you feel?" and value your beliefs, your opinions, and your feelings.

A friend will care about you—as a person.

When we're just learning about our sexual selves and having our first sexual experiences, it really helps to have a partner who is also a caring friend.

Sex vs. Intimacy

Many people think that sex and intimacy are the same. But this is not so. Ideally, of course, emotional intimacy is a vital part of a sexual relationship, but this is not always the case. Some people have sex without emotional intimacy. Many others have intimate relationships that don't include sex. And some people are able to build a lovely blend of the two.

Intimacy means that you feel safe in a relationship—safe enough to be yourself and to be vulnerable with another person—and that this other person feels the same safety and freedom. It means honest communication and nonjudgmental emotional support. Real intimacy isn't instant or easy. It takes time and effort to build.

Being truly intimate with another does not mean constantly baring your soul. It can also mean being comfortable together in silence. It means finding joy in sharing ordinary—as well as extraordinary—moments together.

Sex is not an inevitable part of the ordinary or extraordinary experiences that intimate relationships bring. You can have wonderful feelings of closeness with a variety of people with whom you will never have sex. Intimate friendships—whether these involve friends of the same or the opposite sex or your family members—can be passionate in spirit, feeling, and commitment and can bring a great deal of love, joy, and satisfaction into your life.

With someone who you feel might become a lover or life partner, developing a passionate, intimate friendship is an excellent way to grow into love. In fact, sex—particularly sex too soon in your life or too soon in the relationship—can *interfere* with intimacy if it is used as a shortcut or substitute for all the steps you need to take in order to develop an intimate bond with another person. There are no shortcuts or substitutes for talking, sharing feelings, or taking the time to get to know each other as valuable, distinct individuals and to build solid mutual trust. Substituting sex for any of these vital steps may make true emotional intimacy impossible.

However, intimacy can greatly enhance sexual sharing. While sex with a mysterious, exciting stranger may be a fun fantasy, in real life you may find—when you do feel ready for sex—that sexual sharing in an atmosphere of loving trust and mutual vulnerability is the most rewarding kind of sexual experience you can have.

You may find that each intimate relationship—sexual or not—has a unique and treasured place in your life, in the present or in your loving memories. Developing the capacity to be intimate, comfortable, and caring with others can mean a lifetime of abundance—in love, in friends, and in the very special joy true intimacy can bring.

Growing to be your own person, making your own informed choices, being sensitive to the rights of others to be themselves, and learning to take responsibility for your own actions can greatly enhance your life in many ways—including your sexuality and your relationships on all levels.

With time and personal growth, so much of the pressure, fear, and uncertainty you may be feeling now will fade. In its place may be joy in your uniqueness—your feelings, your fantasies, and your beliefs. There may also be new joy in sharing who you have become with someone else. There will also be the joy of discovering another person in a myriad of ways: talking, touching, laughing, crying, liking, loving, and discovering each other, not only as lovers but also as very special friends!

QUICK SCAN

YOU AND YOUR SEXUALITY

✔ Sexuality is part of who we are; sex is something we do.

✔ Sexual fantasies are normal whether or not you're having sex and can actually reduce sexual tension.

✔ Masturbation is something most people—male or female—do at some point in their lives. It isn't harmful unless it violates your own values and makes you feel terribly guilty or unless it begins to take over your life. But, for most people, it is a pleasurable and healthy choice of sexual activity.

✔ Researchers don't know exactly what makes one person homosexual and another person heterosexual. But it's important to know that sexual orientation is part of who we are, like having blue eyes or brown hair or musical talent. It isn't a choice.

✔ What matters most is not whether you are gay or straight, but whether you're able to love and have non-exploitive relationships with others.

✔ Gender identification—how you see yourself as male or female or somewhere in between—is as much a part of who you are as sexual orientation.

✔ If you don't feel ready to have sex or if your partner is pressuring you, DON'T!

✔ Developing an intimate friendship with another person—which may or may not involve sex at this time—is an excellent way to grow in love. Sex too soon can actually interfere with intimacy. Intimacy isn't just closeness and passion; it's feeling safe with another and free to be truly yourself.

TWELVE

The Truth About Sexually Transmitted Diseases

We had this totally disgusting lecture from some sort of expert in our health class today on all kinds of diseases you can get by having sex. I think she was just trying to scare us. I mean, she spent so much time talking about AIDS—which normal people don't get—right? Also, since things like gonorrhea can be easily cured, or so I've heard, what's the big deal if you get something like that? I think that adults are just trying to scare us into not having sex. Am I right?

Michelle P.

Michelle's view of sexually transmitted diseases (STDs)—also now known as sexually transmitted infections (STIs)—that they always happen to someone else, that they can be easily cured without any harm done, that they're just too disgusting for a nice person to hear about, let alone have—is fairly common, but quite inaccurate.

The most basic fact about sexually transmitted diseases is this: **If you are having sex, you are running the risk of getting sexually transmitted diseases.**

If you want to avoid getting a sexually transmitted disease, you have several choices:

- You can choose to abstain (not have sex at all).
- You can wait to have sex until you're married and then marry someone who is also a virgin—and be faithful to each other.
- You can take all the precautions you possibly can to cut down the risk of getting a sexually transmitted disease.

Preventing sexually transmitted diseases is especially important these days. Even though new combination treatments have extended HIV-infected persons' lifetimes for years, even decades, young people—both men and women—*are* dying from AIDS. Once you have it, there may be treatments, but there is no vaccine and no 100 percent cure.

Genital herpes is also incurable, though not fatal. And even diseases that people take more for granted these days—such as gonorrhea—or perhaps have never heard about—such as chlamydia—can threaten a woman's future fertility by causing pelvic inflammatory disease in her fallopian tubes. Pelvic inflammatory disease (PID) can be very serious, even fatal in some instances.

Particularly in women, a number of sexually transmitted diseases are not easy to detect or to treat.

It's important to know, too, that sexually transmitted diseases can happen to anyone—nice people included. You can have only one sex partner, have sex only occasionally, and keep yourself very clean—and still get a sexually transmitted disease. You can have sex only with someone you love and still be infected with a sexually transmitted disease. Love is not protection, unfortunately, against sexually transmitted diseases.

While it may not be pleasant to think about such possibilities, it's vital to know as much as you can about the risks, symptoms, and treatments of the more common sexually transmitted diseases so that you can decrease your risk of infection and know when to check with your physician for early diagnosis and treatment. (Early treatment is crucial with several forms of STDs.) Since sexually transmitted diseases are at epidemic proportions nationwide, chances are that an STD could happen to you or someone you know. The statistics are shocking:

- Young people ages 13–24 accounted for 26 percent of all new cases of HIV infections in the U.S. in 2010, showing a 22 percent increase from 2008, according to statistics from the Centers for Disease Control (CDC). Of these, most were gay and bisexual males, and more than half of these were African Americans.

- An estimated 60 percent of HIV-positive youth don't know that they are infected, putting them at risk of not only of infecting others, but also developing AIDS and dying at a young age.
- Never heard of AIDS happening to someone young? In 2013, nearly three thousand youths in the U.S. were diagnosed with AIDS, representing 10 percent of those diagnosed that year.
- An estimated 156 youths with AIDS died in 2012.
- Sexually transmitted disease infection rates are highest among young adults 15 to 25 years old.
- There are an estimated two million cases of gonorrhea and three million cases of chlamydia infections each year in all age groups. These two diseases, often undetected and untreated until major symptoms develop, are a leading cause of sterility in young people.
- Teenage girls have the highest rate of gonorrhea in the U.S. Teen boys run a close second. The rate of gonorrhea infection is 20 *times* higher in teen girls than in women over 30, according to statistics from the Centers for Disease Control and Prevention.
- One in four sexually active teens in the United States will become infected with an STD before they turn 20.
- More than five million Americans (and estimates have been much higher) are suffering from genital herpes, with 500,000 new cases each year and, as yet, no cure.

While syphilis and gonorrhea are often the first diseases people think about when sexually transmitted diseases are mentioned, these are much less likely to occur in teens than diseases such as genital herpes or chlamydia, which is the most frequently seen sexually transmitted disease among teenagers.

The following is an overview of some of the troublesome and common sexually transmitted diseases.

AIDS

Can you get AIDS if you're not gay? How do you get it? I mean, can you get it in ways besides having sex, like from swimming pools or if someone with AIDS sneezes near you or something? Can you get AIDS from donating blood? From kissing? I've heard all kinds of rumors and stuff. What's the truth?

Brad A.

What is it?

When people talk about HIV/AIDS these days, they mean two things: infection with the virus that can lead to AIDS (HIV) and the development of AIDS.

According to the Centers for Disease Control, an estimated 62,400 youths were living with HIV in the U.S. at the end of 2012. Of these, 32,000 were undiagnosed, and thus unaware of their infection. As a result, they are not only a threat to others, but also are seriously at risk for going on to develop AIDS because they haven't had the help of the powerful medications that can keep HIV from developing into full-blown AIDS.

The CDC estimates that, left untreated, an HIV infection will progress on to AIDS within 10 years, on the average. Many adults

now being diagnosed with AIDS were actually infected with HIV as adolescents.

AIDS (Acquired Immune Deficiency Syndrome) is a breakdown and failure of the body's immune system and is caused by a virulent strain of a virus called HTLV-III. The virus is usually introduced into the body through intimate sexual contact or by exposure to contaminated blood via a shared hypodermic needle or as a blood transfusion. (The HIV virus is present in the body fluid—primarily blood and semen—of an infected person. And it's possible for someone to have the virus in his or her body fluids without yet having any symptoms.)

According to current research, there is no evidence that you can become infected with the HIV virus through casual contact with an infected person. This means that being in the same room with a person with HIV or AIDS, even if he or she is coughing or sneezing, is not likely to expose you to the infection. However, if a person with AIDS happens to have tuberculosis (a disease that quite often infects people with AIDS) and was coughing, you could be exposed to tuberculosis—but not to AIDS. You cannot acquire HIV/AIDS through hugging, touching, or kissing an infected person on the cheek or closed lips. (It's not yet clear whether the virus can be spread via saliva. So far, no cases have been reported involving the transmission of the HIV virus via French kissing, but, to be safe, until we have more information, it may be best to avoid such kissing with an infected person or someone in a high-risk category.)

You cannot acquire HIV/AIDS by eating a meal or swimming in a pool with someone who has AIDS. (The pool chemicals and water should dilute and kill the virus which, outside the human body, is really quite fragile.) You also cannot get infected with HIV by donating blood. All needles used on blood donors are sterilized and used only once.

How does AIDS destroy a person's health and take his or her life? Once in the bloodstream, the HTLV-III virus attacks and kills a special kind of white blood cell called a *T-cell*. The T-cells are essential to the effective functioning of the body's immune system. Once these T-cells are damaged and depleted, the body is vulnerable to any number of infections and diseases. Some of these, which would be minor or easily cured in a healthy person, such as a yeast infection, are very serious and long-lasting and can even be fatal to a person with AIDS.

Symptoms

Some people can carry the HIV virus and have no symptoms at all. A blood test can detect exposure to the HIV by noting antibodies to the virus in the blood. There is also a new test for the HIV virus using a sample of saliva. This may be especially helpful for those patients who are frightened by needles and blood tests.

It is still too early to tell how many people who have antibodies to the virus go on to develop AIDS. It is possible, even if you don't have any signs of the disease, to transmit the virus to others. So anyone who tests positive is advised to either abstain from sex altogether or, at the very least, use strict safe-sex measures.

Please note: Today there are sophisticated laboratory tests—such as PCR (DNA tests)—to detect HIV very early. Also, there is current research into AIDS prevention, specifically treating people who have been exposed to the HIV virus. All of this is important for a number of

reasons. For example, if a woman is planning a pregnancy or is already pregnant, knowing her HIV status can be crucial to the health of her baby. Researchers have found that giving the drug AZT to HIV-positive pregnant women and to their babies can lower these babies' infection rate significantly—with fewer than 10 percent of these babies being infected with the HIV virus! In terms of prevention for teens and adults, researchers are currently studying a "morning-after treatment" for AIDS exposure. Who would get this? A person who had unsafe sex the night before (as a result of a condom breaking or impulsive sex without protection, with partner who is known to be infected with HIV or who is in a group at high risk for HIV infection). This experimental preventive treatment with the drug AZT to see whether a rapid high dose of this medicine can indeed prevent an individual from becoming infected is still in early stages of research and not available to the general public yet.

Treatment

Doctors treat symptoms and infections associated with AIDS and are sometimes successful in temporarily alleviating these. Until the mid-1990s, the best-known drug used in the treatment of AIDS was AZT. Then, in the mid-1990s, a new group of drugs called *protease inhibitors* was developed. These drugs work in a different way on HIV and have caused many AIDS patients to improve their health very significantly with weight gain and fewer infections. Some have even been able to return to work. Also, some people infected with HIV are long-time survivors, infected with the virus for over fifteen years, and still have not developed AIDS. Ongoing studies are looking at what keeps full-blown AIDS from developing in these survivors.

Researchers are working intensely on testing trial AIDS prevention vaccines. Unfortunately, at the time of this writing there is no vaccine and still no cure for AIDS. Despite so many new (and expensive) drugs, AIDS often leads to an early death.

Special Risk Groups

Anyone who has sex, particularly with more than one partner and without using safe-sex precautions (to be discussed later in this chapter) is at risk for HIV/AIDS infection. At this time, however, some people are at greater risk that others. These include the following:

- Gay and bisexual men—with those between ages 17 and 25 at special risk. A study of young gays by the San Francisco Department of Health's Office of AIDS found that 14 percent of gay and bisexual men between ages 17 and 19 were infected with HIV and that 30 percent of the survey participants reported engaging in unprotected anal intercourse, the highest-risk sexual activity. Teenage gay men under age 19 were as likely to engage in unsafe sex as gay men in their late twenties. These young people told researchers that they didn't feel personally threatened by HIV infection, that they considered it a problem for older gay men.
- *Homeless youth*: These include many teens who are kicked out of their family homes, often because they are gay, lesbian, bisexual or transgender. Their numbers are growing—the Congressional Research Service estimates that there are more than 1 million homeless youths, and between 1 million and 1.7 million runaway/throwaway youths. While an estimated 7–8 percent of adolescents are sex-

ual minorities, these represent 29 percent of homeless youth. And they're in danger—all too often being victimized as they sleep in public places or because they engage in "survival sex" (exchanging sex for food and shelter). Many become involved with older gay men, who are more likely to carry the HIV infection and pass it on to them.

- Intravenous drug users, who may be exposed by shared needles.
- Hemophiliacs and others who require transfusions of blood or blood products. (However, this risk has diminished significantly since 1985, when blood supplies began to be tested for the virus and donors screened more carefully.)
- Those who have sex with any of those in major risk groups. This would include women who have sex with bisexual men, IV drug users, or men who have sex with women exposed to AIDS by drug use or other sex partners. (That is why, these days, sex with a prostitute is particularly risky. Besides having many sexual partners, many female prostitutes are often also IV drug users.)
- Babies of women infected with the virus. As we discussed earlier, considerable progress has been made in prevention of AIDS infection in infants. The result is that there are fewer HIV-infected babies. However, prevention is the key: to receive prenatal preventive care, a woman has to know that she is infected. So testing all pregnant women for the AIDS virus is vital.
- Sexually active teenagers. There are several reasons for this. Studies show that today's teens are more likely to have sex at an early age, to have multiple sex partners as they go through adolescence, and to

neglect safe-sex practices, even when they know better theoretically. The "it can't happen to me" mindset, such a factor in teenage pregnancy in the past, has now, often tragically, become a risk factor for sexually transmitted diseases in teens.

These are just the groups in which HIV/ AIDS is most often seen right now. But everyone who has sex is at risk. And most people infected with HIV or full-blown AIDS are relatively young—a great many in their twenties. Some experts feel that teenagers are the next major risk group. When you're young, it's very easy to feel immortal and that nothing really bad will happen to you or someone you know. Some health educators sadly observe that teens many not take the risk of AIDS seriously until they see their friends and classmates begin to die before their eyes. But, by that time, it may be too late. Be smart. Take precautions NOW.

BACTERIAL VAGINOSIS

I had this fishy kind of creamy discharge (sorry to be gross, but I want you to know what I'm talking about) and my doctor said it was a sexually transmitted disease! I'm really upset because I've only been having safe sex for two months and only with my boyfriend Kyle, who told me he was a virgin, too, when we made love for the first time. The doctor said it was bacterial vaginosis. What is THAT? I was too shy and embarrassed to ask him.

Shelli K.

What is it?

Bacterial vaginosis is a very common vaginal infection that is often, though not always, sexually transmitted. If there is a possibility of sexual transmission, the sex partner should be examined and treated, too, since men can carry and transmit this infection without having any symptoms themselves.

But you can get this infection without having sex. You may be at risk when you're under a lot of stress or have been taking antibiotics or because of poor personal hygiene. This infection is annoying, but not serious.

Symptoms

The primary symptom is a heavy, creamy grayish-white discharge that has a foul, fishy odor. This symptom is most likely to occur in the female partner if the infection has, in fact, been sexually transmitted.

Treatment

This infection can be cured with antibiotics, usually the medication Flagyl (metronidazole) in pill form and sometimes in one dose at your doctor's office.

CHLAMYDIA

For the past week, I've noticed a clear or kind of milky discharge at the tip of my penis, especially in the morning when I wake up. Also, it sort of burns when I urinate. Could this be gonorrhea? My girlfriend hasn't mentioned having any symptoms and I'm afraid to say anything about it to her. What could be the problem?

Gary D.

What is it?

Chlamydia is the number-one sexually transmitted disease in the United States. It is much more common than any other STD, affecting about four million new cases each year. It is estimated that one in ten teen girls is infected. Chlamydia is found most often in sexually active adolescents between ages 15 and 19. This disease is caused by the bacterium *Chlamydia trachomatis* and is usually spread during sexual intercourse with an infected person.

Symptoms

There are quite often no symptoms at all, either in men or women. One recent medical study revealed that some 75 percent of those with chlamydia had no symptoms at all. In the Teenage Clinic at Kaiser Permanente Medical Center in San Francisco, we have routinely tested all girls coming in for routine pelvic exams for chlamydia and found that 15 percent of them were infected—often without being aware of any symptoms. More recently, we have been using a special urine test called NATS (Nucleic Acid Amplification Test Screening)) or urine amplification—a special DNA test that can actually detect DNA strands of the chlamydia organism in the urine. So now woman can be tested for chlamydia without having a pelvic exam. For males, this urine test can screen for chlamydia and even gonorrhea without having a swab inserted in the penis.

Males are more often likely to have symptoms than females. These may include:

- Mild irritation or burning during urination
- A thin milky or clear discharge which is most often evident in the morning.

Some men mistake these symptoms for gonorrhea, but there are some important differences. The incubation period for chlamydia is longer (two or three weeks after exposure) and the discharge is lighter in color. (It is possible to have both gonorrhea and chlamydia at the same time, so if you notice any discharge from the penis, or irritation or discomfort during urination, check with the physician immediately—and let your female partner know about your symptoms so that she can be tested, too.) Chlamydia can also be transmitted between two males. However, since the disease can have more serious consequences in females, we have focused our discussion on heterosexual couples.

Unfortunately, most women do not have symptoms—sometimes not until damage has already been done to their reproductive organs via pelvic infection (pelvic inflammatory disease, or PID), which can occur in undetected, untreated chlamydia. You might ask your doctor to do a test for possible chlamydia if you have vague lower-abdominal pain or find yourself in a special risk category for this disease by answering yes to two or more of the following four questions:

- Are you under 24 years of age?
- Have you had intercourse with a new lover within the past two months?
- Do you use a non-barrier contraceptive? (Barrier contraceptives include the condom and the diaphragm.) Or do you use no contraceptive at all?
- Have you noticed mild bleeding after a gynecological exam or sexual intercourse?

If you are at increased risk, a test for chlamydia as soon as possible is an excellent safeguard for your health and future fertility. Ask your doctor or clinic if the urine screening test is available. After the initial test, plan to get routine follow-up tests for chlamydia twice a year.

Special Risks

Untreated Chlamydia can cause pelvic inflammatory disease (PID) in women — typical symptoms are lower abdominal tenderness or severe pain fever, fatigue, a vaginal discharge, and enlargement of the fallopian tubes — and can cause infertility or later tubal pregnancies due to fallopian tube scarring. It can, in some instances, even be fatal.

In men, untreated Chlamydia can cause inflammation of the major sperm-carrying passage from the testicle to the penis, possibly resulting in infertility.

Chlamydia has also been linked to conjunctivitis (an eye inflammation) and pneumonia in newborn babies whose mothers have the infection. About one-third of pneumonia cases in infants under six months of age are linked with their mothers' chlamydia. And a University of Washington study associated birth-acquired chlamydial infection with severe eye disease in some older children.

Treatment

Antibiotics in a pill form — Azithromycin or doxycycline– are usually prescribed. Azithromycin can be given in one dose at the doctor's office; a prescription for doxycycline would mean taking a pill twice a day for 7 days. In some states, legislation has also been passed that allows the doctor to treat the partner of a patient infected with Chlamydia. This would allow the doctor to give you a prescription for Azithromycin or doxycycline to give to your boyfriend or girlfriend. All treatment would be confidential.

GENITAL HERPES

How do you know if you have herpes? I really need to know! Does any blister on the penis mean herpes, or does it have to be painful? Is there anything that gets rid of these blisters or do you have them forever? Please hurry and let me know!

Scared

What is it?

Herpes progenitalis, or genital herpes, afflicts about one in five Americans age 12 or older. The rate of infection in teens nearly quintipled between 1980 and 1994, with about 4.5 percent of all teens now infected.

Herpes is caused by the herpes simplex type 2 virus, which is related to the virus that causes sores in or near the mouth. Researchers are finding that differences between these two types of herpes virus have narrowed in recent years. Some believe that this — and the growing incidence of genital herpes — may be due to an increase in oral sex, which can transmit herpes viruses of both types from mouth to genitals and back again.

Genital herpes has been called "the sexually transmitted disease without a cure" since its victims tend to suffer recurrent attacks, especially in times of stress. The virus, it seems, never leaves the body, but lodges in nerve tissue until conditions are right, when one's resistance is down, for the next attack.

Symptoms

Symptoms, which first appear 2 to 20 days after exposure (sexual contact with an infected person), include the following:

- Tiny clusters of painful, fluid-filled blisters on the labia, around the vagina, or in the vagina in women; on a man's penis; and possibly, around the anus of both sexes.
- Swollen lymph glands, aching muscles, and fever.

While symptoms usually diminish within a few weeks, the herpes virus lies dormant in the patient's body. Sometimes there is never another active episode of herpes.

Some people who are infected with the genital herpes never have any symptoms, but are still capable of transmitting it to others. In a study at the University of Washington, 636 female college students were tested for herpes. Nine percent were infected and 71 percent of these were completely unaware that they had herpes.

This brings up an important point. If, for any reason, you suspect that you have been exposed or may be at risk for herpes, don't rely on your own observation. Consult your doctor.

More commonly, however, the symptoms do recur, especially when the person's resistance is low due to illness or because of emotional stress. It doesn't take another sexual contact to trigger a repeat attack. Some people can feel recurrence coming on for hours or even a few days before the blisters appear. This burning, tingling, itching sensation is called the *prodrome* and appears in the area to be affected.

During this prodrome, as well as when sores are present, the person with herpes is most likely to infect a sex partner. But it's possible to infect another even when symptoms are not present. Some medical experts feel that regular, continual use of the medication acyclovir may reduce infectiousness. Also, those who are most likely to be infectious—those who have eruptions every four to six weeks—may want to protect sex partners during supposedly dormant times by using a condom. While this doesn't give total protection, it may reduce the risks of transmission.

Special Risks

Genital herpes can cause herpes encephalitis, a virulent, often fatal brain infection in infants born vaginally to mothers who have active cases of genital herpes. This complication can be prevented by Caesarian section delivery when the disease is in an active stage when the mother is due to deliver. Having a herpes infection when the baby is in the womb or having vaginal delivery when the disease is in an inactive stage will *not* infect the baby.

There may be a link, too, between genital herpes and cervical cancer. While this has not been proven conclusively, some studies have shown that women with a history of genital herpes may have an increased cervical cancer risk.

For this reason, a woman with herpes should be particularly cautious and get regular Pap tests. According to the American Cancer Society, cervical cancer is easily detected (via a Pap smear) and treated during its early stages, so the possibly increased risk of getting the disease should be a cause for caution, not panic.

Treatment

At this time, for genital herpes, just as with HIV infection, there is no cure. (A vaccine is currently undergoing clinical trials and may be available soon.) However, the antiviral medication *acyclovir*, taken in pill form, can alleviate symptoms and shorten or prevent recurrences. New research shows that daily use of this drug for three years is safe and effective. In a study of 525 people who had at least six herpes recurrences a year before taking acyclovir, 61 percent were free of symptoms during the third year of acyclovir use. Twenty-five percent of the patients studied were totally symptom-free for the entire three years.

There is also an over-the-counter ointment caller ImmuVir that can relieve painful symptoms of herpes in an hour or less. This anti-viral drug, in tests at Oregon Health Sciences University, shortened the duration of the average of herpes outbreak by about two to three days, and researchers speculate that it may reduce the chances of infecting another person. The drug is available at pharmacies without a prescription.

Note: Avoid the nonprescription self-treatment BHT, available in many health-food stores. This has a number of unpleasant side effects: severe stomach cramps, vomiting, dizziness, and even loss of consciousness when taken on an empty stomach. There is also no reliable evidence that BHT prevents genital herpes outbreaks.

During an outbreak of herpes, aspirin—if you are able to tolerate it—can relieve pain and fever. Cool baths can also provide some relief.

To help decrease recurrences, avoid hot baths and tight clothing. Also, decrease the chocolate, nuts, and seeds in your diet. These contain phenylalanine, which apparently allows viruses to enter body cells more readily. Learning to control stress, following a healthy diet, and getting help to alleviate recurrence—and can make you feel better in general.

GENITAL WARTS

I have these funny, skin-colored, cauliflower-like things around my vagina and near my butt and my boyfriend has the same on his penis. What are these things anyway?

Adrienne W.

What is it?

Genital warts (condylomata acuminata), caused by a variation of the human papilloma virus (HPV), are sexually transmitted. They may occur around the vagina or rectum or on the penis. They may also occur internally on the cervix, in the vagina, or in the urethra in the male. This is the third most common sexually transmitted disease—after chlamydia and gonorrhea—afflicting about one million people every year. Genital warts are three times more common that genital herpes.

These warts are extremely contagious. It is estimated that about *half* of all sexually active adults are infected, but many don't know they have genital warts. A growing number of teens are infected, too.

Symptoms

Genital wart infection has been linked to cervical cancer in women. About 10 to 15 percent of women with untreated genital warts develop cervical cancer. Some 28 percent of women with genital warts show *cervical dysplasia*, or precancerous cell changes in the cervix. One study found that 50 percent of women with invasive cervical cancer also have genital warts.

Any woman with external genital warts should also have a careful internal examination to see if there are warts or if the wart virus is present on the cervix. She should also have a Pap smear at the time and twice yearly thereafter.

Treatment

Removal of the warts by a physician is currently the best available method of treatment. This can be done in one of several ways. Your doctor may apply a topical medication called podophyllin on the warts, giving several follow-up treatments as necessary until the warts are gone, or your doctor may burn the warts off with an electric needle. This may be uncomfortable, but it is a highly effective one-time treatment. Your physician might also use liquid nitrogen to freeze and thus remove the warts. The treatment involves minimal discomfort and is also quick and convenient.

Several recent studies have tested self-administrated topical treatment with good results. Here, the patients applied the prescription medication podofilox to their warts, with promising results. In a study at Sinai Hospital in Detroit of 72 female patients with external genital warts, 75 percent of those given this medication to apply at home found that their warts went away completely. In another study at the University of California at San Francisco, warts cleared completely in 44 percent

of those who used self-administered doses of podofilox.

Stubborn or severe cases of genital warts may be treated by laser or with the anti-cancer drug interferon.

Special Note on HPV Prevention

There is now a vaccine to prevent HPV infection that has been approved by both the Centers for Disease Control and the American Academy of Pediatrics. Given as a series of three injections over a six month period, it is highly recommended for young women between the ages of 9 through 26 years of age, though the best time to get this vaccine is between the ages of 11 and 13, before any genital sexual activity takes place, bringing with it possible exposure to the HPV virus. Though giving this series of injections to girls so young has been controversial, the goal is to immunize as many girls as possible before they become sexually active. The quadrivalent vaccine protects against both genital warts and cervical cancer.

GONORRHEA

What causes gonorrhea? Can you get it from anything besides sexual intercourse? I mean, things like kissing? Or sitting on a germy public toilet seat? I really need to know!

Janet

What Is It?

Gonorrhea is a sexually transmitted disease caused by the bacteria Neisseria Gonorrhea.

This bacteria can usually survive only in the warm, moist environment of the human body. Gonorrhea can occur in the cervix, penis, throat, or rectum, and even in the eye in some cases.

Symptoms

When they occur, symptoms (which usually appear in the male) are evident two to nine days after exposure and can include the following:

- Painful urination and an uncomfortable, thick, yellowish discharge.
- Vaginal or pelvic discomfort.
- A sore throat, rectal pain and itching, and mucus in bowel movements, if the throat and/or rectum have been infected.
- Eye infections in newborn infants of mothers with gonorrhea.

Unfortunately, about 80 percent of affected women have no early symptoms, and later symptoms (such as pelvic or lower abdominal pain) may signal serious complications such as pelvic inflammatory disease.

This is why it's so important to tell your female partner(s) if you are a male with gonorrhea. If you're a sexually active female with multiple partners, a medical exam and gonorrhea and chlamydia cultures and/or tests every three months is a good idea.

At the time of this writing, there are new, more technologically advanced tests that can actually detect gonorrhea in the urine of males and females.

Special Risks

An undetected, untreated case of gonorrhea in a woman can spread from the cervix into the pelvis, infecting the fallopian tubes which lead from the ovaries to the uterus. The resulting abscesses and scar tissue in the tubes can cause blockage and, as a result of this, sterility.

In both men and women, gonorrhea, if untreated, may spread throughout the body, affecting joints (especially knee joints) and even heart valves.

Gonorrhea transmitted from a woman's vagina to her infant's eyes during birth can causes blindness in the child. Although most states have laws requiring hospital personnel to put a special protective antibiotic solution into the eyes of all newborn infants to prevent such a possibility, there are an increasing number of home deliveries these days where this may not be done.

Treatment

Because of the prevalence of penicillin-resistant strains of gonorrhea, all gonorrhea is now treated by new drugs such as *ceftriaxone* by injection and even newer drugs that can be administered by mouth in just one dose.

MOLLUSCUM CONTAGIOSUM

I'm really scared because I have some bubble-like bumps on my inner thighs and near my vulva. They don't itch or hurt, but they're sure ugly and noticeable. What could this be?

Samantha O.

What is it?

Molluscum contagiosum is another sexually transmitted diseases caused by a virus.

Symptoms

Smooth, bubble-like, usually non-itchy bumps on the genitals and/or inner thighs are the usual symptoms. This sexually transmitted disease seems to be seen more often in teens than adults.

Treatment

Treatment must be prompt because these bumps multiply rapidly and don't go away on their own.

With the patient given a local anesthetic, the physician removes each bump with a surgical curette. To avoid infection, this must be done by a physician only and under sterile conditions. There is also a new prescription topical medicine, Aldara, that can be applied to these bumps.

PUBIC LICE

What causes crabs? Do you get them from having sex? Is there any other way you can get them?

Wondering

What is it?

Pubic lice are six-legged parasites (also called *crabs*) that live and lay eggs in the pubic hair. These are usually transmitted sexually, but can also be spread via infected bedding, clothing, towels, and toilet seats.

Symptoms

- Intense itching.
- Visible eggs and lice in the pubic hair.
- Tiny spots of blood on the underwear from sites where the lice have burrowed under the skin.

Treatment

A prescription creme rinse—Nix or Elimite (permethrin) is the usual treatment. However, a nonprescription drug called A-200 (pyrinate), a medicated shampoo for the pubic area, may also be effective when used according to instructions. It is also important to wash bedding, towels, and clothing in very hot water to remove any trace of the lice or their eggs.

A follow-up treatment in a week may be needed: in the meantime, it's vital to abstain from sex to avoid possibly transmitting or becoming reinfested with the lice.

SCABIES

Some kids I know went on a camping trip in the mountains and several came back with something called scabies. Is this something you can get from sleeping in the wild or is it some kind of disease you get from sex?.

Cody Y.

What is it?

Scabies is another parasite disease caused by a mite. It can be transmitted sexually or acquired through close skin-to-skin contact or via infected bedding, clothing, and blankets.

Symptoms

- Intense itching (especially at night).
- Red spots where the mite has burrowed under the skin.
- Raised red or gray burrow lines in the skin.

Genitals, buttocks, breasts, elbows, and hands (especially between the fingers) may all be affected.

Treatment

The prescription creams Elimite (permethrin) or Kwell (lindane) are the most common. Washing clothes and bedding in very hot water and abstaining from sex for at least a week will help make the treatment more effective.

SYPHILIS

Is it true that syphilis will go away, even without treatment? I heard that somewhere. So why do people go for treatments?

Rance G.

What is it?

Syphilis is a sexually transmitted disease caused by a tiny corkscrew-shaped spirochete. While it is usually spread by sexual contact, the disease can also be transmitted from an infected sex organ to an open cut in the skin of another person.

Despite rumors that it is a disease of the past, syphilis is still very much with us and afflicts approximately 30,000 people each year. Although cases of syphilis in the United States are leveling off, there is still a dramatic dispar-

ity in who has syphilis and where it is occurring. Latino and African American youth have a 5 to 6 times greater risk of becoming infected with syphilis than whites, and the incidence is much higher in the southern part of the United States.

Symptoms

Symptoms appear slowly—10 to 90 days after exposure—and in stages. The first-stage symptom is usually a painless sore (called a chancre) on the genitals, rectum, lips, or mouth. This disappears in a week or two. It is followed some weeks or months later by second-stage symptoms, which include a rash spreading all over the body, swollen joints, and a flu-like illness. If you have these symptoms, seek immediate medical help.

Special Risks

Untreated syphilis doesn't just go away. After the second stage, it goes into a latent period that may last for years before the third stage appears. In this stage, the impact on the victim's body becomes tragically apparent, with damage to the nervous system, brain, and/or circulatory systems. This can result in heart and vascular problems, insanity, paralysis, and possibly death.

Syphilis can also be transmitted from a mother to a baby in her womb, causing a number of serious congenital defects including bone deformities, blindness, and facial disfigurement. Women who are pregnant while in the first or second stage of syphilis also have a higher than usual rate of stillbirths.

Treatment

Syphilis is detected by a blood test called the VDLR or RPR and is treated with penicillin injections, or, in the case of penicillin allergy, with other antibiotics. If detected and treated in the early stages, syphilis is curable. If you are sexually active with a number of different sex partners, it's a good idea to get regular blood tests for syphilis.

TINEA CRURIS (JOCK ITCH)

I'm on the varsity basketball team and practice every day. For the past few weeks, I've noticed a scaly, itchy rash in my crotch. The coach says it's "jock rot" and told me to get some cream from the trainer, but now my girlfriend has the same kind of rash. What's happening?

Josh

What is it?

Tinea cruris, or "jock itch," may be caused initially by a fungus that can develop on an unwashed athletic supporter that has been stashed in a closed locker. The fungus may then be transmitted from the supporter to the skin of the man's groin. Then the infection may be transmitted via skin-to-skin (usually sexual) contact. In this instance, it would be classified as a sexually transmitted disease.

Symptoms

The usual symptom is a scaly, itchy rash in the genital area.

Treatment

An over-the-counter drug Lotrimin (Clotrimazole 1%) or Lamisil (Terbinafine 1%)—will

destroy the fungus when used as a directed over a period of time. However, if the rash does not improve within a week, effective prescription drugs are available from your physician.

There are also some things you can do, in addition to help promote healing: dry yourself thoroughly after showering or bathing, and wear cotton underwear and loose-fitting clothing.

TRICHOMONIASIS

What is trich? My girlfriend went to the youth clinic last night because she had some sort of discharge. The doctor told her she had this disease called trich. Also, he prescribed some pills for me. Why should I take these pills? I don't have any problem! What's the big deal?

Ted

What is it?

Trichomoniasis is an inflection of the vagina in women and of the urethra in men. It is caused by *protozoa*, tiny parasites that thrive in moist environments. Although this infection is usually sexually transmitted, it can also be spread via damp washcloths, towels, and bathing suits shared with an infected person.

Symptoms

Symptoms appear 4 to 28 days after exposure. In women, these include the following:

- A frothy, greenish-yellow, foul-smelling discharge.
- Frequent and painful urination.

- Itching.
- Inflammation of the vulva.
- In some, but not all cases, severe lower abdominal pain.

Symptoms are far less noticeable in men — often little more than mild discomfort in the penis — if any symptoms occur at all.

Treatment

The medication Flagyl — in pill form for men and women — is the most common treatment. It is best for both partners to be treated at the same time with a large number of these pills taken all at once. If both are not treated at the same time, sexual intercourse should not be resumed until the other partner has been treated as well.

THE ABCS OF HEPATITIS

Hepatitis, an infection of the liver, occurs in several serious forms, including *hepatitis A* (infectious hepatitis), *hepatitis B* (serum hepatitis), and *hepatitis C* (previously called non-A non-B hepatitis). Now a *hepatitis D* and *hepatitis E* virus have also been described. Most hepatitis viruses are not usually considered sexually transmitted disease, but some forms, especially hepatitis B, can be spread through contact with an infected person and/or by certain sex practices.

Hepatitis A is most often spread by contaminated food and by food handlers who did not wash their hands properly after a bowel movement. However, it can be transmitted sexually, if there is oral-anal contact.

Hepatitis B, like AIDS, is spread by exposure to contaminated body fluids; transfusion of infected blood; shared needles or accidental needle sticks (the latter, a hazard for health care professionals); and sex with an infected person. Hepatitis B can also be transmitted at birth from mother to newborn infant. In some countries, if the mother is not tested for hepatitis B, her child may be infected and not know it until some years later when he or she tests positive during routine school screening tests or a regular exam.

Those at most risk for acquiring hepatitis B via sexual transmission are male homosexuals and male or female heterosexuals who have multiple sex partners. According to one study, a 20 percent incidence of hepatitis B has been found among college students with five or more recent sex partners.

Hepatitis C has, in the past, usually spread through blood transfusion. But today all blood is now screened for hepatitis C before being administered. So now the most common way of becoming infected with hepatitis C is through intravenous drug use and tattoos that are placed without using a sterile needle.

Hepatitis is not a minor problem. It is a serious illness that can be fatal. If you notice symptoms — mild tiredness, exhaustion, loss of appetite, and especially jaundice (yellowing of the skin and the whites of the eyes and dark urine) — call your doctor immediately. If you know someone with hepatitis, avoid close physical relations. If you have had such contact with an infected person, call you doctor. It's important to know what type of hepatitis you have been exposed to, since this will determine your course of treatment.

If You Have Been Exposed to Hepatitis A

Your physician will want to give you an injection of gamma globulin. This may help protect you from acquiring hepatitis A. Today there is a vaccine for hepatitis A. This vaccine is recommended for health-care workers and also for anyone traveling to a country where hepatitis A is very common, usually countries with unclean drinking water. Also, the Hepatitis A vaccine series is now recommended by the American Academy of Pediatrics as part of the routine immunizations for all children and teenagers.

If You Have Been Exposed to Hepatitis B

Your doctor is likely to give you an antibody shot and then a vaccine to protect you. If you are in danger of being exposed to hepatitis B because of medical work or treatments or because of your lifestyle (if you are very sexually active and/or a male homosexual), you might want to look into a vaccination that could protect you from this disease and maybe save your life. Recently, several school districts throughout the country are requiring that all students entering middle school complete the hepatitis B vaccine series.

The vaccine series for hepatitis B consists of three separate injections. The Hepatitis B vaccine series is now also recommended by the American Academy of Pediatrics as part of the routine immunizations for all children and teenagers.

More and more physicians are recommending that all adolescents be immunized against hepatitis B: many colleges are now requiring the complete vaccine series prior to admission.

Avoiding Hepatitis C

There is no vaccine yet to prevent Hepatitis C.

The best way to avoid being exposed to hepatitis C or of not getting infected with hepatitis C is not to use intravenous drugs and be very careful if you are having a tattoo that the equipment used is sterile!

WHAT IS "SAFE SEX"?

Is safe sex really safe? As safe as not having sex at all? What romantic things can you do besides making love . . . or is everything risky now?

Caitlin B.

Many teens wonder what "safe sex" really is—and what kinds of choice it involves. Taking responsibility to protect yourself and your partner from infection with a sexually transmitted disease is vital—and has several levels of safety. What is usually termed "safe sex" should probably really be called "safer sex." Why? Because "safe sex" as usually practiced is much safer than unprotected sex, but it is still not 100 percent safe.

If you want to be 100 percent safe from sexually transmitted diseases, you have three choices:

1. Total abstinence—no sex with anyone.
2. Masturbation (by yourself).
3. Waiting to have sex until you're married—and marrying a virgin or someone who has practiced safe sex and will be faithful to you (and you to him or her) throughout your marriage.

If these three possibilities don't appeal to you, then you need to take responsibility for protecting yourself—and your partner—in situations that carry risks of infection with sexually transmitted diseases.

Ten "Safe Sex" Guidelines

1. *Know what sexual behavior carries risks and what doesn't.* Too many people worry needlessly about catching sexually transmitted diseases from toilet seats, doorknobs, or casual nonsexual contact when they really need to think about—and perhaps change—their sexual choices and practices.

    You need to know, for example, that the more sex partners you have, the greater risk you have of getting a sexually transmitted disease. People in mutually monogamous relationship are at considerably less risk. So are people who are careful about what they do and with whom. It may be more risky to have one or two unprotected sexual experiences than experiences with protection (for example, condoms).

    It's important to know, among sexual activities, which carry more risks than others. The following lists will give you a general idea.

Very Safe Sexual Activities

✔ Kissing with closed lips (dry kissing).
✔ Rubbing against each other while clothed or partially clothed, avoiding direct genital contact and exchange of body fluids
✔ Masturbation (by yourself)
✔ Talking about your sexual feelings and fantasies with each other
✔ Non-genital touching and massage

Reasonably Safe Sex

✔ Sexual intercourse with the man using a condom.
✔ Wet ("French") kissing. New evidence that the AIDS virus can directly infect mucus-membrane cells, such as those found in the mouth or vagina, has been presented. However, experts still consider French kissing a rather low-risk activity since an infected person's saliva contains far less HIV than blood, semen, or vaginal fluids. Just the same, you might think twice about deep kissing someone who is (or might be) in a high-risk group for HIV infection.
✔ Oral sex with latex barriers between the mouth of one partner and the sex organ of the other. This means that a man should wear a condom and a woman needs to put a dental dam (a thin, square piece of latex) on her vulva and vaginal opening.
✔ Mutual masturbation (stimulating each other) with a spermicidal jelly or cream and/or latex rubber gloves.

Unsafe Sex

✔ Sexual intercourse where partners are not protected by condom and spermicide.
✔ Oral sex where a barrier is not used and there is direct mouth-genital contact.
✔ Masturbation with or in the presence of another person where sex toys like vibrators and dildos are shared.

2. *Be selective.* It is vital to be selective not only in terms of partners—if he refuses to wear a condom, don't have sex: if she has had a lot of sex partners or doesn't want

to practice safe sex, don't have sex—but also in what you do. While safe sex rules may sound grim on first reading, stepping back and letting your relationship grow in many other ways and gradually increasing your physical intimacy can make it *better* and more romantic. Think about it. You can have a wonderful time talking, kissing, and caressing each other, gradually building up to sexual involvement with great excitement and anticipation instead of rushing into it because that's the way you've done it before or because you feel it is expected. Taking time to get to know each other first will let you know if you even *like* this person enough to have sex with him or her. With the risks of sexual activity today, it doesn't make sense to have sex with someone who isn't pretty special to you. Also, the better you know and like each other, the easier it will be to talk about safe sex and birth control measures—things that *do* need to be discussed before you ever have sex.

3. *Take the initiative with safe sex practices.* Don't wait for your partner to get around to purchasing a condom or spermicide. Buy some yourself. That way, at least *one of you* will be prepared for *both of you* to have sex.

Condoms are easier to buy than ever and many women are buying them these days. Many stores carry them on open racks. So you can just buy them and have them handy. It may help to know, if you've never bought condoms before, that they come in one size. If you end up having to ask a pharmacist for some and he or she gives you the old "What size?" line, he

or she means the size of the package—for example, a package of 3, 12 or 36.

If a partner is shocked by the fact that you are prepared with safe-sex aids, remind him or her that, these days, it's a smart and loving gesture to be careful and to be prepared in advance for sex. You may explain that you're not implying that he or she strikes you as having a sleazy past or a myriad of unspeakable disease, but that people—including yourself—can have infections without knowing it, and you want to protect your partner as well as yourself. If your partner says that the safe-sex aids will make sex distinctly non-sexy, you might say that feeling safe will allow you to relax and enjoy each other more—and that people can have satisfying safe sex.

4. *Be open-minded about safe sex aids.* If you feel your libido plummet at the mere mention of a condom (let alone a dental dam or rubber gloves!), don't reject these possibilities until you've tried them. Even though it may seem unbelievable to you right now, some people have actually grown to like the soft silky feel of these latex gloved hands or fingers on their genitals. A condom or a dental dam does not have to diminish the pleasures of oral sex. In fact, some young people—particularly males—have told us that they hadn't had the nerve to try oral sex until they used the safe-sex barriers. So these aids may actually expand, rather than limit, your sexual horizons! Also, condoms these days are thinner (and stronger) than they used to be, so sensation isn't dulled nearly as much. So the old line about how wearing

a condom is like wearing a raincoat in the shower isn't really true anymore. Sex can be very pleasurable with a condom and spermicide—even more so than unprotected sex because—even more so than unprotected sex because you're at less risk of getting a sexually transmitted disease.

5. *Be aware of the fact that condoms and spermicides can't prevent* all *types of sexually transmitted diseases.* The condom and other barriers cannot prevent pubic lice, scabies, and, in some instances, genital warts or herpes. To avoid these diseases, you need to avoid sex with someone who shows signs of having these. Take a good look at your partner before you have sex. Taking a shower or bath together first can help make this a bit less obvious and more fun. But if that isn't possible, prolong foreplay and look carefully for any signs of lice, herpes blisters, or warts. That may not sound awfully romantic, but getting these diseases isn't at *all* romantic and, in some instances, can be health-threatening.

6. *Practice good hygiene.* This is a way to avoid getting trichomonas and to make yourself less likely to get or have a recurrence of genital warts or herpes. Don't share towels or washcloths with others. Don't swap clothes—especially damp swimsuits—with another person. Don't wear tight, un-ventilated clothing for long periods, trapping heat and moisture in the genital area. Take regular baths and showers. Wash genital and anal areas before sex. Also, urinating and again washing the genitals after sex may be of some help in preventing some types of sexually transmitted diseases.

7. *If you have suspicious symptoms, seek help* and *tell your partner.* Don't be afraid. County and city health departments, adolescent clinics, free clinics, and youth clinics throughout the nation offer low- or no-cost medical diagnosis and treatment for sexually transmitted diseases. This care is completely confidential and may be given without parental knowledge or consent, in most states, to anyone over age 12. (Check out the laws in your state with the Confidential Care Chart in Chapter 15.) The people who staff these clinics see all kinds of sexually transmitted diseases all the time, know how to treat them, and tend to be quite non-judgmental.

Notifying your sex partner or partners—particularly if they're female and are less likely to have symptoms for diseases such as gonorrhea or chlamydia—is very important. They may not only continue to spread the disease, but may also develop serious complications if they are not treated. Giving them the bad news is not easy, but it is the decent, considerate, responsible thing to do.

If you choose, a health worker will call your partner or partners for you. A staff member will take a list of your contacts and their phone numbers from you, then call these people (without mentioning your name), asking them to come in for examination and treatment.

8. *If you haves a sexually transmitted disease, don't have sex while you're infectious.* This is a very important way to stop the spread of sexually transmitted diseases. Ask your doctor very specifically how long you should abstain from sexual activities. And

then follow his or her guidelines carefully. If you have a chronic condition—such as genital herpes—be especially careful to avoid sex altogether when you're in an active stage and take safe-sex precautions during the times in between.

9. *Get regular checkups.* This is especially important if you're sexually active with several partners. If you just have one partner, a physical and/or gynecological exam once a year will probably be enough. If you have multiple sex partners, plan to have an exam three to four times a year, even if you don't have symptoms of any sexually transmitted diseases. New guidelines suggest that *all* teenage girls who are having sex get tested twice a year for chlamydia. This is an excellent safeguard for your health and fertility and is well worth your time. Regular exams may detect any hidden infections before serious complications arise. The tests are simple: you can get tested for Gonorrhea or Chlamydia with just a urine sample. However, you may need to request tests for chlamydia, gonorrhea or syphilis, and even HIV, since they may not be part of every routine physical or gynecological exam.

10. *Learn as much as you can about sexually transmitted diseases.* These days, ignorance can kill—and there is a lot of ignorance around. For example, a survey of some 860 Massachusetts teens between ages 16 and 19 revealed that while 96 percent of them had heard about AIDS, only 15 percent had changed their sexual behavior to lower their risks. And, in San Francisco, a survey of some 1,326 teens found that their feeling of invulnerabil-

ity to AIDS was growing: 54 percent of those polled said that they weren't worried about getting AIDS, compared to 34 percent in 1985. This lack of worry, unfortunately, is less likely to reflect the security of abstinence and safe-sex practices that it is to point up the fact that too many teens assume that bad things simply happen to other people, never to them.

REMEMBER: IF YOU'RE HAVING SEX, YOU'RE AT RISK FOR SEXUALLY TRANSMITTED DISEASES.

That's a fact. So the more you know about these diseases—how to recognize them and how to prevent them—the better off you'll be. Read this and other books about sexuality. Talk with your doctor. Share your feelings and intentions with your partner. Some of this information may seem distasteful and embarrassing, but it can be health-saving—even lifesaving.

If the current epidemic of sexually transmitted diseases is to be halted, prevention must play a major role. At this time, there is no cure and no preventive vaccine for AIDS. There is, as yet, no definitive cure for genital herpes. And more discoveries are being made all the time about the distressing long-range consequences of other sexually transmitted diseases such as chlamydia and genital warts. Medical research is ongoing, but in the meantime, prevention of sexually transmitted disease in ourselves and our partners is the most valuable defensive weapon we have. Being aware and taking responsibility for safeguarding your own health and that of your partner is a major step toward maturity and growing up to be a healthy, loving, caring person.

QUICK SCAN

THE TRUTH ABOUT SEXUALLY TRANSMITTED DISEASES

✔ If you're having sex, you're at risk for sexually transmitted diseases.

✔ The only true "safe sex" is abstinence or sex with a long-term, mutually monogamous party (and even the latter, if he or she has had previous partners, may be carrying an undiagnosed sexually transmitted disease from a long-ago previous relationship. That's possible with herpes, genital warts or HIV.)

✔ Use safe sex measures every time you have sex!

✔ If you notice any suspicious symptoms—unusual discharges, bumps, blisters, warts or other growths, pain in the abdomen, intense genital itching, tiny spots of blood on your underwear—see your doctor or seek help at a public clinic right away. No STD just goes away on its own. The sooner you get treatment, the better.

✔ **You can legally receive confidential medical care for the diagnosis and treatment of a sexually transmitted disease in most states if you are 12 or older.**

✔ If you're diagnosed with a sexually transmitted disease, tell your partner(s) so that they can be treated, too. It isn't an easy thing to do, but it's the right and loving thing to do.

THIRTEEN

Birth Control:
An Ounce of Prevention

I've heard that it's better to use birth control if you're sexually active, but how active do you have to be to need it? What if you're too nervous to go to a doctor or even talk to your boyfriend about it? Can you get it without your parents finding out? Is it true that you can't get pregnant the first time you have sex? (I really need to know!)

Amber S.

Amber's questions have been echoed by many teens who are confused, scared, and often just plain uninformed about birth control. Too few teens realize the importance of using a reliable method of birth control every time they have sex—*including the first time!* Pregnancy can happen to *anyone* who has sex without using a reliable method of birth control. That's why it's important for you to know as much as possible about contraception, whether or not you're presently sexually active.

A number of studies show that teens are taking big risks by not using reliable methods of birth control consistently or at all. An

unplanned pregnancy can mean not only making difficult choices now—an early marriage, being a single parent, having an abortion, giving a baby up for adoption—but living with the consequences of these choices. The fact is, as hard as it can be to seek and use birth control, doing so is much easier and less embarrassing and distressing than dealing with an unplanned pregnancy.

FIVE LAME EXCUSES FOR NOT USING BIRTH CONTROL

1. *"It isn't romantic."* How romantic is an unplanned pregnancy? How romantic is worrying about pregnancy? Using birth control frees you to enjoy sex more!

2. *"It would be like planning to have sex."* You plan other good things in your life. Why not sex?

3. *"My boyfriend doesn't believe in birth control"* That's fine for him, but *you* need to protect *yourself* against an unplanned pregnancy.

4. *"I'm too embarrassed to talk about it or deal with it."* If you're too embarrassed to admit that you're having sex and that you need to use birth control, maybe you're not ready to have sex.

5. *"Wearing a condom is like taking a shower with a raincoat on. Sex isn't as pleasurable."* Oh, please! Condoms are a vital aid to safer sex as well as birth control and don't have to interfere with sexual sensation. And, of course, there are many other forms of birth control available.

Many teens ask us questions like "Can you get pregnant if…" and add any number of situations to the question. Quite often, if intercourse or ejaculation near the vaginal opening is involved, the answer is yes. The following is a quick guide to circumstances under which it's possible to get pregnant.

YOU *CAN* GET PREGNANT IF…

- You have sexual intercourse without reliable birth control.
- You have unprotected sex at *any* time of the month (even though pregnancy is most likely during ovulation—about two weeks after your last menstrual period—the exact time of ovulation is hard to pinpoint, especially in teens whose cycles aren't well-established).
- You have unprotected sex for the first time or the thousandth time.
- He ejaculates close to your vaginal opening and some semen gets into your vagina.
- You don't have an orgasm or even enjoy sex. While it's true that a man usually would

need to have an orgasm—or "come," as many people call it—to cause a pregnancy, there may be some stray sperm in the lubricating fluid that is secreted when he is sexually aroused. If any of this gets into a woman's vagina, pregnancy could happen. And, of course, a woman doesn't have to have an orgasm or even be aroused in order to get pregnant.

- He "pulls out." The problem is, sperm may be in his lubricating fluid before he comes (see the preceding item), or he may not be able to pull out in time to avoid spilling some semen in your vagina.
- You use a makeshift form of improvised birth control, such as plastic wrap, douching, or standing up immediately after sex. Forget these makeshift methods. Use the real stuff. It works.

TEENS *CAN* GET BIRTH CONTROL

Nonprescription Methods

Condoms (male and female) and spermicidal jelly, cream or foam are generally available over the counter in drugstores, supermarkets, and, in the case of condoms for males, in vending machines in some public restrooms. They are also available at family-planning clinics and at a number of high schools with condom distribution policies.

Prescription Methods

Oral contraceptives (the Pill), Depo-Provera injections, birth control implants, the vaginal ring and hormonal patches are available from your physician or from family-planning clinics (such as Planned

Parenthood) or your local youth clinic or school-based clinic.

Legal Aspects Of Your Access To Birth Control

Contraceptive services are available to minors at clinics in all states. The legal question involved in such services usually does not deal with contraception directly, but with the issue of medical care of a minor without parental consent. Some teens, of course, do have parental consent for contraceptive services. Others don't. Yet these services are, quite often, available to teens without parental consent.

A number of states have *emancipated minor* statutes declaring that legally emancipated minors (for example, those living away from home and/or supporting themselves and making their own decisions, or minors who are married) may give their own consent for medical treatment. A variation of this is the "mature minor" rule, recognized by a number of states, which states that "a minor can effec-

tively consent to medical treatment for himself if he understands the nature of the treatment and it is for his benefit".

Even in states without such rulings, teens can get help. Although clinic personnel may ask a patient's age and whether that patient is emancipated, they will generally not ask for proof. "Our first concern," says one clinic official, "is for the adolescent who needs help." Many echo this sentiment. In fact, the American Medical Association, the American College of Obstetrics and Gynecology, and the American Academy of Pediatrics have all given public support to the issue of contraception for sexually active teenagers.

So birth control information and help are likely to be available to you—if you take the responsibility for seeking it.

WHICH METHODS WORK?

As you will discover in this chapter, there are many methods of birth control. Some

MAKING CHOICES ABOUT BIRTH CONTROL

If You Want	Consider These Methods
Highly effective, continuous protection, with no action from you required after initial insertion	LARC Contraceptives • Implanon Implant • Mirena IUD • ParaGard (copper) IUD
Highly effective, continuous protection, requiring some action from you on a daily, monthly or occasional basis	• Oral contraceptives (the Pill) • Depo Provera (3 month shot) • Vaginal Ring • Patch contraceptive
Effective if used correctly and every time	• Condom with spermicide
Emergency contraception (after unprotected sex or if a condom breaks)	• Plan B One Step (one pill) • ParaGard (copper) IUD
Not recommended for teens	• Barrier Methods like the diaphragm or cervical cap • Natural family planning • Sterilization

are highly effective and require no action on your part except the initial appointment. Others are highly effective and require some action on your part daily, monthly or every few months. Some offer great protection against an unplanned pregnancy, but no protection against sexually transmitted diseases. One method—the condom (male or female condom)—offers good protection against some sexually transmitted diseases and fairly good protection against pregnancy. Other methods are less likely to be a good choice for you at this time in your life—and we'll tell you which methods those are.

Some methods are expensive initially and then cost nothing for several years. Others are regular expenses, either prescription or over-the-counter. Some may be more suitable for you now when life is so busy and privacy so rare. The method you choose may depend on what you can afford—or what is possible for you to get. The right birth control method for you may change a number of times as you grow into adulthood and your lifestyle evolves from dating to marriage to parenthood and beyond. The right method for you will be the one that you will use consistently and that fits your lifestyle.

You might want to take a quick glance at our chart on recommended birth control methods and then read the details in this chapter on all the methods—and why one or the other may or may not be for you—before making up your mind. It's important, of course, to discuss these with your partner, if you're in a long-term, committed relationship, as well as with your physician or a health care provider at your local clinic.

We can only give you information. The best method for *you* is a very personal decision.

Long Acting Reversible Contraceptives (LARC)
What Is It?

Actually, LARC is short for several different contraceptives that all share three major features: first, they are highly effective methods of birth control; second, they require no action or decisions from you for a number of years, except the initial decision to have the device inserted; and third, as of 2015, LARC contraceptives are the birth control method most highly recommended for teens by the American College of Obstetricians and Gynecologists.

There are two types of LARCS with three products used most with teens:

- *Implant:* The implant recommended for teens is the *Implanon*, a thin, flexible plastic rod about the size of a matchstick. It is placed just under the skin on the inner side of your upper arm. Once in place, it is effective in preventing pregnancy for three to four years.

- *IUDs:* These devices are placed into the womb by a medical professional in a very quick, non-surgical procedure. While we used to be leery of the use of IUDs by teens because of the risk of infection with older IUD devices, there are two new IUDs that can work well for teens. One of these is called *Mirena*, which is effective for five to seven years after insertion. The other, called Paragard, is a copper-based IUD that is effective for ten to twelve years after insertion. It is also a very effective form of emergency contraception, preventing pregnancy if it is inserted within five to seven days after unprotected sex.

How Does It Work?

The implant releases a hormone called etonogestrel that prevents pregnancy by suppressing ovulation and also by changing your cervical mucus so that sperm can't pass through to your Fallopian tubes as easily.

The IUDs work in somewhat different ways. *Mirena* releases a hormone called levonogestrel which causes cervical mucus to thicken, blocking sperm from entering the Fallopian tubes to fertilize an egg. The Copper T or ParaGard IUD blocks sperm by a slow release of copper in the uterus which stops sperm and also makes them less able to fertilize an egg and, finally, if an egg is fertilized, the copper makes the lining of the uterus less likely to allow implantation of the fertilized egg. (Pregnancy occurs when the fertilized egg implants itself in the uterine lining.) It should be noted that if an egg is already implanted, an IUD will not abort it.

How Effective Is It?

The implant has a 99% effectiveness rate with less than one pregnancy per 100 women using it. There is some concern that it might not be as effective in women who are seriously overweight or obese. Medical professionals often will not suggest this method for any woman weighing above 190 pounds.

The Mirena IUD is similarly effective, with one pregnancy per 1,000 women during the first year of use and with a 1.1% failure rate over seven years of use.

The ParaGard or Copper T IUD has a less than 1% failure rate in the first year and only two out of 100 women using it for ten years will become pregnant.

Who Can and Can't Use This Method?

The LARC birth control choices are good for those who want a highly effective, reversible, long-lasting method of birth control that does not require any subsequent decisions or actions, like remembering to take a pill daily or getting a shot every three months or putting in a vaginal ring or putting on a patch.

Ideally, a woman choosing an implant will not be significantly overweight. One choosing a hormonal method (the implant and the Mirena) should not have a medical condition or be taking medications that would preclude or interfere with the hormones in the devices. Also, if you have an allergy to copper, the Copper T/ParaGard is not for you.

What Are the Advantages?

Besides being highly effective methods of birth control, the LARC methods have some non-contraceptive advantages. For example, the Mirena can help decrease menstrual bleeding and cramping, and can help if you have endometriosis. In fact, an estimated 20% of those using the device cease having periods by the end of the first year of use. (When the device is removed, periods and fertility resume quickly.) The Copper T/Paragard IUD offers highly effective protection against unplanned pregnancy for women who cannot take the pill or use birth control utilizing hormones—e.g. those who suffer from migraine headaches. The Implanon implant has been found to alleviate heavy menstrual bleeding, cramps and also PMS.

Another advantage that all three of the LARC devices share is that, over time, they are very inexpensive, requiring only a one-time fee rather than ongoing costs. That said, initially, these are more expensive. However, insurance usually covers the cost. If you don't have insurance (or don't want to use your parents' insurance for this), you can find no cost or low cost help at a public health clinic or Planned Parenthood.

The Susan Thompson Buffett Foundation recently pledged a minimum of $200 million to make LARC contraceptives available to women in public health clinics and to promote continued funding of LARC programs nationwide.

What Are The Disadvantages?

Some people are put off by the discomfort of the insertion of the implant and its visibility—both the small bandage necessary in the first few days after insertion and the visibility of the device in the upper arm. This may be significant if you don't want people, like parents, family and classmates, to know.

Some teens are leery of IUDs because they've heard that the insertion is painful. While it's true that it can be very briefly uncomfortable or painful to have the IUD inserted (through your vagina and cervix into your uterus), the procedure is very quick and the discomfort usually doesn't linger. Some doctors use a local anesthetic for implant or IUD insertions, and may give pain medication if the discomfort persists.

Beyond the discomfort of insertion, all of these methods can affect your menstrual periods. In the first few months after insertion of the implant, you may experience some irregular periods or spotting. With the Mirena IUD, you may experience extended days of menstrual bleeding in the first months of use, and then less than usual after that. With the ParaGard IUD, you may experience some cramping, pain or

spotting in the first day or so after insertion. You may also have increased bleeding and cramps during your period initially. However, this usually stops after the first few months. If the pain and bleeding persist, check with your physician for medications that can help reduce the amount of cramping and bleeding.

One shared disadvantage of all three LARCs: while they provide excellent protection against unplanned pregnancy, they do not offer protection against sexually transmitted diseases. So it's important, if you're with a new partner or someone you're not sure is monogamous, that you use a condom—either a male or a female condom—every time you have sex for protection against sexually transmitted diseases.

How Do You Get It?

LARC contraceptives are available from your doctor or a clinic like Planned Parenthood or a public health clinic. All are inserted as minor office procedures. During the implant insertion—usually within seven days of the beginning of your last menstrual period—your skin is numbed with a local anesthetic and the physician makes an incision so tiny (into which he slips the implant) that you don't need a stitch, just a butterfly bandage that is secured by a gauze bandage. The gauze can come off the next day and the butterfly bandage after three days.

The Pill (Oral Contraceptives)
What Is It?

There are many different types of birth control pills ("the Pill"), but most are combinations of synthetic preparations of the hormones estrogen and progesterone. There is also a pill containing only progesterone, but the effectiveness of this "mini-pill" has been shown to be somewhat lower than that of the combination pills. *Triphasic* birth control pills most closely approximate the normal hormonal fluctuations of the menstrual cycle.

How Does it Work?

Oral contraceptives prevent pregnancy in several ways:

- The hormones in these pills prevent the ovaries from releasing an egg each month. If there is no egg, there can be no pregnancy.
- The hormones also affect the lining of the uterus so that if, by some chance, ovulation and fertilization should occur, the egg would have difficulty attaching itself to the uterine lining.
- Progesterone may cause cervical mucus to become thick and difficult for sperm to move through.

How Do You Use It?

Birth control pills, traditionally, have been available in 21- and 28-day packets. If you have a 21-day packet, you will take a pill every day for three weeks with seven days each, generally starting the new packet of pills on the fifth day after your menstrual period begins. If you have a 28-day packet, you will take a pill every day. Seven of these pills, however, are nonfunctional sugar pills. They are included so that you can take a pill every day instead of trying to calculate when you should be starting and stopping your pills.

The triphasic pills are taken on a 28-day schedule—with the hormonal content and combinations changing every seven days. Each different type of pill in the packet is a different color—red for the first seven days, blue for the second week, green for the third week, and yellow for the last week. The yellow pills do not contain hormones at all but are nonfunctional sugar pills, much like the last seven pills in any other 28-day packet.

Pills should be taken at the same time every day. These should also be taken only as directed by a physician. In other words, do not borrow a friend's pills. You must have your own prescription, tailored to your needs.

Among the new birth control pills recently approved by the Federal Drug Administration is Ovcon 35, the first chewable birth control pill (for those who have trouble swallowing pills). This spearmint-flavored, 28 days pill has the same ingredients and works the same way as traditional birth control pills.

Some new options, for girls who decide that they want to have a period only four times a year or maybe not at all, include *Seasonale*, which has an 84 pill packet followed by 7 days of placebo pills during which you would have a period, and *Lybrel* which is taken continuously and suppresses menstruation altogether as long as you take it. This is safe for most women. There is no problem with buildup of uterine lining because these continuous pills prevent ovulation and there is little, if any, buildup of the uterine lining. These pills minimizing or preventing menstrual periods can be a real advantage for girls who have heavy bleeding or severe menstrual cramps.

Some teen girls run into difficulty in their use of the Pill when trying to decide what to do after a relationship ends. After a breakup, they may stop taking the Pill and then, when they meet someone else or get back together

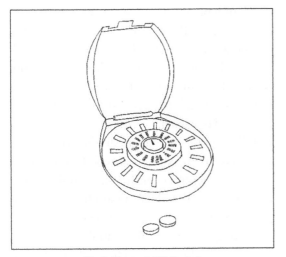

Birth Control Pill Packet

with the boyfriend, either find themselves unprotected for pregnancy or going through a physical readjustment to the Pill. It is best, if your relationship is unstable or has just ended, to keep taking oral contraceptives for several months to ensure continuous contraceptive protection.

How Effective Is It?

Oral contraceptives are very effective, with a failure rate of less than 1 percent. Failures are most likely to happen if:

- You forget to take a pill for one or two (or more) days during your cycle. If that happens, take the forgotten pill as soon as you remember (along with your regular one for that day) and, for the rest of the cycle, use a backup method of birth control—while continuing to take your pills.
- You take the pill regularly but at very different times of the day. Because modern birth control pills have such a low dose of estrogen, having a 24-hour gap can trigger ovula-

tion—and the risk of pregnancy. Try to take your pill at the same time every day and remind yourself by putting your packet next to your toothbrush.

- You're overweight—more than 155 pounds. Talk to your doctor. You may do better with a pill that has a little more estrogen—35 mcg, for example, instead of the usual 25 mcg of estrogen.

Illness can also cause the pill to be less effective. If you're vomiting or having diarrhea, this may affect your absorption of the Pill. Some antibiotics can also decrease the Pill's effectiveness. Check with your physician about this when he or she prescribes antibiotics, and, when in doubt, use backup methods as well as the Pill for the rest of your cycle.

Who Can Use This Method?

The ideal candidate for the Pill is a healthy young woman under 30 who does not smoke. (Many of the side effects of the Pill tend to occur in smokers or women over 35.) Generally, a woman who is menstruating regularly and has well-established cycles and no condition that would preclude use of the Pill may use birth control pills.

Who Should Not Use This Method?

- Heavy smokers.
- Those with a history of high blood pressure, abnormal vaginal bleeding, blood clots, liver disease (such as hepatitis), or cancer in the reproductive system.
- Those with migraine headaches or diabetes who generally are advised to consider other forms of birth control. However, if you really want to take oral contraceptives and

A NOTE OF CAUTION REGARDING BIRTH CONTROL AND SAFE SEX

I'm confused. My doctor said that if I take the Pill, I won't get pregnant. But a friend of mine said I still would have to use a condom or get my boyfriend to use a condom because of the danger of AIDS. My question is: What's the point of taking the Pill if you have to use a condom anyway?

Cheryl H.

Many teens, like Cheryl, are confused about contraceptive options and the necessary use of condoms to help protect against sexually transmitted diseases. While the condom can offer contraceptive protection and decrease one's risk of getting certain sexually transmitted diseases, including the HIV virus that causes AIDS, some want additional protection against pregnancy. Since the Pill is, statistically speaking, a more effective method of birth control than the condom, those for whom preventing pregnancy is an ultrahigh priority will often choose to take the Pill as well as using condoms to get the best overall protection against both pregnancy and sexually transmitted diseases.

There are some young people, of course, whose life circumstances may require contraception, but not necessarily the protection against sexually transmitted diseases that their peers require. These would be young people who are married and monogamous and who have not ever had sex with anyone but each other. Unless that describes you, it's vital to use condoms—either as combination protection against pregnancy and STDs, or in conjunction with other contraceptives.

your doctor agrees, you need to do so under the close supervision of the physician treating your migraines or diabetes.

- Those who must take certain medications known to interfere with the Pill's effectiveness. If you take anticonvulsants (including Phenobarbital), tetracyclines, or similar antibiotics; the antibiotic Rifampin; or the antifungal drug Griseofulvin, discuss this with your physician. You may need to uses another method of birth control.

- If you tend to be forgetful, the Pill may not be for you. To be effective, birth control pills must be taken consistently, on a precise schedule.

What Are the Advantages?
- The Pill is highly effective.
- It is convenient to take and doesn't interfere with sex.
- It may offer some relief from heavy and/or painful menstrual periods.
- Oral contraceptives can significantly reduce

your chances of getting ovarian and uterine cancer.

- The Pill can also reduce your risk of developing fibroid tumors of the uterus, which can cause menstrual problems and, in some cases, infertility.

What Are the Disadvantages?

- Side effects such as spotting between periods, headaches, breast tenderness, and nausea may occur. (These may be due to taking a pill with a hormone balance that is not right for you and may be remedied by switching to another brand of pill with a different hormone concentration—for example, if you have nausea, headaches, or breast tenderness, you may be taking a pill that has too much estrogen for you.)
- If you opt for Lybrel, the "no period" pill, you may still, especially at first, experience some irregular bleeding as your body adjusts to the medication.
- Birth control pills can contribute to high blood pressure, migraine headaches, and changes in blood sugar.
- Very rare but serious side effects include blood clots, strokes, and liver tumors. If you develop a sudden, severe headache unlike any you've ever had before or have pain in your chest or the calves of your legs while taking the Pill, see your doctor immediately.

Risks can be minimized by not smoking and by getting regular medical examinations to make sure that all is well.

Please note: When sizing up the risk of the Pill, do consider the fact that the Pill is quite safe when compared to the risks involved in pregnancy and childbirth, especially if you're young.

How Do You Get It?

Birth control pills are available by prescription only from a physician who has taken a complete medical history and performed a physical examination that will include checking your blood pressure and blood sugar to make sure you don't have any condition that would preclude taking the pill. Under new guidelines, a gynecological examination may not be necessary. In most instances, the doctor will defer the pelvic exam if you are healthy and just prescribe oral contraceptives. However, he or she may want to examine the external genitalia or take a urine test or vaginal swab just to make sure you have no sexually transmitted infections. Annual health checkups are advised.

Depo-provera (Injectable Hormonal Contraception)
What Is It?

Depo-Provera is the first injectable contraceptive available in the United States. Available only from a physician, it is given as a shot in the arm or buttocks and protects against pregnancy for thirteen weeks. About four of these shots per year will give you continuous contraceptive protection.

How Does It Work?

Depo-Provera works much like the Pill in preventing an egg from being released from the ovary.

How Do You Use It?

Once you get the injection, you don't have to do anything for three months. Every three months, you need to get another shot for continuous protection.

How Effective Is It?

Injectable contraceptives are, like oral contraceptives, about 99 percent effective.

Who Can Use This Method?

Most women can use this method if they so desire. The exceptions are listed here.

Who Should Not Use This Method?

- Those with vaginal bleeding without a known cause.
- Those who have had breast cancer (teens with a family history of breast cancer might want to be cautious as well).
- Those with a history of liver-disease, stroke, or blood clots in the legs, or who are allergic to the Depo-Provera injection.
- Those with high blood pressure.

What Are The Advantages?

- Depo-Provera is highly effective in protecting against pregnancy.
- It's a very private method of birth control, with no pills or devices that anyone can discover.
- It's quite convenient, requiring a shot every three months.

What Are The Disadvantages?

- It requires a shot every three months (a problem if you're needle-phobic!).
- It can have side effects such as menstrual changes (heavy periods, no periods, or irregular bleeding or spotting), weight gain, and headaches. (Some side effects diminish with time. Others can be managed with the help of your physician.)
- It can cause reductions in bone mineral density, causing some concern about long term effects in adolescents. One study of teen girls using Depo-Provera found that bone density decreased 3.1% after two years of continuous use. A group of teens *not* using a hormonal method of birth control had an average increase of 9.5% in bone density over the same period of time. Because the adolescent years are an important time for building bone density, you may wish to discuss this with your physician, especially if osteoporosis, or bone loss/thinning of bones, is prevalent in older women in your family. Another recently published study showed that young women who discontinued the use of Depo-Provera experience a complete recovery of bone density, offering some reassurance for the future.

How Do You Get It?

Depo-Provera is available only from a physician and is given as an injection by the doctor or nurse every three months.

Other Combined Homormonal Birth Control Methods (The Vaginal Ring And The Patch)
What is It?

The vaginal ring (NuvaRing) is a round, flexible ring that is inserted in the vagina and stays in place for three weeks, releasing estrogen and progestin hormones that provide protection against pregnancy for one month.

The patch is a transdermal adhesive patch (OrthoEvra) that is put on the skin of the abdomen, upper arm, upper torso or buttocks. This, too, provides a constant flow of hormones protecting against pregnancy much the way the ring does.

How Does It Work?

The ring and the patch work the same way birth control pills and the implant do, with hormones that suppress ovulation and thus protect against pregnancy.

How Do You Use It?

The ring is inserted into the vagina and stays in place for three weeks before being removed for one week to induce menstruation. (This works the way the placebo pills do in a packet of 28 cycle birth control pills.) After this week off, you insert a new ring for another three weeks.

The patch is applied to the skin of your abdomen, upper arm or buttocks and is changed once a week, using one patch for each of three weeks. The fourth week, you don't use any patches at all, during which point you have your period.

How Effective Is It?

The ring has been shown to be 99% effective in studies of adult women. Adolescents have not been studied, however. The patch has also been found to be as effective as other hormonal methods of birth control with one exception: it was not as effective in preventing pregnancy in women who weighed more than 198 pounds.

Who Can Use This Method?

Women who are able to use other hormonal methods—such as the pill—could use these two methods. However, both entail responsibility on your part—remembering

to remove the ring after three weeks and, after you've had your period, insert a new one. And you need to remember to replace the patch after a week and have one week a month of not wearing one while you have your period.

Who Should Not Use This Method?

Besides those who would not be able to use other forms of hormonal contraception, women who should not use these methods would be ones who have difficulty with the idea of inserting the ring once a month or remembering to change the patch once a week for three weeks out of four. Also, if you're prone to skin rashes, irritations or have an allergy to adhesives, the patch may not be for you.

What Are the Advantages?

These methods offer a high level of birth control protection without the need for any action or decision at the time of sexual intercourse.

What Are the Disadvantages?

Like other hormonal birth control methods, the ring and the patch may cause some breast tenderness, headaches, nausea and breakthrough spotting or bleeding, especially at first.

And, like other hormonally-based methods, they are highly effective birth control methods, but do not offer any protection against sexually transmitted infections.

Where Do You Get It?

As with all hormonal birth control methods,

the ring and the patch are prescription only and need to be prescribed by a physician.

The Condom (Male)
What Is It?

The condom is a thin sheath of rubber or animal tissue that is slipped over the erect penis before intercourse. For best results, it is used in combination with spermicidal cream, jelly, or foam.

How Do You Use It?

Roll the condom carefully over the *erect* penis, taking care to leave space at the end for seminal fluid if the condom doesn't come with a receptacle tip. It's also important to hold on to the condom as you're withdrawing from your partner after sex to guard against spilling the collected semen. Do not re-use a condom. Use a fresh one each time you have sex.

How Does It Work?

The condom prevents pregnancy by keeping sperm from entering the vagina. Instead, the semen is deposited in the reservoir tip of the condom or in a space left by the man at the end of the condom. It works best when used in conjunction with spermicides.

Many condoms these days come prelubricated with spermicides. If you're using one that is not prelubricated and you don't need the extras contraceptive protection because your partner is using the Pill or another effective method of birth control, yet you need extra lubrication, *use only those lubricants that are manufactured for sexual use!* These include products such as K-Y jelly. DO NOT use an oil-based lubricant such as Vaseline with a condom, as it can damage the latex

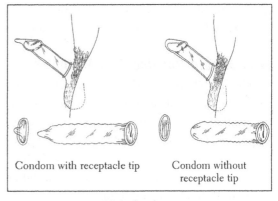

Condom with receptacle tip   Condom without receptacle tip

Male Condoms

material with amazing speed. One study found, for example, that Vaseline Intensive Care Lotion can destroy a condom in five minutes. Baby oil or mineral oil can destroy one in a minute or less!

How Effective Is It?

Condom-user failure rates range from 10 to 20 percent. This percentage can be cut drastically if the man follows the manufacturer's instructions carefully and uses a spermicide in addition to the condom.

For best protection against sexually transmitted diseases—another *very* important use for condoms—it is essential to use those made of *latex*. DO NOT use "natural" or animal tissue condoms, which do not provide adequate protection against STDs. Use only fresh latex condoms. *Fresh* means that you haven't been carrying it in your wallet for weeks or months.

Who Can Use This Method?

Ideally, just about everyone (except those who both have been virgins until now or who have been in a monogamous relationship for five years or more) should use this method to help prevent sexually transmitted diseases— notably AIDS—in addition to pregnancy.

Who Should Not Use This Method?

There isn't anyone who should not use this method. This said, if you are in a long-term, committed relationship, if birth control is very important to you and if you dislike the condom enough to be tempted not to use it "just this once," then you might consider another method. If, however, you're not in a long-term, mutually monogamous relationship, *do* use condoms no matter how inconvenient they might seem to you. Condoms can safeguard you against life- and/or fertility-threatening sexually transmitted diseases as well as against an unplanned pregnancy.

What Are The Advantages?

- The condom is safe, with no adverse side effects.
- It is widely available in drugstores, supermarkets, and restrooms. It is also distributed at some schools.
- Particularly when it is used with vaginal spermicides, it can be a very effective method of birth control.
- The condom offers some protection against AIDS and other sexually transmitted diseases.

What Are The Disadvantages?

- Because the condom needs to be put on the *erect* penis, some people feel it interferes with lovemaking. Others, however, make rolling the condom on simply part of foreplay.
- Some complain that condoms may detract from physical sensations. But many con-

doms today are very thin. Avanti condoms (which are especially thin) and Pleasure Plus condoms (with a special tip designed to be pleasurable for both partners) are made of polyurethane (helpful if you're allergic to latex) and are perhaps the best brands to use if you (or your partner) hate the idea of condoms. (You may be in for a pleasant surprise!)

- The condom can break, spilling semen into the vagina. This is most likely to happen if the man forgets to leave a space at the tip for semen and/or if the condom is old or not of good quality.
- The condom can slip off and spill semen in the vagina. To minimize this possibility, the man should withdraw his penis before he loses his erection and should hold onto the condom as he withdraws.

How Do You Get It?

You can buy condoms anywhere. Drugstore condoms may be fresher and of better quality than those sold in gas stations and restroom vending machines. Condoms are usually displayed on open racks in stores, so you don't have to ask for them. You don't need parental permission to buy them. If you end up having to buy them over a drugstore counter and asking a clerk for them, remember that condoms come in one size. If a clerk asks you "What size?" he or she means the size of the *box*. Condoms typically come in packages of 3, 12 or 36.

The Condom (Female)
What Is It?

It covers the cervix, vagina, and outer lips, acting as a barrier contraceptive and also as a protection against sexually transmitted diseases, including AIDS and genital warts.

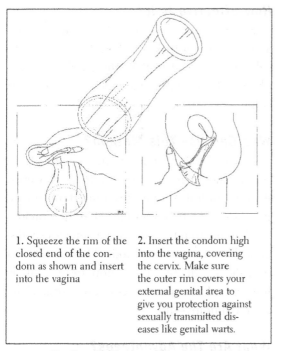

1. Squeeze the rim of the closed end of the condom as shown and insert into the vagina

2. Insert the condom high into the vagina, covering the cervix. Make sure the outer rim covers your external genital area to give you protection against sexually transmitted diseases like genital warts.

The Female Condom: How to Use It

How Do You Use It?

The woman can insert this device (see illustration) into her vagina up to eight hours before sex. Insertion may seem awkward at first, but with some practice it's not difficult at all. Be sure to insert the condom straight into the vagina. Don't twist it. And use plenty of lubrication (spermicidal jelly, cream, or foam or a simple lubricant such as K-Y jelly).

After intercourse, you remove it and throw it in the trash. You need to use a new female condom for every act of intercourse. Do not try to use a male and a female condom at the same time.

How Effective Is It?

The female condom has about a 20 percent failure rate overall, but its effectiveness in preventing pregnancy rises if you're very careful to use it correctly and every time you have sex.

Who Can Use This Method?

Any woman can, but it may be especially useful for women whose male partners refuse to wear condoms or whose lifestyle involves multiple partners and who are at high risk for exposure to sexually transmitted diseases.

Who Should Not Use This Method?

Ideally, there isn't anyone who shouldn't consider this method for protection from sexually transmitted diseases. But if you would be tempted NOT to use it "just this once," another method might work better for you.

What Are The Advantages?

- The female condom can protect a woman whose male partner will not wear condoms.
- It can also protect a woman more completely than a male condom can, since it also covers the outer vaginal area and labia. This is especially important when protecting against HIV, genital warts or herpes infections.

What Are The Disadvantages?

- It can be awkward to insert, at least initially. (Practice helps, so practice before the first time you'll be using it.)
- It isn't quite as effective as methods mentioned earlier in preventing pregnancy—but this effectiveness can be improved by using spermicidal cream or jelly with it.
- You must be very careful when inserting it NOT to tear it with your fingernails.

How Do You Get It?

The Reality female condom is available at most drugstores and some supermarkets and discount stores.

Spermicidal Jelly, Cream And Foam
What Is It?

Spermicidal jelly, cream, and foam are chemical contraceptives that, when inserted into the vagina via tamponlike applicators, kill sperm. Foam will also block sperm trying to enter the cervix. Foam, which comes in a container under pressure (like shaving cream) is generally considered to be the most effective of these spermicides.

How Do You Use It?

You insert the spermicidal foam, jelly, or cream into the vagina with a special applicator that usually comes with the product (see illustration). If you repeat sex in the same day or night, you need to insert a new supply of spermicide into the vagina.

How Does It Work?

Spermicides immobilize and kill sperm cells as they travel up the vagina.

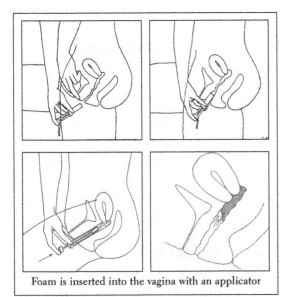

Foam is inserted into the vagina with an applicator

Spermicidal Foam/Jelly: How to Use It

How Effective Is It?

Spermicides vary in effectiveness. Used alone, these birth control methods are considered less effective than the condom or diaphragm. In use without any other device, foam is the most effective spermicide.

Who Can Use This Method?

Anyone not allergic to the chemicals in spermicides can use this method. However, if birth control is especially important to you, it's important to remember that spermicides used alone aren't as effective as previously discussed birth control methods. They also do not provide as effective protection from sexually transmitted infections as condoms—especially male condoms—do.

What Are The Advantages?

- They're readily available at most drugstores and have few side effects (though they can cause vaginal or skin irritations in some people).
- They need to be used only when you have sex.
- Nonoxynol-9, the active ingredient in most spermicides, may help to prevent some sexually transmitted diseases but may also increase the transmission of some sexually transmitted diseases such as HIV (see below)
- These contraceptives, used with a condom or diaphragm, make those methods even more effective.

What Are The Disadvantages?

- Some feel that inserting these into the vagina shortly before intercourse is an inconvenience (but some quite happily incorporate it into foreplay).

- Some feel these are messy, or they are allergic to the chemicals.
- The biggest disadvantages: spermicides, used alone, just aren't as effective as other methods of birth control discussed earlier.
- Nonoxynol-9, the active ingredient in most spermicides, may be irritating to the lining of the vagina or rectum. This irritation can actually cause increased absorption of such viruses as HIV. Therefore, many organizations such as the Centers for Disease Control do not recommend using spermicides with Nonoxynol-9

How Do You Get It?

Spermicides are sold in drugstores, supermarkets, and discount stores.

Natural Family Planning
What Is It?

There are several variations of this method, but all have one goal: helping the woman estimate the days in her monthly cycle when the risk of pregnancy is highest and when sexual intercourse should be avoided.

How Does It Work?

Natural family planning works by alerting couples to the times of highest fertility so that they can avoid intercourse—and probable pregnancy—during those times.

Those who get the best results tend to monitor a combination of body changes during the month: basal body temperature, changes in cervical mucus, and other signs of ovulation. (This method is *not* simply a matter of counting the days since your last period to determine when you're likely to be ovulation.)

How Effective Is It?

Among mature married couples who carefully monitor body changes and are highly motivated enough to abstain from sex during the fertile periods, this method may be helpful—especially if their religious beliefs preclude using any other method. For this group, theoretical effectiveness levels may be as high as 80 to 85 percent.

However, teens are less likely to be able to use this method effectively. Why? Because many teen girls do not yet have regular menstrual cycles—and that is a must if this method is to be effective at all. Also, many young people don't have the patience, motivation, restraint, and tolerance for the periods of abstinence that this method requires. The failure rate of this method among teens can be abysmal—and tragic. It is not recommended for teens.

What Are The Advantages?

- Natural family planning has no method-caused side effects.
- It will reduce one's chances of getting pregnant to 20 to 30 percent vs. 80 percent probability of pregnancy if no contraceptive measures are taken at all.
- It is also the only birth control method that is officially accepted by the Catholic Church.

What Are The Disadvantages?

- It can be risky. No matter how careful one's calculations, ovulation does not always follow regular patterns. Thus, it can be difficult to determine just when it happens from one month to another.
- This method requires a fair amount of sexual

abstinence during "unsafe" days. Patterns of desire do not always coincide with "safe" and "unsafe" days.

NOT RECOMMENDED FOR TEENS

Besides natural family planning, there are several other common birth control methods not recommended for teens (even though they may work very well for your parents or other adults).

- Barrier Methods Like the Diaphragm and Cervical Cap: Both of these are barrier methods that place a latex barrier (either a diaphragm that fits high in your vagina and covers the cervix or a cervical cap that fits over your cervix) between any sperm and your cervical opening. These are used with spermicidal jelly or cream.

    Why don't we recommend it for teens? Because it takes a lot of maturity and responsibility to use this method every time. You also need privacy and planning to use this effectively. Studies with teens have found that it just isn't practical for most—and while the barrier methods are quite effective if used correctly and every time, teens are more likely than adults to not use it consistently. And a diaphragm or cervical cap does you no good at all if it's left in your drawer at home!

- Sterilization: Sterilization is a popular method of birth control for married people who have had all the children they want and for adults, married or single, who have decided that they will never have children.

When the male is sterilized, the procedure is called a *vasectomy*, which involves cutting and tying of the vas deferens (to effectively block the passage of sperm) via a simple operation that may be performed in a doctor's office. This operation is not the same as castration. The male will be able to function just as well sexually and will ejaculate seminal fluid with no sperm in it. However, it may take ten to fifteen ejaculations after the surgery is performed before the ejaculate will be entirely sperm-free.

Sterilization for women is a bit more complicated, involving a brief hospital stay. This procedure, called a *tubal ligation*, means that the fallopian tubes are severed to prevent the passage of the egg from the ovary to the uterus. This operation may be done through a tiny abdominal incision or through the vagina. The tubes may be severed by cutting, by blocking them with special clips, or by sealing them off with electric currents.

Why we don't recommend this for teens: Because it should be considered a permanent form of birth control. Even though some research is being done on reversible methods of sterilization, at this time it must be considered permanent.

Even if you're sure at this point that you don't want children ever, your feelings may change over time, especially if you find yourself in an adult relationship at a different time in your life when having children might be, much to your surprise, suddenly desirable. It's true that some people live perfectly happy lives without having children. But it's better not to make an irrevocable choice in your young adult life—even if you could find a doctor who would perform the procedure when you're still in your teens.

IN AN EMERGENCY

In most cases, sex is *not* an emergency. There is always time for responsible people to take adequate birth control precautions.

However, no matter how responsible you are, accidents or worse can happen. Condoms can break. You suddenly remember that you've been so busy and preoccupied that you've forgotten to take your birth control pills for several days. And, unfortunately, rape and sexual assault can happen. In these instances, what can you do after the fact to prevent pregnancy?

The best known "morning-after" contraceptive is Plan B OneStep, which uses one pill with 15 mg of the hormone levonogestrel. This is *not* an abortion pill. It works by delaying ovulation or stopping sperm from penetrating the egg. It does not abort a fetus.

The sooner that you take Plan B OneStep after unprotected intercourse, the more effective it will be. Taking it within the first 24 hours reduces your risk of pregnancy by 89 percent. If you take it within five days of having had unprotected sex, your risk is still reduced 80–85%.

Fortunately, your chances of getting Plan B OneStep and being able to use it promptly have improved a great deal in the past few years. In 2013, after years of court battles, Plan B OneStep was approved by the U.S. District Courts for *over-the-counter sales without any age restrictions.*

So technically—legally—you should be able to buy it at your local pharmacy, especially at larger stores like CVS. In real life, it's important to know that pharmacists or clerks who have religious objections to this pill or to your buying it can refuse to sell it to you.

However, this "conscience clause" legally requires them to refer you to another store or to another employee at that store who will ring it up for you.

The cost depends on where you buy it, but will usually range from $30–65 with an average of about $49. A generic version of Plan B is expected to come out in 2016. While this is expected to be less expensive, it may not be as widely available as Plan B because the court rulings that prohibit age restriction in buying the product apply only to the brand name Plan B. Age restrictions may be present for the generic product, enabling only those over 17 to buy it over the counter, until these anticipated restrictions are challenged in court.

Although this updated version of Plan B seems to have fewer side effects, about 25 percent of women taking it have feelings of nausea, about 10 percent experience vomiting, and even fewer have fatigue, breast tenderness or dizziness.

Due to the expense and the potential side effects, this isn't something you'd want to use as your regular method of birth control. But, in an emergency, it is highly effective as well as readily available.

Another form of emergency contraception that *can* continue to function as a highly effective method of birth control is the copper IUD, the ParaGard. When inserted into the uterus, it prevents the implantation of a fertilized egg into the uterine lining.

Not all medical professionals are familiar with or willing to prescribe emergency contraception. You can find doctors or clinics in your area by calling the toll-free hotline 1-888-NOT-2-LATE or by going to the website www.not-2-late.com.

Emergency contraception is effective, but it's not meant to function as your regular form of birth control. It's much less stressful to be using a highly effective method of birth control all along if you are sexually active.

QUICK SCAN

BIRTH CONTROL—AN OUNCE OF PREVENTION

✔ If you want to prevent an unwanted pregnancy, you must use a reliable method of birth control every time you have sex, including the first time.

✔ While abstinence is the only 100 percent guaranteed way to prevent pregnancy, highly effective birth control methods like the LARC contraceptives, birth control pills, the Depo-Provera injection, and other hormonal methods such as the vaginal ring or the Patch are very close to 100 percent effective when used correctly.

✔ Unless both you and your partner have never had sexual contact with anyone going into your relationship, or unless you were both tested for various sexually transmitted diseases before becoming sexually involved with each other, you need to use a condom for protection against sexual transmitted diseases, even if you're using one of the highly effective methods of birth control.

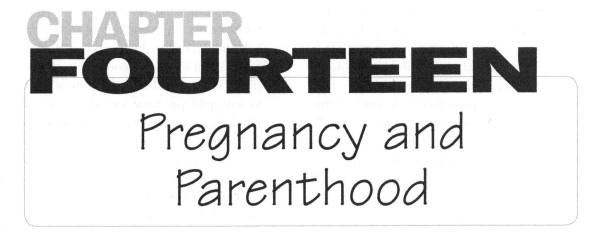

Pregnancy and Parenthood

CONSIDERING PARENTHOOD

I'm 14 years old and I want to have a baby. I try to be very sensible and think of the unfairness it would bring to a child and to my family, but I still want to get pregnant. If I do have a baby, do you think it might be abnormal because I'm so young? Do you think I could take care of it? I'm pretty mature for my age and I've got a way with children. I love kids a lot and I'd be willing to get a job and support my child. I don't know what to do. I want a child very badly, but I want what's best for it.

Anonymous

Something amazing has been happening with teen pregnancy rates since 1990: they're plummeting!

Overall, according to information from Child Trends Databank, teen pregnancy rates declined 51 percent between 1990 and 2010. Teens younger than 15 had the sharpest decline: 66 percent. But 15–17 year olds were close behind, with a 59 percent drop in pregnancy rates. The rate for 18–19 year olds declined 44 percent. This decline happened in all racial and ethnic groups and was a major factor in the 64 percent drop in the abortion rate among teens during that same time period.

There are a lot of theories about why this decline is happening, and there may be many factors involved.

Some believe that better sex education and greater teen knowledge about and access to reliable methods of birth control is a major factor. Some feel that teens are realizing that, with the challenges that the current economy is presenting for young people, they will need as much education and vocational training as possible in order to be competitive in the workplace and be able to support themselves and their families in the future. Still others point to a growing sense of empowerment among young women, who imagine futures that include having fulfilling careers as well as finding joy in marriage and parenthood. Younger women these days are more savvy and realize that a woman can't have it all, all at the same time; but, by taking sensible steps toward an independent future—completing her education before even thinking of becoming a mother—she can have a full and happy life.

Whatever your dreams for your future, parenthood—or nonparenthood—is one of the most important choices you'll ever make. It can affect your life tremendously and, if you're a parent, the life of a child as well. This is a decision that must be made with care, NOT left to chance!

And if it is a conscious choice—as a number of teen pregnancies are—it's important to know what you're choosing for yourself, the father of your baby and, not the least, your child.

Whether you're single or married, in adolescence or young adulthood, there are some vitally important questions to ask yourself if you're thinking about having a baby.

1. *What are my plans for my own future?* Do you have specific educational, career or lifestyle goals? What will it take to achieve them? If you don't have clear-cut goals beyond early parenthood, have you thought realistically about how you will support yourself and your child? If you have only vague ideas about this, think twice. Your parents may not be thrilled—or even able—to help you out. Public assistance does not go far. And the wages that a young person with less than a high school education can earn—even if he or she can get a job—are inadequate for supporting a family, however small. If the marriage seems like the way to go, think twice, too. Teenage couples have a notoriously high divorce rate.

You need to have a viable plan for your future before you even think of bringing a baby into your life. Don't you want your future child to have as good a life as possible? To achieve that goal, you may need to wait until you have a good education, job skills, and at least a minimum amount of financial security. Think about getting a truly marketable skill and at least a high school diploma.

This will give you more choices in life and will help make parenthood, when it comes, an active, positive choice, not something that just happens because you have nothing else to do with your life.

2. *Why do I want a baby?* People have babies for all kinds of reasons, many of them very personal: we're not saying one reason or the other is right or wrong. But if you hear yourself saying things like "I want someone who will love me no matter what!" or "I want people to look up to me," or "I want to prove my love to my boyfriend and for us to be together forever," you may be setting yourself up for disappointment.

It's true that, in many schools, pregnant teens get a lot of attention, and friends may look at you in awe. But once the baby is here and you're tied down with so many responsibilities, your friends may move on to hang out with people who have more ordinary teen lives and fewer, if any, major responsibilities.

A baby isn't proof of love, of manhood, or of womanhood. A baby is a person. You can show love to your boyfriend in a myriad of ways, but, statistically speaking, early parenthood may be more likely to divide you than bring you closer together.

And while babies are wonderful, loving little people, they also make enormous demands on you and on your time, energy, and patience. Parenthood is much, much more about what you can give your child than about what the child can give you.

3. *What do I expect of my baby?* If you envision an invariably angelic, cuddly, cooing, sweet-smelling baby, you may be in for a shock. A baby, especially in the first few months of life, is by necessity self-centered and demanding. A baby is a separate person who may or may not resemble you, who may or may not live up to your dreams for him or her. A baby cannot even help itself, let alone your relationship with its father or your unmet emotional needs.

Could you love a child of either sex? A child who is average or even physically or mentally challenged? What you will give this little person is much more important than what you'll get.

4. *What can I give my baby?* Most of us want the best for our children. Can you offer your baby the best right now? What do we mean by best? We're not talking private schools or trips to Europe or fancy suburban homes. We're talking unconditional love, a fair amount of economic security, freedom from hunger, and, ideally, the emotional support of two parents who are committed to the child and to each other.

The ideal, of course, is not always possible. Many single-parent homes are rich with love, commitment, and caring. But when a family is headed by an unmarried teenager, the children involved start out with some strikes against them. They're more likely to grow up in poverty, more likely to fail in school, and more likely to grow to become teen parents themselves.

Parenthood can be a difficult job for a man or woman of any age. Although a baby may bring you very special joy, you will also have many challenges. In many instances, the child's needs will have to come before yours. The hardships and sacrifices involved are not always easy for anyone, but may be especially hard to take if you're still in the process of growing up and are feeling really needy, too.

5. *Am I ready for the responsibilities of parenthood?* Parenthood is a 24-hour-a-day, 18 year commitment at the very least. But most parents come to realize that their child is forever—and that the emotional commitment to parenting never really ends.

The active parenthood it takes to raise a baby and toddler takes a very special commitment, however. It may involve giving up a lot of personal freedom, curtailing your social life, and being constantly aware of and concerned for your child's needs.

Are you ready to plan most of your current life around a baby? Are you ready to give up the freedom to come and go as you please?

These are important points to consider before you become a parent.

Keep in mind, we're not down on parenthood at all. To the contrary, we see it as one of the most wonderful, challenging, scary, and rewarding life experiences one can have. Because being a parent is probably the most demanding and important job a human being can have, it's important to be truly ready for meeting its challenges and savoring its joys.

IF YOU THINK YOU MIGHT BE PREGNANT

Please help me. I had sex for the first time and did not get my period this month. What's going on? Am I pregnant? I'm only 14 years old and very scared. I'm afraid to tell my mom that I had unprotected sex!

Kris

What if you think you may be pregnant? What are the symptoms?

- A *missed menstrual period.* This is usually, though not always, your first clue that you might be pregnant. However, you may skip a period if you're not eating properly or if you're under a great deal of stress.
- *Fatigue.* You feel tired all the time, even when you've had enough sleep.
- *Breast changes.* Your breasts feel tender and swollen, much like they may feel just before your period, only this feeling doesn't go away after a few days.
- *Urinary and vaginal discharge changes.* These would include more frequent than usual urination and a heavier vaginal discharge.
- *Morning sickness.* This queasiness and nausea can happen at any time of day (especially when you smell food cooking) but it is most likely to strike just as

you're getting out of bed in the morning. This sickness is triggered by HCG (human chorionic gonadotropin), which the fetus produces at an especially high level during the first three months. This is why morning sickness is most likely to occur in early pregnancy.

If you have one or more of these symptoms, do check with your physician. Many people use home pregnancy tests first. That's fine. But then you need to see a physician *right away.* This is important whether your pregnancy is planned or unplanned, wanted or unwanted. You may choose to go to a private physician, an adolescent clinic, a school clinic, a free clinic, or Planned Parenthood. But it's important to get your pregnancy confirmed by a physician. The physician will note changes in the size and firmness of the uterus as well as a bluish hue to the cervix. All of these may be signs of pregnancy.

Once your pregnancy is confirmed, you and your physician or another medical professional at the practice or clinic can discuss your plans. If you plan to continue the pregnancy—whether you will marry the father, be a single parent, or place your baby for adoption—you need to take precautions such as avoiding drugs, alcohol, and other habits so that your baby will get a healthy start to life. If you plan to terminate the pregnancy, the earlier this is done the better. Many clinics will not perform abortions after the first trimester (twelve weeks or beyond). And late abortions are not legal in a number of states. So if you're thinking of having an abortion, you need to seek help sooner rather than later.

What About the Father?

One thing that really upsets me is when people talk about teen pregnancy and they just focus on the teen mother and all her choices. What about the father??? My favorite cousin, who got into a really good college, didn't end up going because his girlfriend got pregnant and she decided to keep the baby and proved that it was his. Even though he wanted her to have an abortion or give the baby up for adoption, she refused. Now he has to pay child support, like forever, for a son he never gets to see and he had to get a job and just go to community college part time instead of Duke. It didn't seem fair that his whole life was changed and he didn't get to make that decision. My aunt thinks she got pregnant on purpose to keep him from going away to college and that the girlfriend hoped he'd marry her, but he's so over her and upset, that's not going to happen. It's so unfair!

Emily K., 15

While Emily's cousin's distress is understandable, a case could be made that he did make a decision in having unprotected sex. These days, especially when three lives can be changed forever by a pregnancy—planned by both or only one or totally unplanned—it doesn't make sense to have sex without a condom. Even if she is on birth control pills, a condom is protection, not only against sexually transmitted infections, but also against one-sided, life-changing decisions about parenthood.

And the impact of teen fatherhood can be life-changing. A recent joint study by researchers at the University of Virginia and the University of Michigan found that boys who became fathers at 17 or younger were less likely, ten years later, to have finished high school and more likely to have lowered job prospects and lower life-time income than their peers who did not become fathers while still in their teens.

Other studies have found that teen fathers tend to have lower self-esteem than their childless peers and tend to come from homes where parents were less educated, had more kids and were more likely to be single parents for at least some of the teens' growing up years. Studies have found, too, that while the self-esteem of teen parents may rise temporarily after the birth of the child, the level of self-esteem plummets once again—in comparison with peers who are not parents—several years after the birth of the child.

So even if one is considering early parenthood to give life meaning and oneself an important role in the world, the fix is temporary. While many teen fathers want very much to be involved in the lives of their children, many aren't able to offer much financial support and may be shut out of the child's life altogether if the couple splits up, child support payments aren't made and/or other people become involved with the two young parents.

What can you do if your girlfriend is, or might be pregnant?

- *Offer your emotional support right away.* Even if there is some doubt about whether you might be the father, support her getting early testing for pregnancy so that a whole range of choices will be available. Some young people, out of fear and denial, wait so long to see a doctor about a suspected pregnancy that the option of abortion just isn't possible. We're not saying that abortion is the top option for everyone, but if it would be something she would seriously consider, the sooner her pregnancy is confirmed, the better. Offering your support emotionally may help to give you more of a voice in subsequent decision-making. In any event, saying to a girl with whom you've had sex "You got pregnant? That's your problem! Goodbye!" isn't right or fair.

■ *Know that you do have the right to establish the fact that you are or are not the father of the baby.* If there's the slightest doubt, it is a good idea to be sure, as being a father and supporting a child both financially and emotionally, is a long, serious, life-changing commitment. A blood test can show if you could possibly be or definitely are not, the father of the child. A DNA test, which is more expensive and has to be done after the baby is born, is much more definitive in establishing paternity.

■ *Make an effort to talk over choices with your girlfriend and your parents to see what choices are available to you.* What plans do both of you have for the future and how would these be affected by early parenthood? What help and resources could your parents and hers offer? Taking an active role right away in talking about options may give you more say in what ultimately happens. But do know that, as important as your preferences might be, the ultimate decision will be hers. While that might not seem entirely fair, she is the one carrying the child and who may give birth or not. Her life is more

profoundly and immediately impacted by the pregnancy.

■ *If she chooses to continue the pregnancy, have the baby and keep it, and you are the father, you have certain responsibilities.* As the father, you are responsible to support your child to the best of your abilities and to see to the child's safety and well-being. You also have a responsibility to be the best parent you can be, despite your youth and limited financial resources. You have not only a responsibility, but also a *right* to know and nurture your child—and this is most likely to happen if you maintain as amicable a relationship as possible with your girlfriend/ex-girlfriend.

■ *If she chooses open adoption, check the laws in your area regarding a father's right to participate in the ongoing process.* In open adoptions, the adoptive parents may be in touch with the birth mother—who may even be able to visit and get to know the child and who even more often will get pictures and regular updates of the child's progress. If you would like to be part of that, too, speak up. The father's involvement is not always automatic, so you need to check the laws in your area and let your wishes be known.

■ *If she wants an abortion and you're against it, your options may be limited.* This can be very painful, especially if you feel strongly that abortion is wrong and/or if you want the baby. However, since her body, health and life are most affected by this pregnancy, her preference is likely to prevail.

■ *If you have decided that you want to get married, read on to the next section!*

From a male perspective, in summary, if you're not ready to become a parent right now, the best choice you can make is preventive—wear a condom whenever you have sex or choose abstinence!

MAKING CHOICES ABOUT A PREGNANCY

A girl who is pregnant—or a young couple facing a pregnancy together—have four choices. It's important to discuss these right away, despite your fear or distress or excitement, as some need to be acted on quickly and some are definitely life-changing.

The four choices are:

- The young couple marries and plans to raise the child together
- The mother decides to give birth and raise the child as a single parent, with or without the involvement of the father
- The baby is given up for adoption
- The pregnancy is terminated by abortion.

No one of these options is right for everybody. Not all will be available or acceptable to everyone. Not one of these is an *easy* option. But one may be best for you, given your unique circumstances.

You may find that those around you have a lot of opinions about what you should do. Some teens have told us that their friends put a lot of pressure on them to keep their babies—and are highly critical of classmates who have abortions or relinquish their babies for adoption. Other teens tell us that their parents (and their boyfriends) often assume abortion is the only option.

While it's important to listen to those who

love you—especially to your parents (whose lives may well be profoundly affected by this decision, too)—it's important to listen to your own feelings, too, and to get professional counseling if you're having difficulty making a decision that feels right for you. Consider the direction you want your life to go, what you could or could not offer as a parent, and talk about this with those close to you. Together, you may work toward making a decision you can live with.

We're not advocating one option above another. We will simply review the four choices that you may be facing, giving you brief information about each choice with comments from teens who have made those choices.

Marriage

Teen marriages, especially those prompted by pregnancy, have a rough time, with a divorce rate twice that of couples even a few years older. However, some teen couples are making it. It helps if you have finished high school and are in your late teens. It helps if your families are supportive. It also helps if you had plans to be married anyway, pregnancy or not. And it helps if both of you have above-average maturity and commitment. Teen couples who make it seem to have a lot of love, a mutual commitment to struggle and share, as well as supportive others: families, friends, counselors, and physicians.

Voices of Experience

Greg and I have always loved each other, but had a hard time right after we were married and our daughter Jennifer was born. He felt left out and jealous when I spent time with the baby. Now that she's a little older and is really attached to him, it's better. We felt pretty trapped at first: Greg as the bread-winner and me as a stay-at-home mother. Finally, my mother agreed to watch the baby several hours a day so I could work part time. Now Greg and I both work, take college courses at night, and share caring for the baby. We're lucky to have parents who help us, our education and skills, a healthy baby, and a wonderful doctor. But it still isn't easy. My school friends have kind of drifted away. I'm very young to be a wife, let alone a mother. Sometimes, even though I'm rarely alone, I get lonely.

Vicki, 17

My marriage only lasted a year and a half. My husband was a nice person, but too restless and young to be married. I had such stars in my eyes when I was 16 and pregnant. I was happy to drop out of high school and say good-bye to my dreams for the future. I thought Joe and I would be happy forever. Now I'm trying to finish high school, get a job, and get off welfare. I really love my child, but I miss my youth and I feel like it is gone forever.

Janelle, 19

Having the Baby and Raising It as a Single Parent

This option has become increasingly common among teens in the last 30 years.

The advantage, of course, is that you can grow to be a parent to your child (quite possibly with help from your own parents and extended family).

Some pitfalls of single parenthood for a teen: the risk of being undereducated and impoverished as well as having difficulties with the daily demands of parenthood. It's very hard to finish school and to get the education you need to adequately support yourself and your child when you have parenting responsibilities at such a young age. (But some young people, particularly those whose parents are supportive of them and/or those who are fiercely determined, do manage to get educated and fully employed.) It can also very hard to give up your freedoms (maybe freedoms you took for granted) when you assume the very adult role of parent at such a young age.

Voice of Experience

My mother takes care of my baby when I'm at school and she'll do the same when I go to community college to study to become a nurse next year. But as soon as I get home from school, the baby is MY responsibility. I fit homework and everything else in between caring for her. Between those two things—school and taking care of my baby—I don't do anything. I don't go out at all anymore. I love my daughter more than anything, but being a mother means a lot of responsibility and loss of freedom. People need to KNOW that beforehand.

Johanna, 17

Having the Baby and Giving It up for Adoption

This used to be one of the most common choices of unmarried mothers, but is less frequently the *first* option chosen these days. Unfortunately, some teens choose this option second—after trying to be a single parent for a time and feeling totally overwhelmed. Then they put their babies up for adoption. Since later relinquishments can be a trauma for both mother and child, and since a child's chances of being adopted decrease as he or she grows out of the infancy stage, it is far preferable to make the choice for adoption either before the baby is born or as soon as possible after birth.

An advantage of choosing adoption, of course, is that your baby has a chance for a new life with a family that wants him or her very much. The primary disadvantage has been that you relinquish your child forever to another family—in many instances, never knowing what has become of him or her. This has been changing, however, with the growing popularity of open adoption.

Open adoption, often arranged through an attorney, means that birth parents can play an active role in choosing adoptive parents. In some open adoptions, birth parents continue to be informed about their child's progress and some even have continued contact with the child. Even in some of the more traditional agency adoptions, there seems to be a more open attitude in terms of the birth mother and adoptive families having more knowledge of each other.

Voice of Experience

I felt a mixture of terrible grief and great relief when I gave my newborn baby boy up for adoption. It was the hardest thing I've ever done. But I feel I gave BOTH of us a chance at life. I know that the two parents who wanted him enough to go through all that screening will give him more than I could right now. It hurts me to admit that, but I know it's true. And I can pick up my life and go to college. If I had kept the baby, that wouldn't have been possible and I might have come to resent the baby for that.

Sandi, 17

Having an Abortion

Despite the storm of controversy surrounding it, abortion *is* legal in the United States as a result of the U.S. Supreme Court's *Roe vs. Wade* decision in 1973. And it *is* an option chosen by many young women. It is estimated that about one-third of abortions in the United States are performed on teenagers.

It's important to know that many people have strong moral issues about abortion, while others feel that it is a reasonable option in a difficult situation. It's also important to know that abortion is NOT a substitute for a responsible use of reliable methods of birth control. It is a legal alternative for pregnant women who feel that their best choice—of several difficult ones—is to terminate the pregnancy.

Women in this position have historically sought abortions whether these were legal or not, and many women have died as the result of illegal abortions performed by incompetent practitioners or of attempts to self-induce an abortion. Making abortions legal has meant that they're safer for you and, in some cases, considerably less expensive.

Abortions may be surgical or medical. The so-called surgical abortions *don't* involve making an incision. The most common type is the vacuum aspiration method. After a local anesthetic is administered, the physician inserts a small tube (connected to a suction device) through the cervix, and the contents of the uterus are, in effect, vacuumed out. This needs to be done by the twelfth week of pregnancy. So-called medical abortions, also done in the first trimester of pregnancy, mean that an injection or pills end the pregnancy.

Although not really a method of abortion, Emergency Contraception, which is a high dose of hormones taken up to 5 days after unprotected vaginal intercourse, can prevent fertilization of the egg by the sperm and prevent a pregnancy from occurring (Chapter 13). A medical form of abortion can be an injection of methotrexate, which is being used as an abortion drug in cities across the United States.

One of the newest methods of abortion is the use of ultrasound to spot a fertilized egg (referred to at this point as a *gestational sac*) a week to ten days after conception. Here the sac, no larger than the head of a match, is removed via a syringe placed in the cervix. The procedure takes two minutes and is less likely to cause bleeding or cramping afterward than the other two methods. Although this technique is quite new, it is an increasingly popular option among women seeking help very soon after unprotected intercourse (sometimes before they have missed a menstrual period).

Women who have first-trimester abortions are usually home the same day and, typically, experience little physical discomfort except perhaps for some brief, menstrual-like cramps.

It is much more difficult—legally, medically, and emotionally—to have an abortion in the second trimester. The health risks are greater, the doctors willing to perform the procedure are fewer, and the expense and pain are considerably more. These abortions are often done using an injection of saline or prostaglandin solution into the uterus, replacing the amniotic fluid. This results in the death of the fetus, followed by labor and delivery of the dead fetus. In many areas, such an abortion is done only in case of dire need, and many states have laws setting time limits—often 20 to 24 weeks of gestation—after which time an abortion may not be performed.

Voices of Experience

I was just relieved afterward. I felt that I was making the right decision. But it's a decision I never want to have to make again. Still, I don't feel guilty or like my life has been scarred by the abortion.

Ellen, 18

I cried afterward even though everyone was very nice and it wasn't physically painful. I wondered what the baby might have been like and if I had made the right decision. One of my girlfriends calls me a "murderer" and won't speak to me. I feel terrible about that. But my parents have helped me a lot. So did the counselor at the clinic. I felt depressed for a time. It still hurts to think about it. Maybe it always will. Still, I feel like I probably made the right decision.

Beth, 17

If you are seriously considering abortion, seek help from your physician or call Planned Parenthood in your area immediately. Your local Planned Parenthood office can give you information about local laws and resources.

WHY FOLLOW-UP MEDICAL CARE IS VITAL—WHATEVER YOUR CHOICE

Whether you choose to continue or to terminate your pregnancy, good follow-up medical care is vital.

If You Are Continuing Your Pregnancy

- Regular visits to your physician or clinic are REALLY important. The doctor needs to monitor your health and your baby's health and growth during the months. As a teen mother, you're physically at high risk. So regular medical care and monitoring is especially important.
- Don't take any drugs—even aspirin—without checking with your doctor first. A number of drugs can be harmful to the baby, especially during the early months of pregnancy when the baby's internal organs, arms and legs, teeth, and eyes and ears are forming. Some physicians caution against drinking beverages containing caffeine—colas, coffee, tea—during pregnancy.
- Stop smoking. Smoking can have harmful, even lethal, effects on a fetus. Women who smoke during pregnancy are twice as likely to miscarry or have a stillborn child or a low-birth-weight infant. Low-birth-weight babies tend to have twice as many physical and mental handicaps as other newborns and are more likely to die in infancy.
- Don't drink alcohol. Abstaining from alcoholic beverages during pregnancy can help protect your baby against fetal alcohol syndrome (FAS) or fetal alcohol effects (FAE). These devastating, alcohol-induced conditions can mean lifelong disabilities, including impaired vision or hearing, facial abnormalities, spinal curvature, lack of coordination, and emotional or behavioral problems. Researchers have found that a woman who has only a few drinks a week may be at risk of having a baby with at least some of the symptoms.
- Eat a balanced diet, take iron and other vitamins as your physician may direct, and exercise. A well-nourished, well-toned body can help make pregnancy and childbirth easier. But, before you try anything on your own, check with your doctor.
- Report troublesome symptoms such as bleeding, swelling or puffiness of your face or limbs, sudden weight gain, blurred vision or a severe headache to your doctor immediately. He or she may be able to prevent these symptoms from growing into serious complications.

If You Are Terminating Your Pregnancy

- Make a follow-up visit to your doctor or Planned Parenthood to discuss your use of a reliable method of birth control. Abortion (along with the three other options) is a difficult choice to make. You don't want to have to face such a situation again.
- While most women indicate that they do not need post-abortion counseling, do consider seeing a therapist if you have persistent depression or other troubling feelings and find it difficult or impossible to discuss these with those close to you.

LIVING WITH YOUR CHOICE

None of the choices we have discussed is easy. But with the support of those you love—as well as medical and mental health professionals when you need them—you can make the best of whatever choice you have made.

If you have chosen to postpone parenthood by having an abortion or giving your baby up for adoption, you have the chance to go on with your life plans now and opt for parenthood later if you choose and feel at last, ready to nurture a child. Yet in a sense, you may feel forever changed by your pregnancy and by your difficult choice. The experience may give you greater will and momentum to go on to accomplish your dreams—and to safeguard them by using a reliable method of birth control.

If you have chosen to embrace parenthood as a single or married parent, you may well have your hands full. Seek help and support from those around you. And, while nurturing your child to the best of your abilities, take some time to nurture yourself: stay in school, get crucial job skills, and equip yourself educationally and emotionally to take the best possible care of yourself and your child. And use a reliable method of birth control so that you don't have another child too soon—before you are physically, financially, or emotionally ready to take on the considerable challenge of two or more small children. (When it comes to small children one plus one does not equal two—but about ten! Give yourself and your child a break!)

Parenthood can be exhilarating and exhausting. It can be one of the most challenging, taxing, painful, and joyous roles you'll ever fill. It's far too important to be left to chance.

QUICK SCAN ✔

PREGNANCY AND PARENTHOOD

✔ Symptoms of pregnancy include a skipped period, fatigue, persistent tenderness and swelling of breasts, heavier vaginal discharge, frequent urination, and morning sickness. If you have some or all of these symptoms, see your doctor. Don't just rely on home pregnancy tests. You need good medical care and advice immediately, whatever decisions you make about your pregnancy.

✔ None of the options you face with an unplanned pregnancy are easy ones. No one option is right for everyone. Seek help from those you love and trust and from medical professionals in making your decision.

✔ Good follow-up medical care, including getting reliable birth control, is important whether you give birth or have an abortion.

✔ Parenthood is one of the most life-changing decisions you'll make. It's too important to be left to chance.

CHAPTER FIFTEEN

Help! When You Need It (And How To Ask For It)

I heard that a girl is supposed to go to a doctor if she has had sex, no matter what her age is. Is that true? WHY? And what can I tell my mom about why I need to go to the doctor? She doesn't know I'm having sex. I only did it twice. Do I still have to go to the doctor?

Courtney L., 16

Please don't take this personally, but I don't like doctors! It's not that I hate them. I've never had a physical exam that I can recall. What can I do not to be afraid of doctors?

Petrified

Going to a doctor may be scary, especially if you have never been in the habit of seeking medical care on a regular basis. However, asking for help when you need it is an excellent health safeguard.

When do you need help? You need to see a physician or another health professional in a number of situations.

IN AN EMERGENCY

An emergency doesn't mean just a serious injury or unmistakable signs of an appendicitis attack. Severe depression and suicidal feelings constitute an emergency. So do symptoms of a serious or potentially serious medical condition—such as diabetes. If, for example, on reading Chapter 10, you noted similarities between your symptoms and those of the medical problems discussed, it is a very good idea to consult a physician.

Don't hope that such symptoms will just go away. Don't adopt an "I'll wait and see!" attitude. In the long run, you'll be far less scared if you seek medical help, testing, and advice. You may find that you do have a special medical need. In that case, you will benefit a great deal from early diagnosis and treatment.

On the other hand, you may find that your condition is not as serious as you had feared. The sooner you find this out, the less time you will spend agonizing over the possibilities.

Many teens, however, are afraid of what the doctor might think of them if they do turn out to be healthy after all. "The doctor will think I'm dumb...hysterical...a hypochondriac...a nuisance..." are often-voiced fears.

While we can't speak for all doctors, we have found that most doctors won't feel this way at all. Your doctor will think that you're wise for being concerned about your body and for seeking help promptly when it seemed that something might be wrong. Your doctor will also be just about as relieved as you are that nothing serious is wrong.

IF YOU'RE SEXUALLY ACTIVE

Both males and females who are sexually active should be aware of the availability of confidential testing and treatment for sexually transmitted diseases and birth control services. Certainly, if you note any symptoms that might mean you have a sexually transmitted disease, do get tested and treated immediately. These diseases *don't* just go away! And even if you have no symptoms, it is important to be tested twice a year for Chlamydia, a sexually transmitted disease that is an epidemic among teens and has become one of the major causes of infertility.

If you are extremely sexually active with multiple sex partners, besides rethinking your lifestyle in view of the fact that some sexually transmitted diseases today are not only health- and fertility-threatening, but also life-threatening, you also need to get routine tests every two to three months for a variety of sexually transmitted diseases.

If you're sexually active, even with one partner, birth control is a concern and you may want to talk with your doctor about the method that would work best for you. Also, particularly if you have or have had multiple

partners, regular testing for sexually transmitted diseases is a necessity for your continued good health. While most sexually active young women tend to have pelvic examinations when they are tested for diseases like Chlamydia and Gonorrhea, that isn't absolutely necessary in all instances. Today, testing for Chlamydia and Gonorrhea (in both males and females) can be performed using a urine sample.

Also, the National Cancer Institute and the American College of Obstetrics and Gynecology recently changed the criteria for screening for cervical cancer: the Pap smear. These new guidelines state that the first Pap smear should be performed three years after a woman begins to have sexual intercourse, or when a woman turns 21 years of age, whichever comes first. So, if a girl has sex for the first time at 16, she would have her first pelvic exam and Pap test at 19. With these new guidelines, routine pelvic exams are being performed much less often on young teens. You can even get birth control pills without having to have a pelvic exam first. However, if you're taking oral contraceptives, your physician may want to see you every six months just to check your weight and blood pressure.

Many teens fear seeking such medical help because they're afraid that a doctor will be judgmental about their sexual activity. Some doctors may be judgmental, but, especially if you seek help from a youth-oriented free clinic or youth clinic, school-based clinic, a family planning service such as Planned Parenthood, or a physician who specializes in adolescent medicine, chances are excellent that you will receive competent and nonjudgmental help. These health-care professionals, who care primarily for adolescents, are likely to be sensitive to your needs and difficult, if not impossible, to shock.

Adolescent-medicine specialists (called *ephebiatricians*) are often physicians with basic training in pediatrics or internal medicine who have done special additional training in the subspecialty of adolescent medicine. They may be found in a number of clinics or in private practice where they may combine practice of adolescent medicine with pediatrics, internal medicine, or another specialty: in some cases, they may see adolescents exclusively. These physicians, who genuinely like and actively choose to work with young people, may be particularly in tune with your feelings and needs.

Of course, there are nonjudgmental doctors in all specialties and settings—from clinics to private practice. If you have bad luck with one doctor, don't give up on finding one who will understand you and help you.

AS PART OF YOUR REGULAR HEALTH MAINTENANCE

Preventative medicine is a growing concept in health care these days, but it isn't really such a new idea. Seeking competent medical advice for relatively minor complaints such as colds or flu may help keep these from becoming major problems and may enable you to care for yourself more effectively.

Routine physical examinations are vitally important, too. If you're under 18, you should have yearly physical examinations. After age 18 and through the twenties, you should have a physical once every two years. Again, whether or not you are sexually active, you should have your first gynecological exam and Pap smear by age 21. If you are having sex, this exam and

test should be done within three years of your first sexual intercourse.

These routine checkups are important. They will enable you and your doctor to spot any possible problems before you experience a major health crisis. These examinations can also help make you more aware of your body and how it works. They offer you an opportunity to ask questions and share ideas with your physician about what you can do to enhance and maintain your health and fitness.

IF YOU HAVE QUESTIONS ABOUT YOUR BODY

A health professional—a doctor, nurse, or nurse practioner—is an excellent person to consult if you have any questions at all about your growth, development, or body in general. "But I'd feel like a total dork!" you may be saying. "I'd hate to bother a person like that with questions they might think are seriously clueless. They might say 'I don't have time for you.'" It could happen that you encounter a health professional who has neither the time not the inclination to answer your questions: if so, he or she is obviously not the person for you. But many of those who treat adolescents—primarily or exclusively—tend to be extremely sensitive to the special needs you may wish to discuss.

LEGAL ASPECTS OF YOUR MEDICAL CARE

One question that many teenagers have (and are almost afraid to ask) is "Can I be treated without my parents' knowledge or consent?" or "Will everything I say here get back to my parents?"

There are instances where you can get medical treatment without parental consent. For example, if you have or feel you might have a sexually transmitted disease or any other reportable communicable disease, you can get medical testing and treatment on our own and on a confidential basis if you're a "mature minor"—age 12 or 14 (depending on the state) or older.

Many states allow minors who are legally *emancipated* (living away from home, supporting themselves, and so forth) or "partially emancipated" (their parents have lost control over them in a certain area) to receive birth control help without parental knowledge or consent. In many places, too, there is recognition of the "mature minor" concept. That means that you are capable of understanding medical treatment and are thus able to give your own consent to it.

In practice, some doctors and/or clinics will take your word for it—without asking for proof—that you're emancipated. Others will be more cautious and ask that you get parental consent or have a parent accompany you. If parental consent would be a problem for you, it's a good idea to find out immediately what the policies of a particular doctor or clinic are while you are considering your health-care alternatives.

Your local Planned Parenthood Clinic can be an excellent source of information on where and how you can get health services. Though much maligned in the current controversies over abortion, Planned Parenthood clinics devote most of their efforts to providing general healthcare and birth control services for women.

In recent years, some states have passed laws requiring parental consent and involvement in certain instances—most notably abortion—that involve a teenager. In every state, this mandatory parental consent can be bypassed via a legal process that your physician or clinic counselor can help you initiate. If you live in a state where such laws exist and, especially if you're pregnant and want to have an abortion, you need to seek help early so that you can either make use of the judicial bypass or get help in telling your parents.

Under ideal circumstances, all of these laws and regulations should not be necessary. Ideally, teens in a crisis would feel they could tell their parents. But the fact, as we all know, is that teens who feel they can talk with their parents, especially in a crisis, will do so on their own without being required by law. And those who can't talk with their parents often have very good reasons for not pursuing communication and seeking support that doesn't exist. Ideally, parents will be involved. Realistically, not everyone has parents who can or will help them through a crisis. But help, often confidential help, *is* available to you.

COMMUNICATING WITH YOUR DOCTOR

I don't know if this is a normal problem or whether it's just me or maybe it's because my doctor is part of an HMO and is totally busy, but this is the problem: by the time I get the nerve to ask him a question or tell him a problem, he's half out the door and I feel really stupid. But at the same time, I'm mad because I'm not getting as much as I should out of seeing my doctor. What can I do?

Frustrated

How much are you supposed to tell a doctor? This doctor I went to when I had a problem with my period asked if I'd ever been pregnant. He also wanted to know if I was sexually active and sort of acted like it would be okay if I had sex with a man OR a woman! What's it to him? Besides, I'm grossed out because I'm not having sex with anybody and he should have known that!

Grossed Out

Good communication with your doctor is vital. There are several ways you can help your doctor—and help yourself at the same time.

- *Be Honest.* Don't lie to your doctor about symptoms, sexual activity, or anything else he or she may ask you. Don't be afraid. Your confidential relationship should be respected. And doctors are notoriously difficult to shock. A doctor is there to help you, not to pass judgment.

  If a doctor asks you a specific question, it may be important to his or her diagnosis. Your lie might make a correct diagnosis more difficult—and vital treatment could be delayed significantly or not given at all. So it's to *your* benefit to be honest.
- *Don't expect your doctor to be a mind reader.* Some doctors are very perceptive and can sense sometimes that you really want to talk about something. Some others, who are still sensitive to your needs, may not know you

well enough to discern this or may get confusing signals from you.

The doctor may be in a tough spot. He or she may realize that you have unexpressed areas of need, buy may also be aware that if he or she seems overly inquisitive, you may be offended. So you can both help each other a bit here. If you want to talk about something but find it difficult, say so: your doctor may be able to help you discuss your concern.

- *Don't be afraid to ask questions.* Asking questions can help you learn and better understand your body and whatever treatment you may be getting. Most doctors would *prefer* that you ask questions. They will probably think that you're intelligent and concerned to ask, not dumb or troublesome.

  Ask about specific treatments, medication, or tests you're getting. Why are these being given? Are there any side effects? How can you help increase the effectiveness of the treatment? How long should you take medications? Will the tests hurt? Will they be expensive?

  Ask about any bodily function or aspect of development that you don't understand. Most doctors will be happy to explain this to you. If you understand your body, it will help the two of you to communicate better and will also help you take better case of yourself.

  If you don't understand a direction or suggestion your doctor has given you, ask him or her to clarify the point. Don't pretend to understand if you really didn't. That's not fair to you. All medical conditions can be explained in plain English, so if your doctor gets carried away with long Latin phrases and other medical jargon, call a halt and ask for an instant replay — in English!

And again, if your doctor is not askable, maybe you need to see a new doctor.

- *Give a good medical history.* This is one of the most important ways you can help your doctor to help you. Some of the questions the doctor might ask will seem dumb, such as ones about your family's medical history, but these can be important, since certain medical conditions can run in families.

If your doctor asks about your sexuality, he or she isn't trying to be nosy or to embarrass you. Your sexual activity, birth control method, possible pregnancy, STD risk, and so forth may all impinge on your health.

Some questions asked may take a little research on your part. You may have to check which immunizations you had had, for example, or look at a calendar and do some counting to recall the first day of your last menstrual period.

What are some of the questions a doctor is likely to ask you?

- What brings you here today?
- How long have you had this (problem or symptom)?
- How old are you?
- Has anyone in your family had cancer? Diabetes? Heart disease? High blood pressure? Allergies? Tuberculosis? Kidney disease? Asthma? Any other serious health problems?
- Do you have any of the following (never, sometimes, or frequently): sore throats, colds, headaches, dizziness, ear infections, constipation, diarrhea, excessive weight loss or gain, excessive thirst, difficulty in concentrating, feelings that trouble you, or suicidal thoughts? Any other troublesome feelings of physical symptoms?
- Have you ever been hospitalized? If so, when? Why?
- How much sleep do you get each night?
- Do you eat a balanced diet? Do you eat breakfast?
- Do you smoke? Drink alcohol? Drink coffee, tea, or colas? In what amounts?
- Have you experimented with drugs or taken drugs on a regular basis? If so, which ones?
- Are you taking any medications now (either prescription or over-the-counter drugs)? If so, what are you taking and for what reason?
- Are you sensitive to any particular drug?
- Are your immunizations up to date? Now there are new recommendations of vaccines for teens. According to the CDC and American Academy of Pediatrics, all teens ages 11 or 12 years and older should receive the Tdap immunization (this is for tetanus, diphtheria and now Pertussis (whooping cough) as well as the immunization to prevent Meningococcal Meningitis. Also, young teen females are now being encouraged to receive the new vaccine series to prevent cervical cancer.
- When did you begin to menstruate?
- Are your periods regular?
- What date did your last period begin?
- How many days do your periods last? Is the flow light, medium, or heavy? (How many pads or tampons do you use per day?)
- Do you have cramps? If so, how long have you had them? How severe are they?
- Do you have nausea with these cramps?
- Do you have premenstrual symptoms (ten-

sion and irritability, weight gain, tender breasts, a bloated feeling, headaches)? How long do these symptoms last?

- Do you ever spot or bleed between periods?
- Are you sexually active?
- If so, what method of birth control do you use? Have you ever had any problems or symptoms stemming from this method?
- Have you ever been pregnant? If so, how long did the pregnancy last and how did it end (abortion, miscarriage, stillbirth, live birth of a premature baby, live birth of a full-term baby)?
- Have you ever had any operations or surgical procedures? If so, why and when?
- Do you have pain when you urinate?
- Have you had any discharge from your penis?

THE PHYSICAL EXAMINATION

I'd like to know what happens during a physical. Do you have to get a blood test? A urine test? What's the difference between a physical for a man and one for a woman? I don't mean to sound ignorant, but I don't think I've ever had a real physical before and now I have to have one before I go to camp and I want to know what to expect.

Robin

The physical examination is, with the medical history, one of the best ways for a physician to assess your health. It's important that the examination be thorough, covering the body quite literally from head to toe. Every physician has his or her own way of performing a complete physical, but there are many similarities. The following rundown will give you a general idea of what to expect.

The General Examination

After you finish talking to the doctor, you will go to an examination room (after stopping off at the bathroom to leave a sample for urinalysis). You will usually be able to undress and put on an examination gown before the doctor knocks on the door, asks if you're ready, and enters the room.

First, the doctor will usually measure your height, weight, blood pressure, and pulse, and perhaps even take your temperature. Then the top-to-toe examination will begin. The thoughtful physician will, as a courtesy to you, only uncover one area of your body at a time, keeping the rest covered. If your doctor doesn't do this and/or makes you feel like "Exhibit A: Nonperson," tell him or her that you're feeling uncomfortable and embarrassed. This is important for you and for the doctor, who may not mean to be thoughtless. Your gentle reminder may help him or her to be more considerate now and in the future.

First, the doctor will examine your skin for any abnormalities—such as any moles that may have increased in size, any rashes, or any signs of bleeding under the skin. Next, he or she will examine your head, starting with your hair. (Some diseases may cause changes in the texture of the hair or significant hair loss.) The doctor will probably examine your ears with an ear speculum, which enables him or her to see into the ear canal. A hearing test may also be included.

The doctor will check your eyes by shining a light into them to check pupil reaction and then will ask you to follow his or here moving finger with your eyes. This enables the doctor to see whether you have any weakness in the eye muscles. He or she may also examine your retina with a special instrument. This test is extremely important, since disorders such as diabetes, high blood pressure, and brain tumors may be, in many cases, diagnosed by examining the retina in this way. The doctor may also check your vision, by asking you to read a special chart on the wall.

In examining your nose, the doctor will look to see whether there are any abnormalities of the nasal bones or the nasal cavity itself. When examining your mouth, the doctor will look carefully at your teeth, gums, tongue, and throat. Although the doctor usually does not have dental training, he or she can tell whether the teeth are in fairly good condition or whether you need immediate dental care. Also, some diseases have symptoms that can appear in the mouth. Moving to your neck, the doctor will feel for an enlargement of the lymph glands or an enlargement or abnormality of the thyroid gland.

Examination of the chest area—breasts, lungs, and heart—follows. The breast examination is now no longer a necessary part of the routine physical examination of the adolescent female. However, breast examinations continue to be important for adult woman over the age of 18. However, if you do have a concern about your breasts or have noted a lump, bump, change in the color or appearance of the skin on your breast, then you should mention this fact to your doctor. In this situation, a thorough breast exam by the physician would be in order.

Then the doctor will listen to your lungs with a stethoscope, checking for any signs of lung disease, such as asthma, which may manifest itself with a wheezing sound, or pneumonia or chronic lung disease, which may have symptoms such as decreased air exchange. The physician will also use the stethoscope to listen to different areas of your heart.

As your doctor begins to examine your abdominal area, it's important to relax, since abdominal muscles can make an accurate examination difficult. In this part of the physical examination, the doctor will check the size of the liver and spleen as well as look for any signs of tenderness of these organs. He or she will also gently examine this area for any evidence of abdominal masses, tumors, or tenderness. The doctor will also probably examine the lower back for any sign of kidney tenderness, which can be a sign of kidney disease. If the doctor touches a ticklish spot, don't' be ashamed to giggle: we all have such spots. You're normal. So giggle, then take a deep breath and try to relax.

Often, in doing the abdominal exam, the doctor may feel or press the area where your bladder is located. It's a good idea, then, to empty your bladder (perhaps after giving a sample for urinalysis) before the examination begins. This is especially true for women, since direct pressure may be placed on the bladder during the pelvic examination.

Examination of the genitals usually follows.

Male Genital Examination

In the male, this includes an examination of the penis to see if there are any abnormalities. If you are uncircumcised, the doctor will check to see if your foreskin retracts easily. He or she will also look for any signs of abnormal growths, such as small skin tumors or genital warts on the penis.

It is very common for the adolescent male to have an erection during the genital exam part of a physical examination. If this happens to you (or if you're just afraid it will and have been avoiding the doctor because of this fear), it may help to know that the physician sees this as a very common, non-specific, automatic reaction—not an indication of sexual interest in him or her! Think about all the erections you have each day that aren't related to any stimulation. This is just another one of those. And your doctor will understand this if it happens in the examination room. This may help to ease, if not totally eradicate, your embarrassment.

The testicles will also be examined for any signs of tumors, unusual pain, or signs of hernia. Here the doctor will ask you to cough or exert pressure (as if you were moving your bowels) to enable him or her to see if there is any evidence of a possible hernia.

Female Pelvic Examination

As we mentioned earlier, the indications for a routine pelvic examination have recently changed and you may not need to have such an exam yet. However, if you have a vaginal discharge, do not have the availability of a urine screen for Chlamydia and or Gonorrhea, or have a concern about the appearance of your genitals or have reached the age at which a Pap smear is indicated, you may need to have a gynecologic exam.

The doctor will first examine the labia for any signs of growths, cysts, rashes, or other irritations. Then he or she will put a gloved finger into your vagina to ascertain which size *spec-*

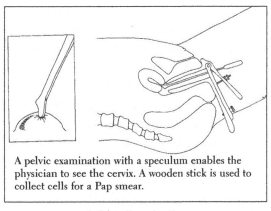

A pelvic examination with a speculum enables the physician to see the cervix. A wooden stick is used to collect cells for a Pap smear.

A Pelvic Examination

ulum may be needed. This instrument, which helps the doctor to see and examine your cervix, comes in a variety of sizes, from infant to adult size. Before inserting the speculum, the doctor may warm it with water and then gently insert it into your vagina, taking great care not to hurt or pinch you.

With the speculum in place, the doctor can see the cervix clearly and can note any abnormalities, such as redness, erosion, cysts, polyps, or irritation. A bluish hue to the cervix may indicate pregnancy.

A *Pap test* will be done with the speculum still in place. The doctor will insert a very small, specially designed wooden applicator to obtain a small sample of the superficial lining around the mouth of the cervix. (Or, to get a better sampling, he or she will put a small, soft brush into the cervical os, or opening.) This procedure does *not* involve cutting, but simply gentle scraping, and it is painless. After obtaining the sample, the doctor places the spatula/applicator on a slide and sends it to a pathologist for examination.

The Pap test is important, since it can detect changes in the superficial cells, which can reflect changes in the cervix itself. These changes may vary from inflammatory changes that happen with a vaginal infection such as trichomonas, to abnormal cells that may be a sign of cervical cancer. This cancer is quite treatable if caught early, and regular Pap tests can detect such cancer early. As we have mentioned earlier, the age at which the first Pap smear needs to be performed has changed from at the onset of sexual activity to three years after the first episode of vaginal intercourse. Also, if a Pap smear microscopically shows signs of genital warts on the cervix, you will be called back for a laser treatment to remove these. This is important, since the virus that causes genital warts has been linked to cervical cancer.

This test is usually not done during menstruation, so if you are scheduled for a physical examination and get your period, let the physician know. He or she may want to reschedule your exam or your Pap test. However, if you're experiencing pelvic pain, it's important to get

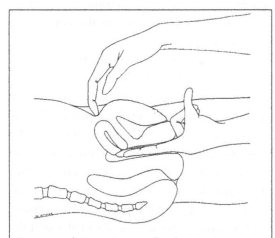

During a pelvic examination, the physician inserts two fingers into the vagina and feels the uterus through the abdomen

Bi-Manual Pelvic Exam

an exam whether of not you're on your period. At the end of the Pap smear, the doctor may also put a cotton swab in the cervix to test for chlamydia and gonorrhea. A new urine test for chlamydia and gonorrhea, called the LCR or urine DNA amplification test, is simple and does not require a pelvic exam. However, it involves very new technology, so not all doctors do the test.

After the Pap test, the doctor gently removes the speculum from the vagina and begins the bimanual examination of the uterus and ovaries. He or she will insert one or two fingers into the vagina until they touch the cervix while placing his or her other hand on the abdomen above the uterus. In this way, the doctor can examine the uterus for position, shape, size, and tenderness. He or she will examine the ovaries for enlargement, cysts, tumors, or tenderness in much the same way.

If a woman has a uterus that is tipped toward the back, the doctor may need to insert a second finger into the rectum (with one remaining in the vagina) to adequately examine the uterus. If you're tense, this can be painful, so do try to relax.

Relaxation is important for the whole pelvic examination. If you're tense, it can be uncomfortable, If you breathe deeply, even closing your eyes, and try to relax, the procedure should not cause any real discomfort. Most doctors try to be as gentle and considerate of your feelings as possible during this examination.

Rectal Examination

Good news: a rectal examination is no longer considered a routine part of a physical exam of an adolescent. However, if you have a specific complaint such as blood in the stools or itching which could be a sign of hemorrhoids or cracks in the skin around the rectum such as rectal or anal fissures, a rectal examination would be necessary. A prostate exam which is normally a component of the physical exam for adult and older males, is no longer necessary for teen males unless specific symptoms (like a discharge from the penis) justify a digital exam of the rectum

Continuing the General Examination

After a thorough check of your genital organs and rectum, the doctor will look carefully at your extremities—your arms, legs, hands, and feet—for any sign of joint swelling or bone deformities, and will often examine your back (spine) for any signs of abnormal curvature, since scoliosis can be a problem for a number of teenagers.

A neurological examination, where the doctor checks your reflexes, coordination, sensory and motor functions as well as cranial nerves, may conclude the physical examination.

Lab Tests

Certain lab tests—blood and urine—may follow, if they didn't precede the examination. The urinalysis, of course, is painless and can help detect a number of problems such a kidney disease, urinary infections, and diabetes. The blood test may be a bit painful and scary for some, but it is very brief and is an important way of checking for anemia and other blood disorders.

These two tests are done routinely when you have a physical examination. There may be other lab tests—for example, for gonorrhea, chlamydia, or syphilis—that your doctor may suggest or that you may request. These diseases may not be detected during the regular examination and lab tests. The test for syphilis is a blood test—either the traditional VDLR or the newer RPR. The tests for both gonorrhea and chlamydia are cultures taken with a cotton-tipped applicator from possible sites of infection, such as the penis, cervix, rectum, mouth, or throat. These tests re a very good idea if you're sexually active with multiple partners and/or you have had any unusual symptoms that may indicate you have been infected with one of these sexually transmitted diseases. Also, if you think you may be pregnant, you will need to request a special test.

Vaccinations

There are some pivotal times between the ages of 11 and 18 when you need to get certain vaccinations, intended to protect you from some serious, even life-threatening, diseases. You've been familiar with vaccinations since you got poked and prodded just before starting kindergarten.

By the time you're 11 or 12, there is a whole new group of vaccinations you need to have. If you're past that age and haven't had this group of vaccines, talk to your doctor about getting them today—no matter how much you hate needles. Your health, even your life, may depend to it!

These include:

- *HPV Vaccine*: This is the vaccine to protect you against the Human Papillomavirus, which can cause not only genital warts, but is also a factor in cervical cancer. Though we discussed this in Chapter Two, we want to emphasize here that *both* boys and girls need to get this vaccine—and ages 11 or 12 are the ideal time. The vaccine can protect you best if you get it before you engage in any kind of sexual activity. If you're older and didn't get the series of three injections at the beginning of puberty, get these shots now! You need to have the entire series of three. (The age range recommended is 9–26, but obviously the younger you get the vaccine, the better protected you will be!)

- *DPT (Diphtheria, Pertussis, Tetanus):* It's likely that you haven't had this vaccine since you were five and about to start kindergarten. Well, guess what? Its effectiveness is probably beginning to wear off and you don't want to be unprotected. Pertussis (or whooping cough) is on the rise because of so many people losing immunity to the disease. If you have respiratory disorders like asthma or are around babies or small children—those much younger siblings or little niece or nephew—it's especially important that you get this immunization. Pertussis can be very serious—even fatal—in babies.

- *Meningococcal Conjugate Vaccine:* This vaccine protects you against meningococcal disease, which is a leading cause of bacterial meningitis, an infection around the brain and spinal cord that can be spread when people are in close contact—like crowded classrooms, college dorms or military barracks. For that reason, the first vaccination is usually given before a young person starts junior high, with a booster shot given between the ages of 16–18 to keep the college or military bound young adult safe. It's a vaccine well worth getting. Bacterial meningitis can be fatal, and some survivors still suffer devastating disabilities like the loss of limbs, brain damage, seizure disorders, strokes or deafness. So this vaccine is something to take very seriously—especially in remembering that age-16 booster shot! A recent survey showed that while 78 percent of 11 or 12 year olds get the initial vaccination, fewer than 30 percent of 16–18 year olds get the booster shot. Ask your doctor about that second dose!

- *Flu Vaccine:* Particularly if you have a chronic medical condition or if you simply don't want to be sidelined with a nasty case of flu, do remember to get your annual flu shot as early in the fall term as the vaccines are available!

GETTING HELP FROM MEDICAL WEB SITES

I've found some great health Web sites that tell me everything I need to know about medical and health stuff. My mom still insists I have to go have a physical and see my doctor once a year. What I want to know is, why? Everything I want to know, I can find on the internet. It's not like my doctor likes to spend all that much time explaining things to me anyway. How can I convince my mom to agree with me?

Tyler

The wealth of information available on the internet is one of the true wonders of the dawning new century! As you will see in the appendix, we're big fans of medical and health-oriented Web sites. These can be a really helpful source of information for people of all ages.

However, just as books (even this one) can't substitute for a thorough examination and personalized advice from your own doctor, so the health Web sites can't substitute for in-person medical help. Ideally, information you get from a Web site or support you get from a chat group will supplement information you get from your doctor or bring up questions you can ask your doctor at the next visit!

Also, keep in mind that information you get from the internet or from books is, by necessity, quite general. For the most specific and personally useful advice and information, there's no substitute for your own physician!

GETTING HELP FOR YOUR MENTAL HEALTH

> My parents are going to make me see a shrink because my school counselor told them my grades are dropping and they all think I'm down because of my parents' divorce last year. The only thing I know is I don't want to see a shrink! What can I do about this?
>
> B. G.

Getting help from a mental health professional may be even harder for you to imagine and to do than seeing a physician for a physical problem. It's even more difficult when going to see a mental health professional—a psychiatrist, licensed clinical social worker, or marriage/family therapist—is not *your* choice, but someone else's. You may worry about what your friends would think if they ever found out. You may find it unnerving—at least at first—to talk about feelings that aren't even that clear to you with an adult you don't know. And you may wonder how talking to someone like that would be helpful when, after all, you do have friends who will listen.

For many crises and problems in your life, those who love you—your friends and your family—will be all the help you need. But it can be useful, too, to spend some time with a professional who can help you work through feelings and difficult situations when no one close to you has been able to help.

Why Do People See Therapists Anyway?

Most people see professional therapists after they've reached a point in their lives when old ways of handling feelings and difficult times aren't working anymore, or when changes or conflicts have caused an emotional crisis, or when someone close to them insists that they see a therapist. You might want to think about seeing a mental health professional if:

- You're feeling depressed and/or irritable most of the day, every day for more than two weeks.
- You've lost interest and pleasure in things you used to enjoy.
- You're having trouble concentrating—and maybe your grades have suddenly started dropping.
- A change in eating habits has led to a significant weight loss or gain (a change of 5 percent of body weight or more in a one-month period).
- You've been withdrawing from your friends or driving them away with your angry outbursts or relentless irritability.
- You're experiencing a change in sleep habits—either being unable to sleep or wanting to sleep all the time.
- You're feeling persistent fatigue and your physician has found no physical reason for this.
- You experience feelings of worthlessness or

persistent guilt or overwhelming hopelessness on a daily basis.

- You have recurring thoughts of death and suicide, perhaps even imagining a specific plan for committing suicide or even attempting suicide.
- You feel that you need to talk with someone about a problem that you're too embarrassed or afraid to bring up with your parent or even your friends.

All of these are very good reasons to see a therapist. But who *are* these people and how do you find one who's right for you?

Who Are These Mental Health Professionals?

There are several varieties of mental health professionals. The type you choose may depend on your particular problem or the therapy you would like to have or what kind of care your insurance company covers.

Who are these therapists and how do they differ?

- *Psychiatrist.* This is a medical doctor with specialized post-medical school training in treating mental and emotional illnesses. He or she can treat people with mild to severe disorders who may require medications such as anti-depressants. But this doesn't mean that you can't get these medications if your therapist is not a psychiatrist. Most non-physician mental health professionals have cooperative relationships with psychiatrists who will see their patients for a one-time medication evaluation and write prescriptions as needed, with occasional follow-up visits. If you're thinking of going to a

psychiatrist, look for one who is certified by the American Board of Psychiatry and Neurology, which means that he or she has had special training in psychiatry and has passed a series of special exams to determine his or her competence in the field.

- *Psychologist.* This doctoral-level professional usually has a Ph.D or Psy.D in clinical or counseling psychology. To be licensed as a psychologist, this person must have completed four to six years of graduate study plus several more years of supervised clinical study plus several more years of supervised clinical training (a total of 3,000 hours) and must have passed a special licensing exam in order to practice. Psychologists are qualified to treat emotional problems and disorders. They are also generally experienced in testing and assessment, which can be useful when extensive testing is required, needed, or suggested as part of your treatment.
- *Licensed Marriage and Family Therapists (MFT, MFCC).* This professional has at least a master's degree in clinical or counseling psychology, and a number have doctorates. This therapist has had two to six years of graduate level training (at least two years for a Master's, four to six years for a Ph.D or Psy.D) followed by a required number of hours of supervised clinical work. These hours required vary greatly by state—from 1,000 post degree hours in Arizona to 3,000 post degree hours in California to as many as 5,000 hours in other states. (We're talking at least several years of doing therapy under the close scrutiny of a clinical supervisor.) This type of therapist may do well with individual emotional problems, or may be able

to help you communicate better with your parents or other family members.

- *Clinical Social Worker (MSW, LCSW).* This professional also has at least a master's degree—and some have doctoral-level degrees—in clinical social work or psychology. He or she is especially trained to evaluate and work with emotional problems in a social context. Licensed clinical social workers, like other mental health professionals, have had supervised clinical experience and have passed state licensing examinations.

How Do You Find a Therapist?

If you're feeling suicidal and need help quickly, call your local suicide prevention center or hotline for help and referral for therapy.

If your situation is distressing, but not a suicidal emergency, you might seek a referral from:

- Your physician.
- Local branches of national associations for mental health professionals: American Psychological Association (psychologists), American Psychiatric Association (psychiatrists), the American Association for Marriage and Family Therapists (MFTs), or the Academy of Certified Social Workers (MSWs, LCSWs).
- The graduate psychology department of a local university or the alumni affairs department of the nearest graduate professional school of psychology.
- A friend or relative who has had therapy and whose therapist may be able to refer you to a colleague.
- Your local family service agency (see your telephone white pages) or your family's HMO or employee assistance program (EAP).

Once you have the name of one or more possible therapists make an appointment to see if you might work well together. Don't get discouraged if you find that the first therapist you talk with just isn't for you. Don't stop looking. Mental health professionals, despite having much in common professionally, have different personalities and styles of working. Finding the right therapist for you may be easy—the first one may feel right—or it may take a little more time. But it will happen.

While it's common to feel a little uneasy if you've never had therapy before, you will know, deep down, whether a particular therapist will work well with you. Some questions to ask yourself:

- Does this person listen well?
- Does he or she encourage you to work at seeking your own solutions (instead of claiming to have all the answers)?
- Do you feel that, once you get over the initial uneasiness about being in therapy, you could work with this person?

If you answer yes to these, then you may well have a good match.

What to Expect And How to Make the Most of Therapy

- *You can expect confidentiality.* If you're getting individual therapy, your therapist is not going to tell your parents anything and everything. Psychotherapists of all kinds follow certain ethical and professional codes, and one of the most important of these is confidentiality. In most states, this applies even if you're a minor (see Chart 20 for details about your state).

There are only a few instances where a therapist is bound by law to break confidentiality: first, if you are in immediate danger of harming yourself—for example, if you are suicidal and have a plan, the therapist may notify your family so that they can also help protect your life at this time. The therapist is also obligated by law to report to the proper authorities anything you may tell him or here about physical or sexual abuse. Also, in some states, the therapist also has a duty to warn a potential victim or victims if you appear to pose a serious threat to the life of another. In all other instances, however, what you say to a therapist will (and must) stay between the two of you.

■ *You can expect therapy to be relatively brief in duration.* Except in very unusual cases, people aren't in therapy continuously for years and years. Many HMOs authorize about 20 visits—which may translate into five months of treatment, tops. You may be in therapy a little longer or considerably less, depending on your problem or issues. But therapists these days are trained to make the most of the relatively short time you will have together. (This fact may help make the idea of therapy more appealing to you, especially if you're feeling forced to get help.)

■ *You can expect that there will be times when you feel worse on the way to getting better.* While you're in therapy, you may be exploring some very painful feelings. These are not caused by therapy. They come up in therapy because this is a safe place to let them happen. These are the feelings that may be interfering with your life in a number of ways. By facing and working through these painful feelings in therapy, you will begin to heal and to feel better.

How do you make the most of therapy?

■ *Give your therapy (and your therapist) a fair chance.* It takes time and effort to make changes in your life—from minor ones to major ones. Therapy isn't going to give you all the answers or change your life all at once. It's hard work—and that hard work is mostly yours (or your family's, if you're getting family therapy). The therapist works hard to help and encourage you, but you're the one who makes the changes and develops the insights. If you bail out after one or two sessions and announce that therapy isn't for you, you're not giving therapy—or *yourself*—a fair chance.

■ *Make a commitment to work constructively, even if being in therapy isn't your choice.* It can feel awful to feel forced to go see a therapist. You may be, quite justifiably, angry that you're being seen as the one with the problems when, really, it's your family that's all screwed up. You may well be right—and it may not take your therapist long to see that you are right and suggest family therapy. However, even if you're stuck with individual therapy you don't especially want, you've got the listening ear of a trained professional and an opportunity to gain some insights and, perhaps, to make some changes that *you* want to make. As long as you have to go, you might as well get something out of it for yourself. It can be tempting to sulk and refuse to talk in sessions, but that may not be as useful as telling the therapist how angry you are to be there and how you feel about your family or life situation or anything else you would like to talk about. Don't worry about hurting the therapist's feelings or shocking him or her. Mental health professionals have been trained to do just fine with angry patients and most have heard just about everything, so, like physicians, they are pretty hard to shock. It's also a good idea to resist the temptation to just blow off appointments and not show up. Think about it this way: most therapy these days is pretty brief, so you won't be doing this for a long time. Why not show up and see if it might help you in ways you want?

- *Don't try to impress your therapist—either with how bad you are or how blameless you are.* This is one relationship where it's important to be real. You can say whatever you want and express feelings you might not share even with friends, in a safe and confidential place. If you spend most of your time trying to convince the therapist that you're totally bad or that all your troubles are someone else's fault, you're missing a chance to take the power to improve your own life.
- *Be open to the possibility of change.* We're not talking about therapy changing your whole personality or essentially who you are. What it can help you to change are patterns of feelings, thoughts, and beliefs you have about yourself and the world that could be keeping you from being the best *you* possible.

This can mean growing to feel better about yourself. It can mean learning new communication skills so that you can discuss issues with your parents (and others) without huge and pointless arguments. It can also mean learning the skill to say no to those you love, or to risk being different from your friends when you need to be.

Good therapy is all about helping you build the insight, courage, strength, and resourcefulness to hope and to plan for and make changes that will make a wonderful difference in your life, in small and in major ways.

GROWING TOWARD A HEALTHY FUTURE

You, your physician and/or your therapist are ideally a team working in unison to keep your body and/or mind as healthy as possible. You are the most important member of this health-care team. Many people make the mistake of casting the doctor or therapist into the role of guardian of their health and wellbeing, giving him or her all the responsibility. But a doctor can only diagnose, treat and advise. A therapist can advise, gently guide you toward new insights, listen to you, and support you emotionally during painful times. But *you're* the one who does the daily work to take good care of your health and to make beneficial physical and emotional changes.

You live in your body and you're the person most responsible for its care. Your body *is* you. And do you really want anyone else trying to make the choices that are yours alone?

You can make many choices that will influence your health. We have looked at many of them in this book. Some of the choices enabling you to safeguard your health include the following:

- Understanding your body's growth and functions.
- Eating a balanced diet and exercising regularly.

- Abstaining from harmful habits such as smoking, drug use, and alcohol use.
- Learning to manage stress and deal with other troublesome feelings in constructive ways.
- Accepting and caring for your special medical needs—so you can be free to do what you like and need to do.
- Using care and common sense when you make sexual choices. The dangers of irresponsible sex have escalated significantly in recent years. Making the right choices and taking proper precautions can be health-enhancing, even lifesaving!

- Asking for help when you need it—whether this is help from a parent, a friend, a health-care provider, or a therapist. Sometimes, asking for help is a greater sign of strength and courage than trying to ignore a problem

We hope that this book has given you some vital information and new ideas about some of your health needs and choices. We wish you a full, healthy, and happy life. But only *you* can make this wish reality!

QUICK SCAN ✔

HELP! WHEN YOU NEED IT (AND HOW TO ASK FOR IT)

✔ Both males and females who are sexually active need to be aware of the availability of confidential testing and treatment for sexually transmitted diseases and birth control services.

✔ If you're under 18, you should have yearly physical examinations. After 18 and through your twenties, you should have a physical once every two years.

✔ You can get valuable medical information on the Internet. However, this is no substitute for the personal care and information you need from your own physician.

✔ Take good care of your body with regular exercise, a healthy diet, good stress management, regular medical checkups and using common sense when you make sexual and other lifestyle choices. Making wise choices can be health-enhancing, even life-saving!

APPENDIX
Help! Where To Find It

Recent studies show that teens prefer to get information about their health and other concerns online and that their most trusted sites are those connected with government agencies and research universities. So we've concentrated on finding the best of those sites, as well as those with good reputations for helping teens. Please note, as you read through this, that some crisis lines now offer texting or instant messaging services as well as telephone support, understanding that this new generation of teens is often more comfortable expressing their feelings in text form.

To contact us with a question or comment, please go to Dr. Kathy McCoy's website www.drkathymccoy.com and click on the "Teen Transitions" button at the bottom of the Home page.

Here's our list. We hope this is helpful to you and your friends!

ALCOHOL AND SUBSTANCE ABUSE

Alanon-Alateen
For teens with an alcoholic parent—meetings local and online
www.al-anon.alateen.org

Substance Abuse and Mental Health Services Administration (SAMHSA)
National Alcohol and Drugs Helpline (and also on-site link to treatment locations)
Helpline: 1-800-662-4357 (available 24/7)
www.samhsa.gov

The Cool Spot
www.thecoolspot.gov

National Institute on Drug Abuse
www.nida.nih.gov

CHILD ABUSE/DOMESTIC VIOLENCE HOTLINES

National Child Abuse Hotline: 1-800-422-4453

National Domestic Violence Hotline 1-800-799-SAFE (7233)

CHRONIC HEALTH CONDITIONS

www.diabetes.org

www.epilepsy.com

Note: You can get information about other chronic medical conditions at the General Health sites listed.

CYBERSAFETY, CYBER-BULLYING/CYBERSEXUAL ABUSE

www.stopbullying.gov

www.nationalcac.org/prevention/internet-safety-kids.html

www.NetSmartz.org/Teens

www.endrevengeporn.org

www.undox.me (for help in getting "revenge porn" pictures removed)

DATING ABUSE AND DATE RAPE

Love Is Respect
Hotline: 1-866-331-9474

Text "LOVEIS" to 22522

www.loveisrespect.org

EATING DISORDERS

National Eating Disorders Association (NEDA)
This site not only offers help and information about eating disorders, but also offers a terrific safe, confidential interactive community for teens and young adults called Proud 2BME that offers the latest on healthy attitudes about weight, food, health and style for teens and young adults.

Helpline: 1-800-931-2237

www.nationaleatingdisorders.org

www.Proud2BME.org

Emergency Contraception Helpline
1-888-NOT-2-LATE
www.not-2-late.com

GENERAL HEALTH WEBSITES

Centers for Disease Control
www.cdc.com

National Institutes of Health
www.nih.gov

The Mayo Clinic
www.mayoclinic.com

WebMD
http://teens.webmd.com

LESBIAN, GAY, BISEXUAL, TRANSGENDER AND QUESTIONING YOUTH

The Trevor Project
Comprehensive site for teens, with a variety of services from information and resources to telephone, online chat, text and social networking support.

www.thetrevorproject.org

Trevor Lifeline: 1-866-488-7386

Trevor Chat: Free, confidential instant messaging, access via website

Trevor Text: Confidential, live help via text messaging. This service is available on Fridays from 4 pm to 8 pm ET and 1 pm to 5 pm PT. To access this service, text the word "TREVOR" to 1-202-304-1200 (standard text messaging rates apply).

Trevor Space: Social networking site for lesbian, gay, bisexual, transgender and questioning youth ages 13-24. Access this through the website above.

Trevor Support Center: Find answers to frequently asked questions and explore resources related to sexual orientation, gender identity and more.

LYRIC Lavender Youth
www.lyric.org

PFLAG (Parents and Friends of Lesbians and Gays)
www.pflag.org

GLBT National Help Centers
www.glbthotline.org

This site includes a resources database with 15,000 listings of social and support groups, gay-friendly religious organizations, sports leagues, and student groups. It also provides access to GLBT-friendly doctors, lawyers and counseling professionals.

Hotline: 1-888-843-4564

The Hotline is available Monday through Friday 1 pm—9 pm PT and 4 pm to midnight, ET. On Saturdays, it is available from 9 am—2 pm PT and noon to 5 pm ET.

MENTAL HEALTH

Medline Plus—Teen Mental Health
www.nim.nih.gov/medlineplus/teenmentalhealth

RAPE, ABUSE, INCEST

RAINN—Rape, Abuse, Incest National Network
Offers online hotline and link to find local help.

Online hotline offers instant messaging and online chat support one-on-one with a trained RAINN support specialist. This service is available 24/7. It is safe and confidential; you are never asked to reveal your identity.

www.online.rainn.org

SEXUALITY/SEX EDUCATION

Advocates for Youth
www.advocatesforyouth.org

SEXUALLY TRANSMITTED DISEASES

Centers for Disease Control and Prevention
Voice Information
(Sexually transmitted diseases, HIV and TB
Information)

1-800-232-3228

Toll-free, 24 hours a day, 7 days a week

SUICIDE PREVENTION

National Suicide Prevention Lifeline
1-800-273-8255, available 24/7

www.suicidepreventionlifeline.org

Hopeline (for those with depression who are
not actively suicidal)
1-800-394-4673

TEEN HEALTH WEBSITES

www.kidshealth.org/teen

www.teenhealthfx.com

www.teenhealthissues.org

www.teensource.org (has helpline and referral
to local clinics)

www.teenwire.org

www.goaskalice.columbia.edu (Columbia
University health site for teens)

About The Authors

Kathy McCoy, Ph.D., is an award-winning author of more than a dozen books, most recently *Purr Therapy: What Timmy and Marina Taught Me About Life, Love and Loss*; *Making Peace With Your Adult Children and Aging and Other Surprises*. She is also a psychotherapist in private practice, specializing in parent/teen communication, marital and family conflicts, as well as working with clients of all ages suffering from anxiety and depression.

A former columnist for *Seventeen* and a former editor of *'TEEN* Magazine, she has written many articles for national magazines, newspapers and professional journals such as *Redbook, Readers Digest, The New York Times, Family Circle, Woman's Day, Ladies Home Journal, Glamour, TV Guide* and *The Journal of Clinical Child Psychology*.

A frequent guest on national television shows, Dr. McCoy has made numerous appearances on *The Today Show*, has been featured twice on *Oprah*, and has appeared on a number of other national and local television and radio shows. She has also appeared frequently on the pages of *USA Today* as an expert on

adolescent issues. Most recently she has been interviewed as an expert for the teen magazines *Girls Life* and *Girlfriend*, U.S. News and World Report, Psychology Today and online publications such as The Huffington Post, AARP.com and Today.com.

Dr. McCoy writes a popular blog "Living Fully in Midlife and Beyond," and hosts the podcast "Living Fully with Dr. Kathy McCoy," available on iTunes, Stitcher Radio and Podcastpedia.

Her website is www.drkathymccoy.com

Charles Wibbelsman, M.D., the award-winning author of four books and the former "Dear Doctor" columnist for *'TEEN* Magazine, is a nationally prominent adolescent medicine specialist. In addition to serving as chairman of the chiefs of adolescent medicine for the Permanente Medical Group of Northern California, he was chief of the Teenage Clinic at Kaiser Permanente, San Francisco and is a clinical professor of Pediatrics at the University of California, San Francisco Medical School.

He was a member of the Committee on Adolescence for the American Academy of Pediatrics. He also has served on the Board of the Society for Adolescent Medicine, and on the San Francisco Superintendent of Schools Advisory Committee. He is a recent Past President of The San Francisco Medical Society. He is now on the Board of Directors for Larkin Street Youth Services in San Francisco, a nonprofit organization that offers shelter and education to homeless teens and youth.

Dr. Wibbelsman is also a popular guest on national television shows, including *The Today Show* and *Oprah*. He has appeared weekly on San Francisco's KRON television station's *The Morning Show* for several years, and frequently appears in medical educational broadcasts for physician training.

Index